P9-EJU-488

A *Jerry Baker* Good Health Book

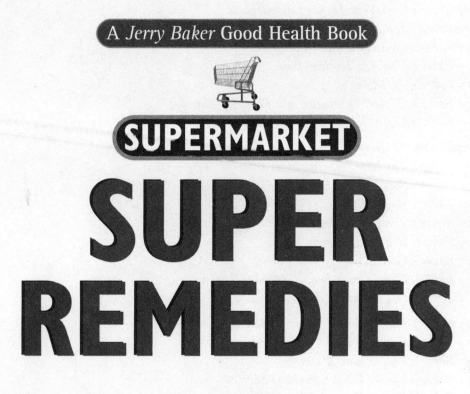

SUPERMARKET
SUPER REMEDIES

www.jerrybaker.com

Other Jerry Baker Books:

Jerry Baker's Grow Younger, Live Longer
Healing Remedies Hiding in Your Kitchen
Jerry Baker's Cure Your Lethal Lifestyle
Jerry Baker's Top 25 Homemade Healers
Healing Fixers Mixers & Elixirs
Jerry Baker's The New Healing Foods
Jerry Baker's Anti-Pain Plan
Jerry Baker's Oddball Ointments and Powerful Potions
Jerry Baker's Giant Book of Kitchen Counter Cures

Grandma Putt's Green Thumb Magic
Jerry Baker's The New Impatient Gardener
Jerry Baker's Supermarket Super Gardens
Jerry Baker's Bug Off!
Jerry Baker's Terrific Garden Tonics!
Jerry Baker's Backyard Problem Solver
Jerry Baker's Green Grass Magic
Jerry Baker's Great Green Book of Garden Secrets
Jerry Baker's Old-Time Gardening Wisdom

Jerry Baker's Backyard Birdscaping Bonanza
Jerry Baker's Backyard Bird Feeding Bonanza
Jerry Baker's Year-Round Bloomers
Jerry Baker's Flower Garden Problem Solver
Jerry Baker's Perfect Perennials!

Jerry Baker's Vital Vinegar Cookbook "Cures"
Jerry Baker's Live Rich, Spend Smart, and Enjoy Your Retirement
Jerry Baker's Vinegar: The King of All Cures!
Jerry Baker's Fix It Fast and Make It Last
Jerry Baker's Solve It with Vinegar!
America's Best Practical Problem Solvers
Jerry Baker's Can the Clutter
Grandma Putt's Old-Time Vinegar, Garlic, and 101 More Problem Solvers
Jerry Baker's Supermarket Super Products

To order any of the above, or for more information on Jerry Baker's amazing home, health, and garden tips, tricks, and tonics, please write to:

Jerry Baker, P.O. Box 1001, Wixom, MI 48393

Or visit Jerry Baker online at:

jerrybaker.com

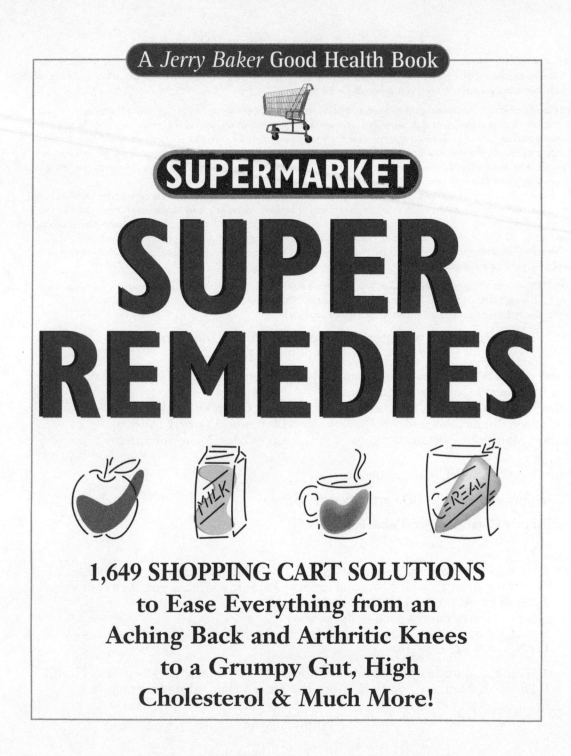

A *Jerry Baker* Good Health Book

SUPERMARKET

SUPER REMEDIES

**1,649 SHOPPING CART SOLUTIONS
to Ease Everything from an
Aching Back and Arthritic Knees
to a Grumpy Gut, High
Cholesterol & Much More!**

Copyright © 2006 by Jerry Baker

All rights reserved. No part of this book may be reproduced or transmitted in any form or by any means, including, but not limited to, photocopying, recording, electronically, via the Internet, or by any other information storage or retrieval system, without the express written permission of the Publisher.

NOTICE—All efforts have been made to ensure accuracy. This is a reference volume only, not a medical manual. Although the information presented may help you make informed decisions about your health, it is not intended as a substitute for prescribed medical treatment. If you have a medical problem, please seek competent medical help immediately. Jerry Baker assumes no responsibility or liability for any injuries, damages, or losses incurred during the use of or as a result of following this information, ideas, opinions, procedures, directions, and suggestions contained in this book. The Author and Publisher also expressly disclaim all representations and warranties relating to and/or arising out of the information.

Herbal research is still in its infancy, and the interaction between herbs and pharmaceutical products remains largely unknown. Herbal remedies and nutraceuticals can have effects similar to those of pharmaceutical products. As a result, they are not without risk. They can interact with each other or with conventional medications, and some people may experience an allergic reaction or other adverse effects when starting an herbal or nutraceutical regimen. That's why you should always check with your doctor before you use them.

Women who are pregnant or breastfeeding and children under age 18 should not use herbal or nutraceutical products without their doctor's specific recommendation.

IMPORTANT—Study all directions carefully before taking any action based on the information and advice presented in this book. When using any commercial product, always read and follow label directions. When reference is made to any trade or brand name, no endorsement by Jerry Baker is implied, nor is any discrimination intended.

Published by American Master Products, Inc./Jerry Baker

Kim Adam Gasior, Publisher

A Jerry Baker Good Health Book and a Blackberry Cottage Production

Editorial: Ellen Michaud, Blackberry Cottage Productions, Ltd.

Author: Matthew Hoffman

Design: Jane Colby, Nest Publishing Resources

Book Composition: Wayne F. Michaud

Illustrator: Wayne F. Michaud

Copy Editor: Jane Sherman

Printed in the United States of America

Illustrations copyright © 2005 by Wayne F. Michaud

Publisher's Cataloging-in-Publication

Baker, Jerry.
   Jerry Baker's supermarket super remedies : 1,649 shopping cart solutions to ease everything from an aching back and arthritic knees to a grumpy gut, high cholesterol & much more! / [edited by Matthew Hoffman].
   p. cm. — (Jerry Baker's good health series)
   Includes index.
   ISBN 978-0-922433-63-6

   1. Traditional medicine. 2. Medicine, Popular. 3. Naturopathy. 4. Self-care, Health.
   I. Hoffman, Matthew, 1959- II. Title. III. Title: Supermarket super remedies.

RC81.B2315 2005   615.8'8
                                     QBI05-200105

                        28 30 29 27   hardcover

Contents

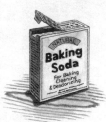

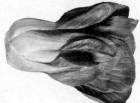

Contents

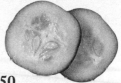
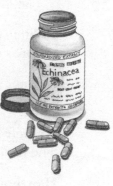

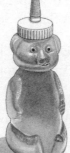

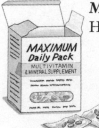
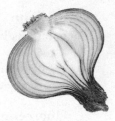

Contents

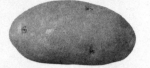
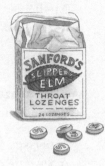
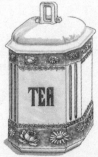

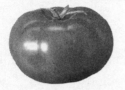
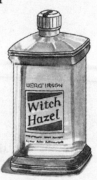
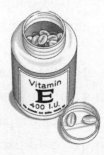

Contents xi

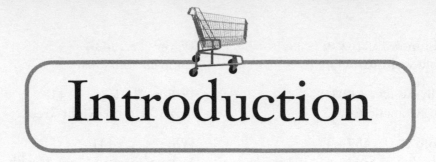

Introduction

Have you looked around your local supermarket lately? I mean *really* looked around?

If you're like me, you make out a shopping list at home and then just run in, grab what you need, zip through the checkout line, and run back out. Heck, I rarely even give my car's engine time to cool off before I'm on my way again. But when my friend Matthew Hoffman and I recently had a discussion about how supermarkets had changed over the past couple of years, I decided to take a look for myself—and boy, am I glad I did!

It turns out that all of those extra aisles that had popped up while I wasn't looking contain more vitamins, minerals, herbal supplements, and other preparations than you can shake a stick at. Hot wraps, cold packs, antihistamines, healing teas, soothing salves—if there's a home remedy for something that ails you, it looks like they've got it!

What's more, supermarkets have stocked up on all those healthful, healing foods that researchers have been pushing us to eat to prevent or relieve most health problems. Blueberries that keep your memory sharp, fish that eases the aches and pains of arthritis, vegetables that clear a stuffy nose—even spices that calm a cranky gut!

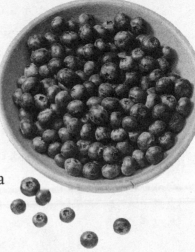

I tell you, a lightbulb went on in my head as I walked down the aisles! As soon as I checked out, I threw my bags in the car and zoomed home to call Matthew. We kicked around a few ideas and then talked about putting together a brand new book.

To start, I asked him to gather a list of the top home remedies, then browse the aisles in a bunch of different supermarkets to see how many of the treatments he could find. And you know what he discovered? The majority of today's supermarkets have more than 1,649 super remedies sitting right on their shelves.

That's right, 1,649!

Surprised? I sure was. Matthew's research revealed that hundreds of top health treatments are as close to us as our local supermarkets!

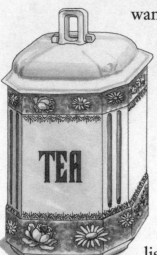

Needless to say, for a couple of natural, down-to-earth guys like Matthew and me, this was big news—and we wanted to share it with everyone. So we packed the latest word on all those healing teas, tonics, foods, salves, and other things into this book, then topped it off with suggestions from 124 doctors and other health practitioners for the most effective ways to use them.

Now it's your turn to check 'em out. Then, the next time you make a grocery list and head for the supermarket, take a list of your most common health complaints and this book with you as well. With these supermarket super remedies in hand, I guarantee that you won't be complaining for long!

Jerry Baker

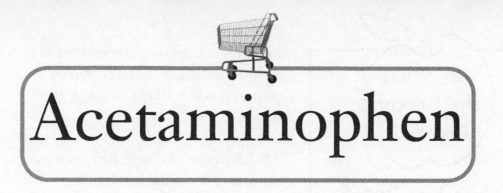

Acetaminophen

RELIEF FOR ALL AGES

You may think that over-the-counter painkillers are as alike as peas in a pod, but acetaminophen, the active ingredient in products such as Tylenol, is in a class by itself. It knocks out pain just as effectively as aspirin or ibuprofen but is less likely to have nasty side effects. Better yet, every member of your family can use it, even the kids. Here's what we mean.

Earache. When you're plagued by an ear infection, reach for the acetaminophen. It quickly eases pain and helps control the fever that often accompanies infections. Follow the label directions.

ON THE SHELF

✓ **Tylenol**

✓ **Feverall**

✓ **Aspirin-Free Excedrin Caplets**

Flu. When preventive measures fail and you're felled by the flu, make yourself as comfortable as you can. Take acetaminophen to fight the fever and ease the aches while you rest and drink lots of fluids.

Bruises. Don't take aspirin when an injury turns you black and blue. Even though it's a great remedy for pain, aspirin reduces the ability of blood to clot normally, which could result in even more bruising in the days following the injury. Aceta-

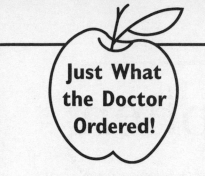

Just What the Doctor Ordered!

Take a Bite Out of Mouth Pain

If there's anything more painful than burning your mouth with sizzling cheese when you take a bite of hot pizza, it's accidentally biting your tongue or cheek while you're eating. Here's how to help the pain in a hurry.

1. Press the area with a gauze pad or a clean wash-cloth to stop any bleeding.

2. Put an ice cube in your mouth and let it rest against the painful area.

3. Take acetaminophen.

4. Dab on some Orabase or other mouth gel to protect the area and help it heal.

minophen is a better choice because it has the same painkilling properties as aspirin but is less likely to cause additional bleeding or bruising.

■ **Shiners.** The next time you have a black eye, leave the steak in the refrigerator and take acetaminophen. It will reduce throbbing without increasing internal bleeding (and making your shiner worse) the way aspirin can, says Donald Schwartz, M.D.

■ **Headache.** Nearly everyone gets headaches sometimes. It's worth checking with your doctor if you get them all the time, or if the pain interferes with your activities, but you'll probably be able to manage most of them on your own. The vast majority (about 95 percent) are "primary" headaches, which means they aren't caused by some dangerous underlying illness. It's fine to take acetaminophen for temporary relief, but keep in mind that painkillers won't eliminate any underlying problems that may be present.

■ **Aches and pains.** We all know what a long day working in the yard can do to your muscles and joints. The next time you've overdone it, pop some acetaminophen. You'll probably start feeling better within a few hours.

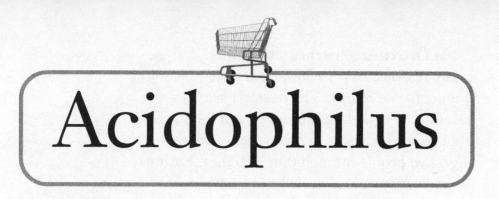

Acidophilus

BACTERIA YOU CAN BANK ON

Did you ever look at pond water under a microscope when you were in high school? It's fascinating (scary is more like it) to see how many microscopic organisms can wiggle around in one muddy drop. If you could take a look inside your own intestine, the view would be even more striking. Your digestive tract is literally swarming with organisms, including acidophilus, a good bug that's so effective at preventing and stopping disease that it's been called a living drug. Take a look below and you'll see why.

■ **Vaginitis.** Acidophilus crowds out the bad bugs that cause vaginitis and restores the acid-alkaline balance (pH) of the vagina so fewer infections can occur in the future. In fact, simply eating 8 ounces of yogurt containing live, active cultures of these beneficial bacteria can result in a significant decrease in infections, says Tori Hudson, N.D.

Cream the Cankers

Canker sores aren't as ugly as cold sores because they occur inside the mouth, but what they lack in visibility, they make up for in sheer pain. One of the most effective treatments for cankers is to eat yogurt twice a day. Just be sure to choose a brand that has live, active acidophilus cultures, because that's what kills the bacteria that cause the sores.

■ **Diarrhea.** Diarrhea strikes for many reasons, so it's acidophilus-rich yogurt to the rescue. The bacteria are essential for good digestion and can fend off attacks by organisms that cause all sorts of digestive problems, including diarrhea. Eating some yogurt daily is probably a smart idea.

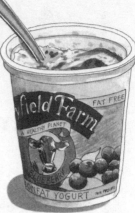

■ **Gas.** If you're bothered by intestinal gas, take acidophilus supplements one to three times daily on an empty stomach. Look for capsules or liquid products with at least 500 billion colony-forming units (cpu), then follow the label directions. Be sure to refrigerate any product you purchase.

■ **Cancer.** Animal research suggests that acidophilus and other organisms in yogurt may decrease the risk of breast, colon, and liver tumors triggered by carcinogens. "Although we have to conduct clinical human trials, the relationship between active cultures in yogurt and the reduced risk of breast and colon cancers looks very promising," says yogurt researcher Ian Rowland, Ph.D. That's certainly a good reason to eat it regularly.

ON THE SHELF

✓ **Live-culture yogurt**
✓ **Kefir**
✓ **Cultured buttermilk**
✓ **Sweet acidophilus milk**

■ **Antibiotic side effects.** Taking acidophilus can help reduce the side effects of antibiotics, which can kill off good bacteria along with the bad.

■ **Travel troubles.** When you're traveling abroad, don't forget to pack the acidophilus tablets. They stock your intestine with good bacteria, which will combat any bad ones you may pick up on your trip.

Acidophilus

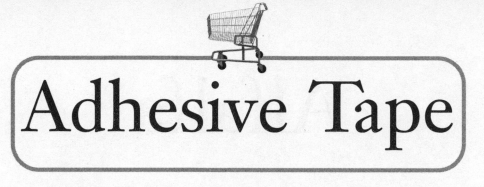

Adhesive Tape

A STICKY SOLUTION TO LITTLE PROBLEMS

Never underestimate the power of that little roll of white tape in your medicine chest. Check this out.

■ **Corns.** To banish a corn, cover it with ordinary adhesive tape. The tape will seal in moisture and help nudge fresh cells to the skin's surface. Eventually, the cells that make up the corn will fall off.

■ **Prickers.** Ouch! Those tiny cactus spines can really get under your skin. Apply a strip of adhesive tape across the stickers, then pull it off. The spines will come along for the ride.

■ **Warts.** The next time you have a wart, find a nice birch tree, cut off a strip of bark, and soak it until it softens. Next, use adhesive tape to fasten the bark directly to your wart. Birch bark contains salicylates, the basis for some FDA-approved wart treatments.

Just What the Doctor Ordered!

Tape Tip!

Here's a quick way to coax a splinter out of your skin using adhesive tape and a raw potato. Tape a potato slice over the splinter and leave it in place overnight. You'll be able to pluck it out easily in the morning.

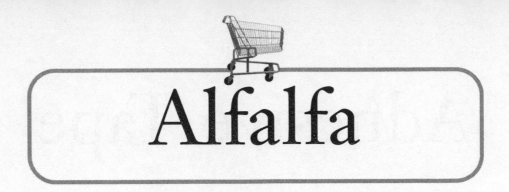

Alfalfa

IT'S ONE GREAT GRASS

Most of the alfalfa grown in the United States is sold for horse and cow chow, but supermarkets are also beginning to stock up on it. And that's good! Here's what it can do.

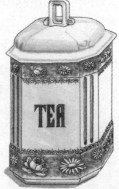

Soothing Sips

ALFALFA AXES ACHES

Feeling a little achy? Combine 1 teaspoon each of alfalfa and dried red clover blossoms, crushed, and add them to 1 cup of boiling water. Steep for 5 minutes, then strain out the herbs and sip. Add 1 teaspoon of honey, if you want, to sweeten it up a bit.

■ **Anemia.** An easy way to boost your iron levels is to sip alfalfa tea. Steep 1 heaping teaspoon in 1 cup of boiling water for 20 minutes, then strain. Drink a cup two or three times a day.

■ **Dragon breath.** Alfalfa is rich in chlorophyll, which can make your breath as fresh as a daisy. Drink up to three cups of alfalfa tea daily or take alfalfa tablets.

■ **Constipation.** Sip alfalfa tea when you're bothered by constipation. It will get you moving—and some doctors think that may also prevent bad breath, since toxins from waste build up and are exhaled through the lungs and mouth.

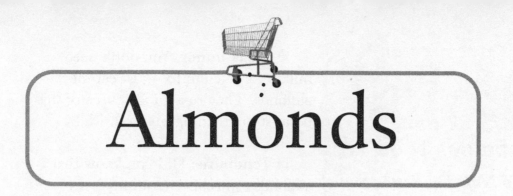

Almonds

MIRACLE MUNCHIES

Almonds are almost the perfect snack. Nothing's more convenient, because you can buy them shelled and ready to eat—by the handful or added to hot cereal or even ice cream. They're jam-packed with essential nutrients. Best of all, they're rich in essential fats that you can't do without. Almonds are so good for you, in fact, that they're almost like little pills that go "crunch." Take a look below and you'll see why.

■ **High cholesterol.** Studies have shown that eating almonds can lower cholesterol. Along with other nuts, they're rich in monounsaturated fat, which can lower levels of harmful low-density lipoprotein (LDL) cholesterol. Try a handful a day for heart health.

■ **Dry skin.** The essential fatty acids in almonds are essential to skin health, since fatty acid deficiency can leave skin looking dried out and wrinkled. Be sure to eat one serving of almonds every day, especially if you suffer from wintertime itch due to dry weather or heated indoor air.

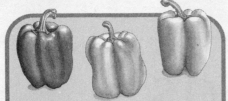

Fabulous Food Fix

Go Nuts for Better Sex

In India, almonds are valued as aphrodisiacs, perhaps because they contain the amino acid arginine, which promotes blood flow to the genitals by aiding in the production of nitric oxide. In fact, arginine is now widely used in modern-day sex-enhancing products such as ArginMax, a dietary supplement that also includes ginseng (an herb touted for energy enhancement) and ginkgo. In studies, women with low libido who took ArginMax for a month reported increased desire, and most men who tried it reported better erections.

■ **Weak bones.** You don't need milk for a calcium fix—just eat more almonds. They're a good source of this bone-strengthening mineral.

■ **Tendinitis.** Did you know that almonds can relieve tendinitis? It's true. They're one of nature's best sources of vitamin E, an anti-inflammatory nutrient that can reduce swelling, says Andrew Lucking, N.D. The fatty acids and E in ½ cup of almonds will help keep inflammation in check. Eat some daily.

■ **Frostbite.** If you're ever frostbitten, plan on eating like a squirrel. That means nuts—lots of them. Their abundant supply of vitamin E is crucial for repairing damaged skin. Eat ¼ cup a day until your skin's completely healed.

■ **Dull skin.** For a super-simple skin cleanser, you can't beat this: Grind shelled almonds to a fine powder in a blender or coffee grinder. Wet your face and rub the almond powder into your skin, then rinse. It will keep your skin soft and squeaky clean.

■ **Heart attack.** Research at major medical schools has shown that eating a handful of almonds five or more times a week cut study participants' heart attack risk in half compared with folks who never eat them.

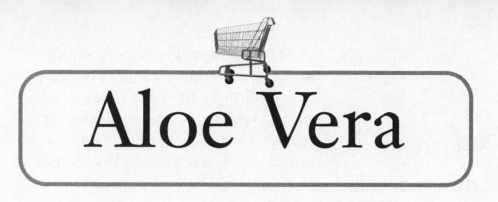

Aloe Vera

NATURE'S ALL-PURPOSE GEL

If you want to see nature's idea of an all-in-one medicine chest, take a look at that fleshy-leafed plant on your windowsill. For centuries, gel from the aloe vera plant has been used for healing. Modern doctors still take aloe seriously—and for a lot of good reasons.

■ **Athlete's foot.** Aloe vera is simply miraculous for healing skin, especially the cracks and blisters of athlete's foot. If you have a plant handy, break off a big leaf, mash it into an ointment or gel, and rub it on your feet.

■ **Burns.** Aloe is often called the burn plant because it inhibits the action of a pain-producing peptide and helps healing and skin growth. If you buy an aloe cream or processed gel, be sure it contains at least 70 percent aloe. Or just keep an aloe plant nearby. When you need to, simply break off a leaf, split it open, and rub the soothing juice over the burn.

■ **Inflamed gums.** Aloe gel heals all tissues, including gum tissue. Simply slice open a leaf, dip a cotton swab into the gel, and apply it to your gums. Don't eat or drink for a half hour afterward—and don't take aloe internally if you're pregnant.

Soothing Sips

SQUEEZE AND SOOTHE

Aloe is especially good for ulcers because it coats irritated tissues and may promote faster healing. You may be able to find aloe juice at a supermarket with a health food section, or, if you grow aloe at home to treat minor injuries, just break open a leaf and squeeze some juice into your mouth. You can take it up to a couple of times a day.

■ **Heartburn.** The juice from this succulent desert plant can take the sting out of heartburn by coating the esophagus and keeping stomach acid where it belongs. Drink ½ cup of juice once or twice a day between meals. Discontinue if your symptoms worsen or persist.

■ **Frostbite.** If you're ever unlucky enough to get frostbite, apply aloe vera gel (after seeing your doctor, of course). It will help your skin heal more quickly, and it inhibits germs that can cause infection.

■ **Shingles.** If you have shingles, you already know how the pain can linger even after the blisters heal. Try smearing on a paste made by blending a smidgen of red pepper with 1 tablespoon of aloe vera gel (or more, if the mixture feels too hot). The capsaicin in the pepper helps reduce substance P, a pain-producing chemical that your body releases during shingles outbreaks. Note that it may take about six weeks to work, and be sure to apply the mixture with a cotton swab so you don't burn your fingers.

■ **Hemorrhoids.** Aloe gel is one of the most soothing treatments for hemorrhoid pain. Apply a little to your finger and dab it directly on the tender spots. It may help the tissue heal more quickly, and it lubricates the area so there's less irritation.

10

Aloe Vera

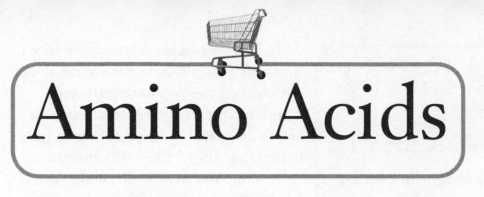

Amino Acids

IT'S A MEAN OLD WORLD WITHOUT THEM

You don't need a degree in chemistry to understand why amino acids are so important. Protein is among the major components of your body's tissues, and amino acids, all 20 of them, are protein's building blocks. You won't literally turn to Jell-O and collapse into a mushy heap if you don't get enough amino acids, but you might as well, because they play a key role in literally thousands of reactions in your body. What can amino acids do for you? Check out the conditions below—plus the chapter on arginine on page 24.

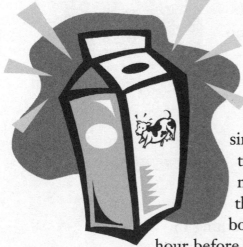

■ **Insomnia.** Oats have long been used to soothe the nerves and treat insomnia, and adding milk further invites drowsiness, since it's loaded with tryptophan, the amino acid necessary to make the brain chemical that controls sleep patterns. Mix up a bowl of oatmeal with milk and enjoy it an hour before bed.

ON THE SHELF

✓ Beef

✓ Poultry

✓ Fish and shellfish

✓ Eggs

✓ Milk

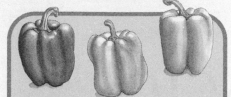

Fabulous Food Fix

Cabbage Clobbers Heartburn

A head of cabbage will help you get ahead of heartburn. It's loaded with glutamine, an amino acid that appears to promote healing in the digestive tract. Studies show that people who eat cabbage several times a week may be less likely to experience heartburn than those who never eat it. If the strong flavor of cabbage isn't to your taste, there's an alternative. Buy powdered glutamine, mix 1 teaspoon in a glass of water, and drink it once a day.

■ **Tired muscles.** Have you noticed that your muscles don't have as much pep as they used to? Pop some carnitine. This amino acid, abundant in red meat and dairy products, helps deliver oxygen to muscles. Take 250 to 500 milligrams twice daily. You may need to take up to 1,000 milligrams to increase your walking distance by 75 percent. "This amount is about twice as high as normal recommendations, so talk with a nutritionally oriented doctor before supplementing," suggests Ronald Steriti, N.D., Ph.D.

■ **Herpes.** The amino acid arginine can be a real problem if you have herpes. Arginine, which is found in nuts, seeds, chocolate, coconut, and sardines, helps the virus replicate, says Judith Boice, N.D. You can fight back with another amino acid called lysine. Found in lentils, legumes, black beans, wheat germ, and seafood, it seems to help discourage herpes outbreaks.

■ **Underactive thyroid.** Here's something to try if your thyroid gland isn't functioning as well as it

Amino Acids

should. The thyroid uses tyrosine, an amino acid available in supplement form, to produce thyroid hormone. Talk to your doctor before you try anything that may affect your thyroid function, however—especially if you're taking medication.

■ **Ulcers.** Glutamine is an amino acid that nourishes the protective cells in the stomach lining and helps speed the healing of ulcers. The suggested dose is 500 milligrams once a day.

■ **Angina.** Carnitine, an amino that's abundant in red meat, may help strengthen the heart muscle. Some doctors advise patients with angina to take 500 milligrams of carnitine a day.

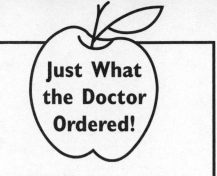

Just What the Doctor Ordered!

Bird Banishes Blues

If you need a little lift, try a turkey sandwich. Tryptophan, an amino acid abundant in turkey, converts to serotonin in the brain. This natural chemical works as a neurotransmitter and a hormone to enhance your mood. You can also get tryptophan from other meats, fish, and dairy products.

■ **PMS.** When you're plagued by premenstrual syndrome, sit down to a bowl of pasta. A diet rich in carbohydrates, such as pasta and whole wheat bread, helps increase your levels of tryptophan, which in turn produces serotonin, a brain chemical that elevates your mood.

Amino Acids

13

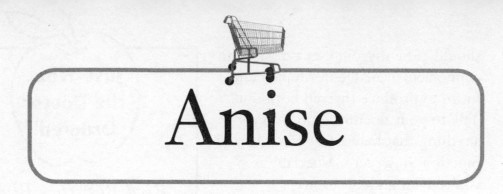

Anise

A CANDY-FLAVORED CURE

Since the time of the ancient Egyptians, fragrant aniseed has proved its worth in the medicine chest as well as in the kitchen. Here's how to use it.

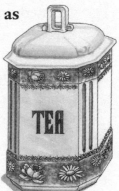

■ **Coughs.** The next time you have a bothersome cough, sip a cup of anise tea—it's an excellent bronchodilator that can make "dry," unproductive coughs productive, says Jamison Starbuck, N.D.

■ **Cranky gut I.** Anise contains a chemical compound called anethole, which settles the stomach. Try it after big meals when your digestive system is a bit overloaded.

■ **Cranky gut II.** Another way to quell indigestion—and enjoy a little zip at the same time—is to sip Pernod, a flavorful liqueur made from anise. It settles the stomach, reduces gas, and sweetens the breath.

■ **Queasiness.** You can combine anise with angelica to quell nausea. Simmer 1 tablespoon of angelica stems and roots in 2 cups of water for 20 minutes. Add 1 teaspoon of aniseed, then strain and take by tablespoonfuls every half hour until your stomach settles. You can have up to two cups a day.

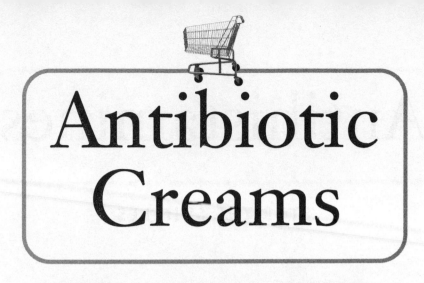

Antibiotic Creams

BALMS THAT BANISH THE BUGS

A mere 60 years ago, humans were almost entirely at the mercy of bacteria, but antibiotics changed all that. These days, you can walk into any pharmacy or supermarket and find a variety of antibiotic creams, which are among the strongest, most effective medicines you can buy. Here's what they can do.

■ **Earlobe pain.** If you have any kind of pain after having an ear pierced—for an earring, that is—apply an antibiotic cream at least two or three times a day for several days. Your earlobe is loaded with bacteria, and some may have gotten into the wrong place.

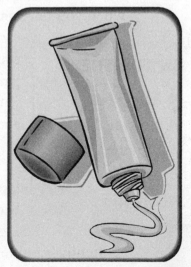

■ **Chafing.** Chafed skin is always vulnerable to infection. When something has rubbed you the wrong way, apply a triple antibiotic cream once or twice a day for a few days.

15

Antihistamines

STOP THE SNIFFLES

As soon as you hear the prefix *anti-*, you know you're dealing with something that opposes something else. That's not a bad quality when the "something else" is histamine, a body chemical that causes congestion, watery eyes, and other allergy or hay fever symptoms. Antihistamines, as the name suggests, are drugs that prevent histamine from doing its thing—and that means rapid relief. Here's how to use them.

■ **Earache.** Over-the-counter antihistamines often help when you have an earache because they decrease secretions that can block the Eustachian tube—and a buildup of pressure in the tube is what causes a lot of the pain. If you have high blood pressure, check with your doctor or pharmacist before taking antihistamines.

ON THE SHELF

✓ **AllerMax**
✓ **Benadryl**
✓ **Dramamine**
✓ **Allegra**
✓ **Claritin**

■ **Hives.** Hives can fade within minutes or last for days or even weeks—but you can fight back. Start with the first line of defense by taking an over-the-counter antihistamine such as diphenhydramine (Benadryl). In most cases, it will ease the reaction. Follow the label directions.

16

■ **Allergies I.** To get a jump on hay fever, take 250 to 500 milligrams of quercetin (a bioflavonoid-antihistamine) twice a day between meals, beginning in February.

■ **Allergies II.** For allergies, a good alternative to antihistamine drugs is to take the herb nettle, which has antihistamine-like effects, suggests Robert Ivker, D.O. Take 300 milligrams in capsule form three times daily. If your allergies worsen while you're using the herb, stop taking it immediately.

■ **Allergies III.** The most important B vitamin for folks with allergies is pantothenic acid. It works like an antihistamine and reduces levels of cortisol, the stress hormone that can spark or worsen allergy attacks. For relief from sneezing and congestion, take up to 100 milligrams of pantothenic acid a day after each meal.

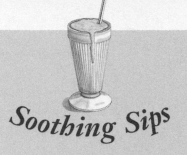

Soothing Sips

BREW SOME RELIEF

While some garden plants may be the root of your problem when you're rashy or congested, others can be your remedy. Chamomile is one of the best antihistamines around, and drinking chamomile tea will also help you sleep. As long as you're not allergic to ragweed, steep 1 to 2 teaspoons of dried flowers in a cup of hot water for 10 minutes, strain, and sip before bedtime.

■ **Pinkeye.** Over-the-counter antihistamines can help reduce the itching and swelling of pinkeye. Follow the label directions.

■ **Poison ivy.** Remember the icky pink stuff your mother smeared all over you after you got home from camp? Calamine lotion is the usual treatment for poison ivy rashes, but antihistamines may work even better because they block itch-causing histamines from the inside out. Follow package directions or ask your pharmacist about the proper dose.

Antihistamines

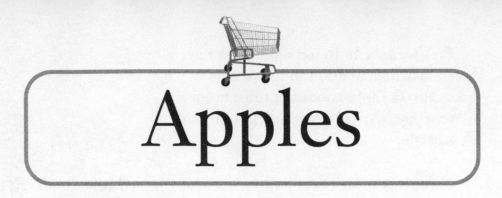

Apples

HEALTH FROM THE GARDEN OF EATIN'

You don't hear the expression "An apple a day keeps the doctor away" very much anymore, probably because apples are considered to be relative lightweights on the nutritional scale. But emerging research may breathe new life into the old cliché: Scientists have recently learned that apples contain a host of nutrients and phytochemicals that could very well leave doctors with a little more time on their hands. Here's why.

■ **High cholesterol.** You should definitely eat more apples if you have high cholesterol. They contain pectin, a type of fiber that binds to cholesterol and keeps it from getting into the blood. In one study, pectin lowered participants' cholesterol by as much as 16 percent. That's important because high blood levels of cholesterol are what contribute to cement-like deposits that form on artery walls and restrict blood flow.

■ **Hot flashes.** Munch on apples, and you'll have fewer blasts from your internal furnace during menopause. Apples contain naturally occurring plant sterols called phytoestrogens, which aren't as powerful as human estrogens but have a similar effect, according to Cornell University researchers, so they may help cool hot flashes triggered by fluctuating hormones.

■ **Queasiness.** There's a good reason that doctors often recommend applesauce for people whose stomachs are flip-flopping. Along with other bland foods, such as plain rice or toast, apples are easy to digest and give your body the nutrition it needs while your stomach's recovering.

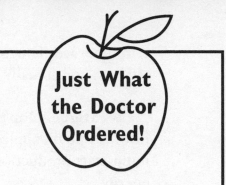

Just What the Doctor Ordered!

Whiten and Brighten

Apples, celery, and other crunchy foods can help polish away tooth stains safely, says Robert Henry, D.M.D. Give 'em a try!

■ **Diarrhea.** The next time diarrhea keeps you confined to the bathroom, remember the acronym BRAT. It stands for bananas, rice, applesauce, and toast—bland and binding foods that help you recover.

■ **Allergies.** Eating an apple a day is an easy way to help you survive allergy season. Apples contain quercetin, a potent bioflavonoid-antihistamine combo that reduces allergy symptoms.

■ **Joint pain.** The next time your joints are hurting—or better yet, before the pain starts—eat a few apples. They contain the trace element boron, which can relieve joint pain and stiffness and actually appears to protect against arthritis.

■ **Fatigue.** Don't let fatigue make your metabolism drag; just load up on apples. They provide malic acid, which helps jump-start production of ATP—the stuff that gives your cells energy.

■ **Dragon breath.** At the buffet table, head for the apples and other fruits and bypass the high-protein snacks if you want to get a jump on bad breath. Protein-rich foods invite odor-causing bacteria in, while crunchy crudités can cleanse your breath.

■ **IBS.** Apples and pears are among the best remedies for irritable bowel syndrome (IBS) because they're loaded with fiber, which helps tame intestinal spasms and encourages regular bowel move-ments. They're also easy to snack on as you go about your daily activities.

Bug Off!

The next time a bee gets in your bonnet (or anywhere else), hustle into the kitchen and grab an apple. It contains a chemical compound that may help inhibit the release of histamine, the body chemical that causes itching when you've been stung.

■ **Stroke.** A study showed that men and women who munched an apple every day had a lower risk of ischemic stroke (the kind caused by a blood clot blocking an artery in the brain) than those who were half-hearted in their pursuit of the Isaac Newton special.

■ **Cancer.** If cancer runs in your family, you should definitely make an effort to eat more apples.

Apples

The quercetin they contain appears to fight cancer, possibly by deactivating carcinogens.

■ **Diabetes.** You can't go wrong with apples if you have diabetes. The soluble fiber pectin slows the absorption of nutrients into the bloodstream, helping to keep blood sugar under control.

■ **Gum disease.** Apples contain compounds that inhibit the gum-destroying enzymes secreted by oral bacteria, so crunch an apple a day to help clean your mouth between brushings.

■ **High blood pressure.** Potassium prevents thickening of the artery walls and works in conjunction with sodium, an electrolyte, to regulate your body's fluid levels. Those levels are important because excess fluid in your arteries can elevate your blood pressure. Fortunately, apples are excellent potassium sources. Add them to your diet regularly.

■ **Constipation.** In hospitals, a mixture of applesauce, prunes, and bran is frequently given to patients with constipation. The soluble fiber in apples keeps stools soft so they pass more easily through the colon, while bran provides bulk from insoluble fiber and decreases pressure on the colon walls. And, of course, prunes are well known for their laxative effect. If you want to give it a try, mix four to six chopped prunes with 1 tablespoon of bran and ½ cup of applesauce and eat it just before bed.

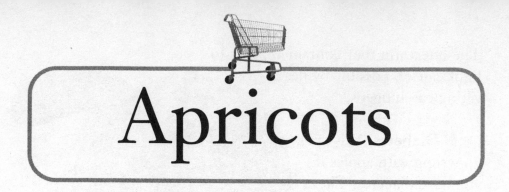

Apricots

GOLDEN GLOBES OF GOODNESS

The bright yellow hue of these fruits indicates that there's more lurking under their skin than a slightly sweet flavor. Apricots—think of them as miniature peaches without the fuzz—are loaded with powerful chemicals that can keep you healthy year after year. Here's how they do it.

Head Off Hives

Food allergies are a lot more common than you might think, and apricots are sometimes the culprits. If you're susceptible to hives and are allergic to aspirin, you may want to avoid apricots. They contain salicylate, the active ingredient in aspirin, which can trigger outbreaks of hives in some people.

■ **Stroke.** The potassium in apricots helps reduce the risk of stroke. In a Harvard study of more than 40,000 men, those who got the most potassium had about 40 percent less chance of having strokes than those who consumed the least.

■ **High blood pressure.** Everyone who's at risk for high blood pressure should eat more apricots, since their potassium may reduce that risk. How much potassium does a 3½-ounce serving of dried apricots offer? Close to 1,400 milligrams—three times the amount found in a banana.

■ **Anemia.** Millions of American women don't get enough iron in their diets, putting them at risk for anemia. Dried apricots are loaded with iron, a mineral that improves the ability of blood to carry energy-giving oxygen to cells.

■ **Aging skin.** The main ingredients in many prescription skin-care drugs, such as tretinoin (Retin-A), are retinoids, a group of natural and synthetic substances that includes vitamin A. Since apricots are rich in beta-carotene, which converts to vitamin A in the body, you can get some of the same anti-aging skin benefits by having some every day.

■ **Cancer.** Nature has created an array of anticancer compounds, and they're free for the taking—as long as you put apricots and other fruits and vegetables on your plate. Apricots were named to the *University of California, Berkeley, Wellness Letter*'s list of top 10 beta-carotene sources. It turns out that just three apricots supply more than half of the vitamin A you need daily. Apricots are also rich in chemical compounds such as lycopene, a powerful antioxidant that can help stop cancer before it starts.

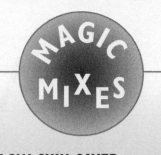

YELLOW SKIN SAVER
You can make your own moisturizer without leaving the kitchen by mixing equal parts of honey and milk and blending in some apricots. Use this homemade combo as a head-to-toe body lotion, then rinse off the excess. The blend feels wonderful, and you can keep it in the refrigerator and massage it into your skin whenever you want.

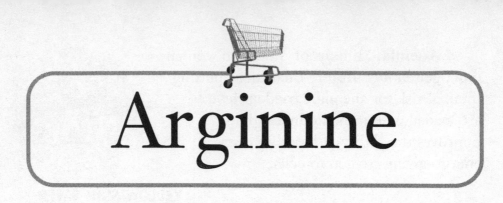

Arginine

A BRICK WITH KICK

Nutritionists talk a lot about the importance of protein, but it's amino acids, the individual "bricks" that make up protein, that deliver a real health-saving effect. One of these aminos, arginine, has gotten a lot of attention in recent years because studies show that it can strengthen the heart, increase energy, and (unless you're taking Viagra) even give your sex life an exciting little boost. Take a look.

ON THE SHELF

✓ **Milk and cheese**
✓ **Beef and poultry**
✓ **Chocolate**
✓ **Fish**
✓ **Nuts**

■ **Heart disease.** Arginine, like the drug nitroglycerin, helps relax artery walls and keep the vessels open. In fact, supplemental arginine has been shown to prolong the time people can exercise before chest pain kicks in, which is significant because exercise reduces cholesterol, blood pressure, stress, and weight—all risk factors for heart disease. Take 1,000 milligrams two or three times daily.

■ **Low libido.** Almonds are highly prized aphrodisiacs in India, perhaps because the arginine they contain is necessary for the production of nitric oxide, which promotes blood flow to the genitals. In one study, women with low libido who took an arginine supplement for a month reported increased desire. Take 1,000 milligrams once or twice daily.

■ **Angina.** Energy bars aren't just for scarfing on the trail anymore—instead, they may help you get on the trail in the first place. A Stanford University cardiologist has developed a first-of-its-kind energy bar called HeartBar, which contains heart-healthy (and angina-reducing) ingredients such as arginine, antioxidants, oat fiber, and fruit pectins. Studies with heart patients have shown that the bar increases the ability to exercise without angina.

■ **Bladder leaks.** Millions of Americans, especially women, experience urinary incontinence. If you have trouble with bladder control, scan your supermarket's supplement aisle for formulas that contain arginine. Naturally found in meat and other high-protein foods, arginine is converted to nitric oxide in the body, which helps prevent the bladder from going into spasm. This can prevent those sudden (and embarrassing) "gotta go" situations. Doctors who recommend

Just What the Doctor Ordered!

Aminos for the Heart

Arginine's cousin, carnitine, is an amino acid abundant in red meat that may help strengthen the heart muscle. Doctors sometimes advise patients with angina to take combination supplements of arginine and carnitine; the usual dose is 1,000 milligrams of L-arginine and 500 milligrams of L-carnitine two or three times daily. If you already have a heart condition or are taking prescription medications, of course, talk to your doctor before taking any supplement.

25

Arginine

arginine for bladder control usually suggest starting with 1,000 milligrams a day.

■ **Erection problems.** Men who have difficulty getting erections should consider taking extra arginine. The nitric oxide formed from arginine helps widen blood vessels, allowing blood to flow freely to the penis. Beans and peanut butter are just two of the many foods that contain this amino acid, but to be sure you get enough, consider taking a supplement. A third of men who take it notice erections returning within just 2 hours. Or, as long as you don't have high blood pressure, take a look at ArginMax, a widely available combination supplement that includes arginine, ginkgo, and ginseng. Studies show that it improves erections in nearly 90 percent of men who try it. You may have to take the full dose of six capsules daily for three to four weeks to see benefits. Consult your doctor first if you're taking any medications, and don't take ArginMax if you're using Viagra.

Head Off Herpes

If you've been infected with herpesvirus, you should avoid nuts, seeds, chocolate, coconut, and sardines. The arginine in these foods helps the virus replicate, says Judith Boice, N.D. Instead, fill up on lentils, legumes, black beans, wheat germ, and seafood, all of which are loaded with lysine, another amino acid that seems to help discourage herpes outbreaks.

Arginine

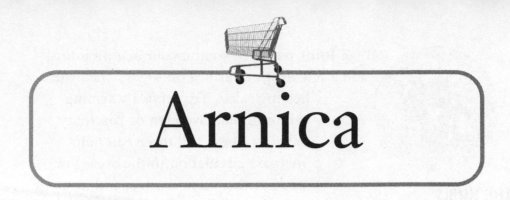

Arnica

RELIEF FROM LIFE'S HARD KNOCKS

If you had to choose one herbal remedy to include in your first-aid kit, it would probably be arnica. Some folks feel that when used alone or with traditional remedies, arnica basically jump-starts the body's natural healing mechanisms. Whatever the cause of your discomfort, arnica may be just the thing for rapid relief. Remember, though, not to use it on areas of broken skin.

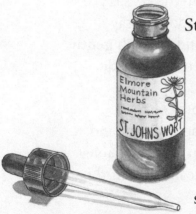

■ **Back pain.** A combination of arnica oil, St. John's wort oil, and castor oil can help quell nerve pain caused by back injuries. Combine equal parts of each oil and gently massage the mixture onto the nerve track, beginning at your buttocks and continuing down the back of each leg. If you have a disk problem, massage the oil into that area as well.

Take the Kick Out of Toe Pain

To quickly relieve the throbbing pain of a stubbed toe, combine 6 to 12 drops of arnica oil with a few tablespoons of olive or almond oil. Mix well and apply it a couple of times a day.

27

■ **Joint pain.** To soothe your aching joints, add a few drops of arnica oil to your favorite healing salve. Try using a warming wintergreen, lavender, or rosemary salve as a base. All three can help increase circulation to the area. For each ½ teaspoon of salve, add three or four drops of arnica oil and apply to sore joints three or four times a day.

■ **Muscle pain.** Arnica gel is an excellent first-aid ointment for sore muscles, especially when mixed with several drops of St. John's wort oil. Apply it frequently wherever it hurts.

■ **Foot aches.** Native American healing traditions say you should rub your feet every morning and evening to ease the burdens they carry. Try using four or five drops of arnica oil for your foot massage. Simply shake the oil into the palm of your hand and rub gently for a few minutes, moving from your toes up to your ankle.

■ **Sprains.** Many naturally oriented doctors consider extracts of arnica to be effective for controlling bruising and swelling from a sprain. Look for it in gel form or add 1 tablespoon of tincture to 2 cups of water, soak a clean cloth in the solution, and apply it directly to the sore spot.

■ **Frozen shoulder.** If you've had a shoulder injury, you may be able to keep your shoulder from freezing just by using arnica gel at the first hint of pain. Apply it liberally to the sore area several times a day.

CUT THE KINKS
A great way to take the kinks out of sore muscles is to apply your own muscle soother. Chop or crumble fresh or dried arnica, add enough water to make a paste, and spread the mixture over the area. Wrap loosely with gauze and leave the paste on for about 20 minutes, then rinse it off.

28

Arnica

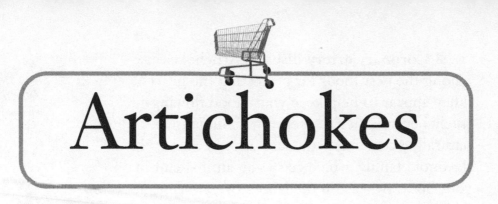

Artichokes

FORTIFY DIGESTION, HEAL THE HEART

We should all tip our hats to the first human who looked at the spiny, finger-stabbing artichoke and decided there was something hidden in all that armor that was truly delicious. Artichokes aren't the easiest food to eat, but they're worth the effort. Apart from their rich, almost creamy taste, they offer some healing benefits that you simply can't get anywhere else. Take a look.

■ **Bloating.** If you have problems with fluid retention, be sure to include artichokes on the menu. They act as natural diuretics to help remove excess fluid from the body.

■ **IBS.** In one study, people with irritable bowel syndrome (IBS) who took capsules of artichoke leaf extract twice daily for six weeks were able to significantly reduce their crampy constipation and diarrhea. If you prefer, you can take a liquid extract.

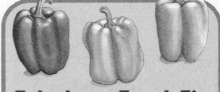

Fabulous Food Fix

Fight the Fumes

Flatulence is a natural, albeit uncomfortable and sometimes embarrassing, fact of life. You can't eliminate it entirely, but you can reduce gas levels by eating artichokes. They contain fructo-oligosaccharides (FOS), indigestible dietary sugars that feed the naturally present "friendly" bacteria that facilitate digestion.

■ **Coronary artery disease.** Artichokes are among the best foods for protecting the heart. They appear to help keep your blood flowing freely because they're packed with luteolin, a naturally occurring plant substance in the flavonoid family, which acts as an antioxidant in your body. At least in the laboratory, concentrated luteolin taken from artichokes prevents the oxidation of bad low-density lipoprotein (LDL) cholesterol. Oxidation makes cholesterol gummy, lazy, and very eager to find a resting place on your artery walls, which in turn makes arteries narrower and ripe for clogging.

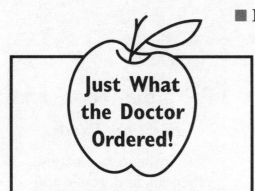

■ **High cholesterol.** Artichokes are full of cynarin, which has been shown to reduce cholesterol production. Cynarin may have benefits for your skin, too. In an Italian study, researchers found that it helped protect collagen, the connective tissue that holds your cells together, against sun damage.

■ **Cancer.** Cleveland researchers have been pursuing the cancer-prevention benefits of another artichoke ingredient, silymarin. At least in the lab, silymarin seems to forestall cancer development at several stages.

■ **Cranky gut.** For good bowel function, you need a constant parade of fiber-rich fruits and vegetables in your diet—and artichokes really wave the fiber flag!

Just What the Doctor Ordered!

'Chokes for Digestion

Dealing with digestive difficulties? Unless you have gallbladder problems, have an artichoke. It's a cholagogue, a vegetable that stimulates the production of bile, which is an emulsifier that aids fat digestion.

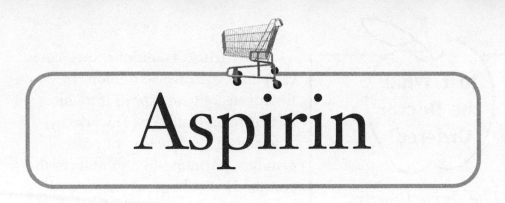

Aspirin

THE ALL-PURPOSE PILL

Aspirin has been a medicine-chest staple for more than 100 years, and its range of medical benefits just keeps on growing. Sure, it's a great analgesic and anti-inflammatory, but that's just the beginning. Aspirin is among the best over-the-counter drugs for arthritis, headache, and dozens of other conditions besides. Here's what it can do for you.

■ **Bee stings.** When you're stung, the first thing you need to do is get that stinger out. Then wet the site and rub an aspirin tablet over it to control inflammation and ease the pain.

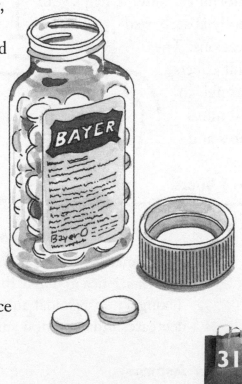

■ **Razor bumps.** To keep your bikini line from looking like a minefield of razor bumps and infected hair follicles, use shaving gel, leave it on for a few minutes, and shave with a wet razor. In addition, spritz the area with water in which you've dissolved two aspirin tablets and a drop of glycerin to reduce redness and swelling.

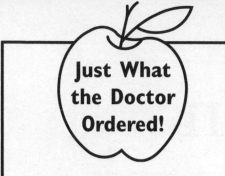

Just What the Doctor Ordered!

The Java Bonus

The combination of 130 milligrams of caffeine (about 1½ cups of coffee) and two aspirin tablets relieves a headache 40 percent better than aspirin alone, according to the National Headache Foundation. In addition to starting your motor in the mornings, caffeine helps your body absorb medications. The full effects are felt in 30 minutes and last for 3 to 5 hours.

■ **Arthritis.** Traditional medicine can't cure arthritis, so millions of Americans rely on aspirin to reduce joint pain and stiffness. It works by blocking the production of prostaglandins, hormone-like substances in your body that help regulate blood pressure, fluid balance, and temperature (among other body functions) and are often implicated in inflammation and pain. Talk to your doctor about the dose that's right for you.

■ **Bursitis.** Most cases of bursitis heal by themselves in 7 to 10 days. You'll feel better in the meantime if you take aspirin to reduce inflammation and pain. Follow the label directions.

■ **Menstrual pain.** Aspirin blocks the effects of chemicals that cause uterine contractions, which is why it's one of the best treatments for menstrual pain. Follow the label directions.

■ **Sciatica.** Nerve inflammation is behind the excruciating pain of sciatica and disk injuries, says David Borenstein, M.D. Taking a nonsteroidal anti-inflammatory drug such as aspirin decreases inflammation surrounding the disk and nerve.

Natural Aspirin

Wearing a copper bracelet has never been scientifically shown to do much of anything for arthritis pain, but here's a traditional treatment that really does seem to help. Native American healers recommend wearing a bracelet of willow root. It works because willow contains salicin, which is similar to the active ingredient in aspirin. When salicin is absorbed through the skin, it may help reduce the inflammation that causes the pain.

■ **Heart attack.** Because aspirin has an anti-clotting effect, it lowers your risk of developing a blood clot that can trigger a heart attack. Many people take half a regular aspirin or one low-dose (81 milligrams) aspirin a day as a preventive. There are some side effects, though: Aspirin can irritate the stomach and cause bleeding in some people, and it can even increase your risk of stroke. Talk to your doctor before you start taking aspirin regularly.

■ **Shingles.** Take two aspirin the next time you have a shingles outbreak. It won't always eliminate the pain, but it will reduce it to more manageable levels.

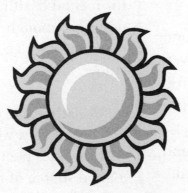

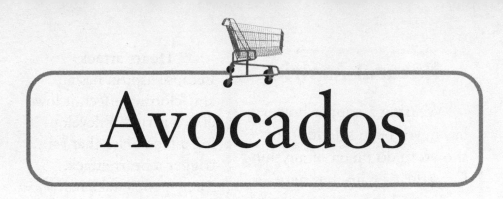

Avocados

FOOD THAT FIGHTS BACK

It's easy to understand why avocados have gotten a bad reputation. For one thing, they contain more calories than just about any other fruit. They're also loaded with fat, with up to 30 grams each. Don't let any of this scare you off, though. Eaten in moderation, avocados are among the best foods for preventing disease—and they have some extra benefits you may not be aware of.

Mood Food

Feeling down? Avocado contains tryptophan, an amino acid that's ultimately converted into serotonin, a "feel good" brain chemical. In one study, when women who were depressed feasted on tryptophan-rich foods, such as avocado, turkey, chicken, fish, dairy products, soybeans, and nuts, their depression eased.

■ **Mental problems.** Avocados are a good source of folate (folic acid), a B vitamin that's essential for mental health. In fact, if you don't get enough folate, your brain could atrophy, according to one study.

■ **Fatigue.** If you've been tired and achy lately, whip up a salad that includes plenty of avocado. It's a good source of magnesium, the mineral used by cells to stave off fatigue and ease muscle pain.

34

■ **High blood pressure.** It's hard to resist lightly salted chips and guacamole—and why should you? The avocado in guacamole is packed with potassium, a mineral that helps keep all the other minerals in balance and is vital for lowering blood pressure, says Jeremy Appleton, N.D.

■ **High cholesterol I.** Researchers at the University of California, Los Angeles, have found that avocados (at least those grown in California) boast 76 milligrams of beta-sitosterol in a 3½-ounce portion. This plant compound can inhibit the absorption of cholesterol from your intestines, so you'll have less in your bloodstream, reducing your risk of heart disease. What's more, animal studies have shown that beta-sitosterol inhibits the growth of cancerous tumors. Not a bad reason to stick them on your menu.

■ **High cholesterol II.** The fat in avocados is mainly unsaturated. It helps lower levels of low-density lipoprotein (LDL) cholesterol—the bad kind—while maintaining levels of high-density lipoprotein (HDL) cholesterol—the good kind. Dozens of studies have linked unsaturated fat to a reduced risk of ticker trouble. Researchers in Australia asked a

MAGIC MIXES

FRUITY SKIN SAVER
You'd be hard pressed to find a more emollient fruit than avocado. Its high fat content makes it an ideal base for a facial mask. Mash half an avocado, then add ½ teaspoon of vitamin E oil and 1 tablespoon of plain yogurt. Mix well and apply it to your face, paying close attention to the fine lines around your eyes and mouth. Leave it on for 20 minutes, then rinse off with warm water.

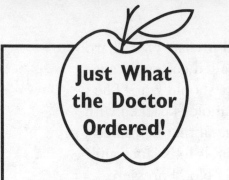

Just What the Doctor Ordered!

More Oil, Better Sex

Over time, the vagina's natural lubrication tends to diminish, and even slight dryness can make intercourse irritating or downright painful. You can spend a fortune on commercial products, or you can take matters into your own hands for a fraction of the cost. The solution? Apply lubricating avocado oil. It's completely natural, and it feels good, too. Many women also find that having a massage with soothing oil helps them relax prior to intercourse—and avocado oil is one of the best.

group of women ages 37 to 58 to follow a high-carbohydrate, low-fat diet for three weeks and a diet rich in unsaturated fat from avocados for another three weeks. Depending on how much the women weighed, they ate ½ to 1½ avocados daily. When the participants were on the avocado diet, their total cholesterol levels dropped by 8 percent on average, compared with just 4 percent when they followed the high-carb, low-fat plan.

■ **Stressed tresses.** For deep conditioning that fights the effects of heat, smog, and fog, mash half an avocado with ¼ cup of mayonnaise—the real mayo with eggs and oil in it. Apply it to your scalp first, massaging it in well, then comb out to the ends of your hair. Cover with a shower cap, then wrap a hot, wet towel around your head and relax for 30 minutes or longer.

■ **Overweight.** An 18-month study at Brigham and Women's Hospital in Boston compared a diet rich in unsaturated fat with a low-fat diet. Those on the high-fat plan were allowed about 45 grams of fat a day, mostly from foods such as avocados, nuts, and olive oil. The group on the low-fat diet received only 25 grams a day. A year later, the low-fat group had a net loss of 6 pounds, while the high-fat folks had a net loss of 11!

Avocados

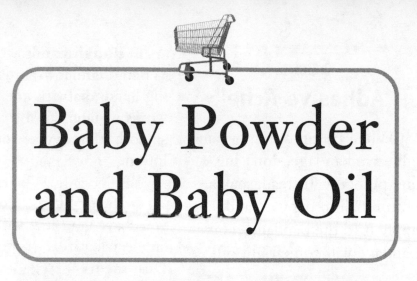

Baby Powder and Baby Oil

TRICKS TO SOOTHE AND SOFTEN

The same qualities that make baby oil and baby powder perfect for a baby's delicate skin will pay off when you're dealing with your own hide. They're soft, gentle, completely nontoxic—and effective in ways you've probably never thought about.

■ **Dry lips.** When your lips are cracked and dry, rub on a small amount of baby oil.

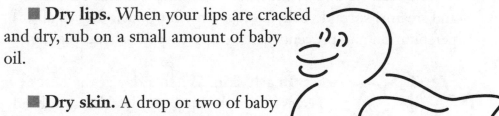

■ **Dry skin.** A drop or two of baby oil in your bathwater will leave your skin feeling soft and fresh.

■ **Chafing.** If you're getting chafed, dust on some baby powder to help the skin surfaces glide smoothly over each other. Use a cotton ball to apply enough powder to lightly cover the irritated area; the best time is after bathing and before dressing.

37

Stop "Adhesive Ache"

When trying to remove an adhesive bandage, don't tug and pull at it. Instead, soak a cotton ball in baby oil and apply it to the bandage. The bandage will come right off.

■ **Rough hands.** When it comes to softening hands, baby powder works wonders. Just smooth it on as you would lotion.

■ **Razor burns.** Do you shave your legs with an electric razor? Dust them with baby powder first to prevent friction burns.

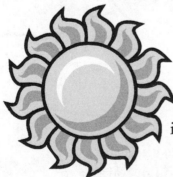

■ **Stinky shoes.** To keep your shoes (especially hardworking sneakers) dry, comfortable, and smelling fresh, dust the insides with baby powder.

■ **Stuck-in-bed syndrome.** When the weather turns hot and steamy, sprinkle baby powder on your bedclothes to absorb perspiration and prevent that sticking-to-your-sheets feeling.

■ **Beach skin.** When a day at the beach leaves you with damp, sandy skin from head to toe, sprinkle yourself with baby powder. It will absorb the moisture, and the sand will all but fall off—which will help prevent irritation later.

Baby Powder and Baby Oil

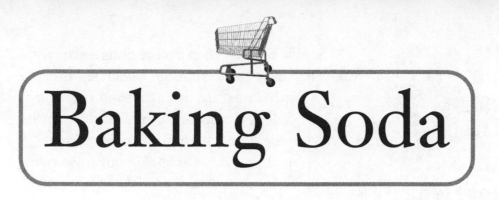

Baking Soda

ONE POWERFUL POWDER

Does anyone actually use baking soda in cooking anymore? Entire Web sites are devoted to new and creative uses for this ubiquitous kitchen ingredient, so don't be fooled by its low cost or its down-home profile. Baking soda is much more than a baking (and deodorizing) product. Doctors recommend it for all sorts of conditions—and for good reason.

■ **Gum disease.** If you want to clear up a persistent case of gingivitis, try this inexpensive yet very effective remedy. Shake about 1 teaspoon of baking soda into a small dish and drizzle in just enough hydrogen peroxide to make a paste. Then work it gently under the gum line with your toothbrush. Leave the paste on for a few minutes, says Sara Grossi, D.D.S., then rinse your mouth.

■ **Poison ivy.** The next time you have a close encounter with poison ivy, bathe in baking soda. Dump ½ cup into lukewarm bathwater and soak for a while.

Fabulous Food Fix
White and Bright

Fresh strawberry juice is said to whiten teeth over time. Paint the juice on your teeth and leave it there for 5 minutes, then rinse with warm water with a pinch of baking soda added.

MAGIC MIXES

Stuffy nose. When you're congested, you can wash away that irritating, thickened mucus with a mixture of 1 teaspoon of baking soda to 1 pint of warm water. Use it in a nasal douche or Water Pik with a nasal nozzle to irrigate your nose two to four times a day.

Shingles. A leisurely soak in a tub of lukewarm water spiked with baking soda will ease the discomfort of shingles.

Sunburn. Did you know you can take away the pain of sunburn with a baking soda soak? Fill your tub with cool to lukewarm water, add some baking soda, and soak for as long as you like.

QUELL THE SMELL
Here's a recipe for dusting powder to quell foot odor: Combine 2 parts powdered calendula flowers with 1 part each powdered slippery elm, lavender flowers, and aluminum-free baking soda. Sprinkle on your feet before putting on your socks and shoes.

Smelly feet. You can soothe irritation and reduce odor by powdering your feet with baking soda to absorb perspiration.

B.O. Baking soda keeps your fridge odor-free, so why not you? Use it as a dusting powder or body rub, or sprinkle a handful in your bath.

Calluses. To soften and loosen callused skin, periodically soak your feet in a pan of water to which you've

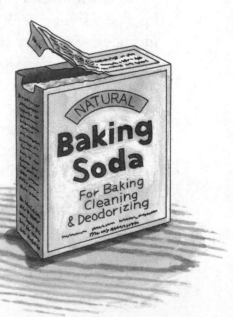

added a teaspoon of baking soda. As the callus softens, gently rub it away a bit at a time with a pumice stone or emery board. Follow up with lotion or cream to soften your feet. (This remedy is not appropriate for people with diabetes, who may have poor circulation in their feet and thus may injure their skin.)

■ **Canker sores.** You can lower mouth acidity with baking soda to reduce the discomfort of canker sores. Just add 1 to 2 teaspoons of baking soda to a quart of warm water, swish it around in your mouth, and spit it out.

■ **Tooth stains.** Toothpastes made with baking soda can help lighten tea, coffee, and other surface stains. Or you can use the stuff straight out of the box. Just pour a little in your hand, add a drop or two of water, and dip your wet toothbrush into the powdery paste.

■ **Pizza mouth.** The next time you have a mouth burn—from eating a steamy slice of pizza, for example—rinse your mouth with a baking soda solution. It will reduce acidity, which is important because mouth acids cause additional pain, and their levels rise quickly after burns or other injuries. Add a level teaspoon of baking soda to an 8-ounce glass of water. Swish the solution around in your mouth a couple of times a day until the discomfort is gone.

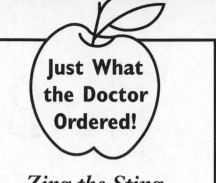

Just What the Doctor Ordered!

Zing the Sting

Bee stings release acidic venom, and baking soda is a well-known alkaline substance that can neutralize the reaction in a jiffy. Simply pour a little baking soda into your hand and add enough water to make a paste. Smear it on your sting and leave it there for at least 20 minutes to reduce pain, swelling, and redness.

Bananas

THE TROPICAL CURE

You may think bananas are just something to hold up an ice cream sundae, but researchers have found that this popular fruit has some magic under its skin. Here's a sampling.

■ **Low libido.** Need an instant libido lifter? Take a whiff of banana nut bread. According to studies from the Smell and Taste Treatment and Research Foundation, women who smelled the aroma of banana nut bread had an increase in vaginal lubrication as well as libido.

■ **Diarrhea.** When you have diarrhea, it's best to eat bland and binding foods. Bananas, along with rice, applesauce, and toast, are easy to digest and will help you recover.

■ **High blood pressure.** Potassium counterbalances sodium and helps reduce excess fluid in your body, which will lower your blood pressure. To get plenty of potassium, eat plenty of bananas.

PMS. An over-the-counter product called PMS Escape reduces premenstrual cravings for sweets and eases anger and depression, but it's also a mild diuretic that can deplete potassium. If you're using this or similar remedies, eat a banana daily to restore normal potassium levels. Bananas also supply vitamin B_6, which may reduce PMS-related mood swings, breast tenderness, and bloating.

Weak bones. The Framingham Heart Study found that women whose diets were rich in bananas and other potassium-rich foods had denser bones in their spines and hips than women with potassium-poor diets. Work these sunny fruits into your diet on a regular basis.

Ulcers. When a banana is dried and pulverized, it helps fortify the mucosal lining of the stomach and promote healing of ulcers, according to researchers in India. The dose used in the study was two capsules of banana powder taken four times a day for two months.

Dull skin I. Here's a facial you'll go bananas for: Puree one banana and one avocado in a blender. Apply the mixture to your skin and leave it on for at least 20 minutes, then rinse with warm water and pat dry. If you have dry skin, follow up with a moisturizer.

MAGIC MIXES

HAIR YOU GO
This mixture is just the ticket for dry, frizzy, or damaged hair. Mash half a ripe banana and half a ripe avocado in a bowl. Add 1 tablespoon of extra-virgin olive oil and three drops of lemon oil. Mix everything together and work the mixture into your dry hair. Cover your hair with a shower cap, wait 60 minutes or so, and shampoo as usual. For badly damaged hair, repeat this treatment up to three times a week until the bounce and shine return.

■ **Dull skin II.** Want an even simpler skin treatment? Just mash a banana and add 1 tablespoon of honey. Cover your face with the mixture, let it sit for 15 minutes, and rinse with warm water.

■ **Nighttime restlessness.** Having trouble sleeping through the night? Eat a few bananas during the day. Their abundant potassium encourages deep, restful sleep.

■ **Plantar warts.** You can remove painful plantar warts with banana peels. At bedtime, tape a piece of banana peel, inner side down, over the wart. Cover the peel with a bandage or a tight sock and leave it on overnight. Repeat the process each night until the wart is gone; it shouldn't take more than two or three treatments.

■ **Heart attack.** The B vitamins in bananas can go a long way toward protecting your heart. In a study of 80,000 healthy professional women, those whose diets included the most vitamin B_6 and folate (another B vitamin) were the least likely to have heart attacks. So whatever your risk level, have a banana.

■ **Cancer.** Bananas contain a chemical compound, called glutathione, that neutralizes free radicals, natural molecules in the body that cause cell damage. Studies suggest that glutathione helps prevent cancers of the mouth and pharynx.

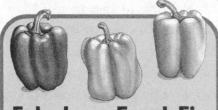

Fabulous Food Fix

Go For the Green

A banana that's a bit underripe—that is, still a little green at the tip—produces half the glycemic response of a ripe banana. In other words, it's less likely to cause a spike in your blood sugar, which is especially important if you have diabetes, says Thomas Wolever, Ph.D.

Bananas

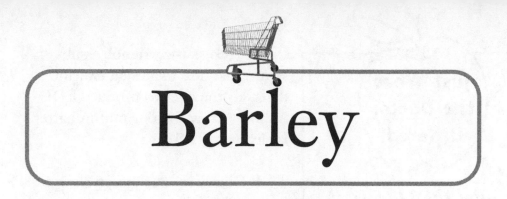

Barley

A GREAT GRAIN

Americans have never been very big on barley, perhaps because it has a strong, almost musky taste. Once you learn what barley can do for your heart—indeed, for just about every part of your body—though, you may decide that a thick bowl of barley soup is just what the doctor ordered.

■ **High cholesterol.** You're not likely to find this remedy at Starbucks—at least not yet—but one study comparing muffins made with hulled barley to ordinary, low-fiber ones made from refined wheat found that the barley muffins were cholesterol-flattening champs. They reduced artery-clog-ging LDL cholesterol by 12 percent, which can translate into a 20 percent reduction in heart disease risk. Barley contains beta-glucan, a type of fiber that many studies have shown to lower cholesterol by trapping some fat and cholesterol from foods and ushering them out of your body before they can be absorbed.

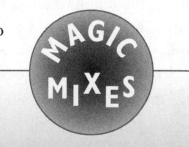

SOAK AND SAY "AH!"
To relieve itching and restore the proper pH of your skin, add 1 cup of apple cider vinegar and 1 cup of barley flour to a tepid bath. Don't worry, the vinegar smell will dissipate quickly!

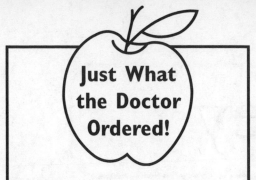

Just What the Doctor Ordered!

Quiet the Queasies

If dining out at the local greasy spoon leads to nausea, sipping barley water is the ideal "dessert." It contains catechins, which help calm your stomach. Boil a small handful of pearl barley in 1 quart of water for an hour. Strain the liquid, then add 1/2 cup of it to 1/2 cup of warm milk. Try to eat the cooked barley, too, since it may help counter any accompanying indigestion and diarrhea.

Plus, it boasts tocotrienol, a substance that deactivates an enzyme that tells the liver to produce LDL. Adding barley to your muffin batter is clearly a good idea!

■ **Diarrhea.** Barley can slow intestinal motion and curb diarrhea. To make it tasty, prepare pearl barley according to the package directions and add 1 cup to beef broth. The mixture replaces lost fluids and electrolytes in addition to calming your intestinal turmoil.

■ **High blood pressure.** A lot of nutrition information is couched in caveats, and you've probably heard them all. Well, here's a fact: When researchers at Texas A&M University tested the effect of barley bran flour, barley oil capsules, or wheat flour on men and women as part of a low-fat diet, they found that those who got either kind of barley significantly lowered their blood pressure.

■ **Diabetes.** At the University of California, Davis, researchers gave men meals made with regular pasta or pasta with barley flour. The men who had the barley pasta didn't produce as much insulin (a hormone that plays a role in diabetes) as did those who ate the other pasta.

Barley

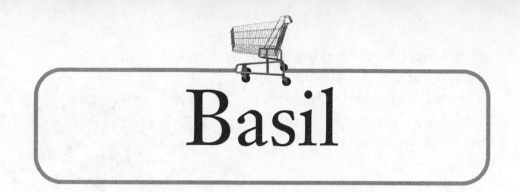

Basil

MORE THAN JUST A SPICE

The strong scent and pungent flavor of basil are signs that it can do a world of good. In fact, it contains concentrated chemical compounds that may fight cancer, ulcers, and dozens of other conditions besides. Here's how it can help you.

■ **Drug-induced ulcers.** Researchers in India tested the oil from basil leaves and found that it reduces the ulcer-producing activity of aspirin and alcohol. If you use either on a regular basis, your stomach will no doubt appreciate it if you add the herb to your evening meal whenever you can.

■ **Sprains.** Put pesto on the menu. There's good evidence that basil helps fight inflammation and swelling.

■ **Warts.** Basil contains several antiviral compounds that make warts disappear. Just crush a few basil leaves, place them right on the wart, and cover the area with a bandage. Change the dressing every day, and the wart should disappear within a week.

■ **Gas.** If beans and other starchy foods make you gassy, simply top your dish with a sprinkling of basil. It's a carminative herb, a fancy way of saying that it helps reduce gas.

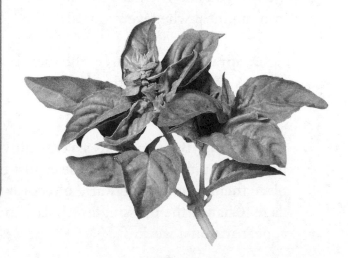

■ **Queasiness.** Basil contains aromatic, camphor-bearing oil that makes for a pleasant-tasting anti-nausea tea. Simply steep 1 teaspoon of leaves in a cup of boiling water for 15 minutes, then strain and sip.

■ **Cancer.** One compound in basil, called eugenol, increases production of antioxidants and may be helpful in preventing colon cancer.

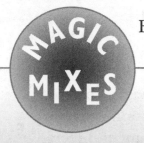

MAGIC MIXES

STEAM AWAY CONGESTION
The next time your sinuses start pounding, try an herbal steam. Boil a few cups of water and add 2 to 3 teaspoons of basil and a few drops of eucalyptus oil. Then carefully put the pot on a table or counter, drape a towel over your head to trap the steam, lean over the pot (but not so close that you burn your face), and breathe deeply. Inhale the steam through your nose and exhale through your mouth, Repeat for 10 to 15 minutes two or three times a day.

Beans

DISEASE-LICKIN' LEGUMES

Beans are the ultimate power food, low in fat and high in protein, vitamins, and minerals. That's reason enough right there to add more beans to your diet, but there's something else: Study after study has shown that beans are loaded with biologically active substances that can, quite literally, save your life. Here's how.

■ **Heart disease.** A study of 12,000 Americans ages 25 to 75 presented at an American Heart Association conference showed that people who ate a variety of legumes several times a week had a 19 percent lower risk of heart disease than those who ate legumes less than once a week. Researchers believe that both the protein and fiber in legumes may help hearts stay healthy.

■ **CFS.** According to Ralph Ofcarcik, Ph.D., good nutrition may be the single most important strategy for whipping chronic fatigue syndrome (CFS). "Since the immune system is functioning at less than an optimum

Fabulous Food Fix
Legumes for Lovin'

Good news for men: If erections don't come as easily or as quickly as you'd like, eat more beans. They contain arginine, an amino acid that helps blood flow freely to the penis.

49

Disarm the Gas Grenades

On the scale of gas-producing foods, beans are almost off the chart. What you may not know is that these foods cause trouble mainly for people who don't eat them very often. Adding beans to your menu more frequently will often cut down on excess emissions—and that's good news for everyone!

Here's another helpful hint: The Japanese seaweed kombu reduces beans' odoriferous by-products, thanks to a chemical compound called glutamic acid. Add a little kombu to beans or other gas-producing foods while they're cooking.

level," he says, "it makes good sense to focus on 'nutrient-dense,' or unprocessed, foods." Beans are among your best bets.

■ **Back pain.** Beans are a nearly perfect food when you have disk pain. They're jam-packed with protein, the nutrient that your body needs to repair damaged disks and ligaments. Also, unlike meat, dairy products, and some other high-protein foods, beans don't stimulate the production of pain-causing inflammatory chemicals in your body.

■ **Constipation.** Beans are Mother Nature's laxative. Eat ½ cup a day to keep constipation at bay.

■ **Diabetes.** There is a movement among desert Native Americans to return to their original diets, which typically included a lot of beans. These low-fat, low-sugar, high–complex-carbohydrate foods are more healthful than today's highly processed, packaged foods. Studies have shown that people on such a diet in Arizona and Australia have more stable blood sugar levels than most of us who eat a "normal" diet. There shouldn't be any reason why you can't add a serving a day.

Beans

■ **Ear noise.** You may need to eat more beans if you have the annoying ringing in your ears known as tinnitus. Beans are rich in magnesium, a mineral that can promote better circulation in the inner ear. Try adding ½ cup to your meals regularly and see what happens.

■ **Herpes.** If you have herpes, eat more lentils, black beans, and other legumes. They're loaded with lysine, an amino acid that seems to help discourage herpes outbreaks.

■ **Stress.** If your life is in overdrive, it's vital to include beans in your diet. They provide a bushel of pantothenic acid, which is critical for keeping your adrenal glands up to snuff when they may be maxed out, depleting your energy, says Jamison Starbuck, N.D.

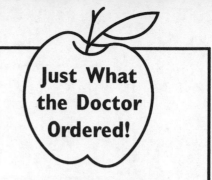

Just What the Doctor Ordered!

No More Sniffles

If you find that you keep getting cold after cold, add more beans to your plate. They're loaded with zinc, a mineral that appears to prevent colds, either by stopping the cold virus from reproducing or because they increase the body's immune response.

■ **High cholesterol.** Just ½ cup of cooked beans kicks in 3 to 6 grams of fiber, both the insoluble type (a colon cancer fighter) and the soluble type (a cholesterol controller). A study at the University of Kentucky found that eating 1 cup of canned beans in tomato sauce daily for three weeks lowered cholesterol in middle-aged men by about 10 percent.

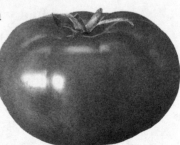

■ **Fatigue.** Beans release carbohydrates into your bloodstream slowly and can keep your energy humming at peak capacity. "Beans will sustain you longer than a food such as a potato, which quickly releases its carbohydrates," says Kim Galeaz, R.D.

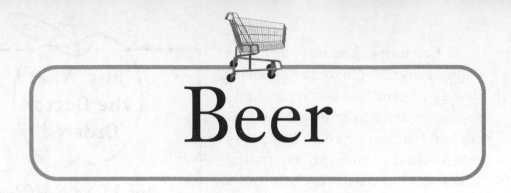

Beer

SALUBRIOUS SUDS!

The next time you hoist a cold one, you may want to give a little toast to good health. Wine gets all the headlines, but beer, from the lowest-calorie "lites" to the creamiest of stouts, has some benefits you may not have heard about.

■ **Circulatory problems.** Studies have shown that quaffing one or two beers a day will reduce your likelihood of having a stroke, heart problems, or other vascular diseases. *The American Journal of Cardiology* reports that the ethanol in alcoholic beverages is what lowers risk.

■ **Flaky scalp.** Hops is the herb that flavors beer, and Native Americans use it as a cure for dandruff (among other things), according to Gary Null, Ph.D. You don't need to comb the fields and woods for hops, however; just shampoo your hair with beer or add a good squirt of the "suds" to your regular shampoo.

■ **Stress.** After a long, hard day, relax in a beer bath to soothe your spirit and soften your skin. Just pour three bottles of brew into a tub of water, settle in, and think lovely thoughts!

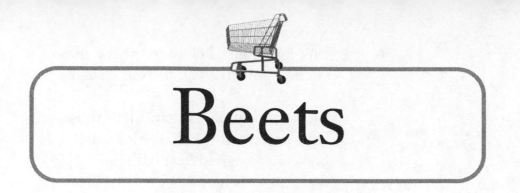

Beets

Don't think for a minute that those gnarly-looking roots with the crimson interiors are only good for making borscht. Beets are delicious pickled, roasted, and boiled—and that blood-red hue is produced by a high-powered plant pigment that has some remarkable healing powers. Take a look.

■ **Heart problems.** Betacyanin, the compound that gives beets their rich color, may help cells take in more oxygen, so eating fresh beets or freshly grated beetroot in salads could literally give your heart a breath of fresh air.

■ **Cancer.** Beets are loaded with anticancer compounds. Mainly, they're high in antioxidants, chemical compounds that prevent harmful oxygen molecules in the body from damaging cells and setting the stage for cancer. What's more, the betacyanin in beets may help inhibit normal, healthy cells from mutating into cancer cells. In one study, researchers tested beet juice, along with the juices of other fruits and vegetables, against common cancer-causing agents. They discovered that beet juice ranked close to the top in preventing potentially cancerous changes.

■ **High blood sugar.** All of those high-protein, low-carbohydrate diet books have started beet bashing. Somehow, their authors got the idea that beets are loaded with sugars that raise blood sugar and insulin and cause insulin resistance and even diabetes. Wrong. The sugars in beets are absorbed fairly slowly into the bloodstream. In fact, a cup of cooked beets packs about the same amount of carbohydrates as a slice of whole wheat bread—and raises your blood sugar even more slowly.

■ **Heart attack.** Just 1 cup of fresh beets delivers one-third of your daily requirement for folate, the B vitamin noted for keeping homocysteine in check so that it can't set you up for a heart attack. (Getting enough folate also dramatically reduces the chances of neural tube birth defects.)

■ **Constipation.** Beets are a good source of fiber, delivering about 3 grams in each cupful. Most Americans get only half the recommended 20 to 35 grams of fiber needed daily for good bowel function, and constipation makes you feel tired, cranky, and irritable. Who needs it? Have a glass of water, eat your beets, and get a move on!

Soothing Sips

JUICE AND DIGEST

Because the liver and gallbladder are intimately involved with digestion, it makes sense that food therapies can help them work a little better. A traditional way to help the gallbladder work more efficiently is to drink beet juice. Blend a few cooked beets with other vegetables, such as celery, parsley, or carrots, and drink about two cups a day, says Rowan Hamilton, Dip.Phyt.

Beets

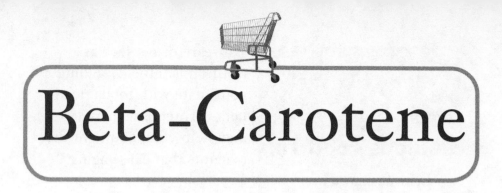

Beta-Carotene

IT'S ALL IN THE COLOR

The brilliant pigments that color fruits and vegetables belong to a large chemical family known as carotenoids. One of them, beta-carotene, is the plant-based building block for vitamin A and one of the most powerful plant chemicals ever studied. Should you make an effort to eat a kaleidoscope of colorful foods? Absolutely!

■ **Vision problems.** Carrots are good for your eyes, and so are other orange and yellow vegetables and fruits, since they're all rich sources of beta-carotene. Add two or three servings of carrots, squash, or pumpkin to your menu, along with plenty of greens, every day.

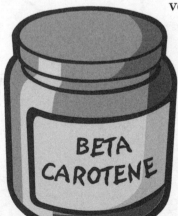

ON THE SHELF
✓ **Sweet potatoes**
✓ **Carrots**
✓ **Kale**
✓ **Spinach**
✓ **Winter squash**

■ **Aging skin.** Vitamin A, which is crucial for skin health, is one of a family of natural and synthetic substances known as retinoids, the primary ingredients in prescription

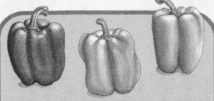

Fabulous Food Fix

Less Breast Pain

Millions of American women cope with breast pain, especially around the time of their periods. Fruits and vegetables that are rich in beta-carotene appear to prevent breast pain in some women, so add as many to your diet as you can!

skin-care drugs such as tretinoin (Retin-A). Filling your plate with foods rich in beta-carotene, such as carrots, may help your skin fight the oxidants that cause aging.

■ **Colds.** Don't take colds lying down. Load up on carrots and other foods rich in beta-carotene. They boost your immune system as it gears up to battle offending germs. They also battle free radicals, those pesky oxygen molecules that damage tissues throughout your body—including cells in your immune system.

■ **Cancer.** Researchers have long known that people who eat the most beta-carotene–rich fruits and vegetables have the lowest risk of lung cancer. One study of nonsmokers found that people who ate the most vegetables could lower their lung cancer risk by 25 percent. Significantly, this effect is not found with beta-carotene supplements!

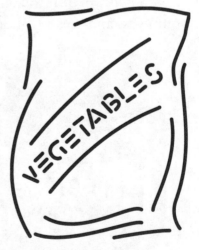

Beta-Carotene

Bioflavonoids

HEAD-TO-TOE PROTECTION

Forget the fancy chemical name: The *bio-* in bioflavonoids tells you that these plant chemicals—found in apples, onions, grapes, and even red wine—are all about life. They're powerful antioxidants, meaning that they prevent oxygen-like molecules in the body from causing cell damage that can trigger some of our most serious health threats. What else can bioflavonoids do for you?

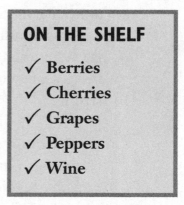

■ **Ulcers.** Most ulcers are caused by *Helicobacter pylori*, a nasty bacterium that essentially drills holes in the stomach and intestinal walls and allows powerful acids to damage tender tissues. You can fight back by eating fruits and vegetables. Their bioflavonoid content squelches the growth of bacteria.

■ **Heart disease.** Why is it that Europeans have so much less heart disease than Americans? The credit, at least in part, goes to red

ON THE SHELF

- ✓ Berries
- ✓ Cherries
- ✓ Grapes
- ✓ Peppers
- ✓ Wine

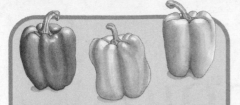

Fabulous Food Fix

Eat and Breathe Better

You can fight asthma by eating an apple a day. Apples contain quercetin, a potent bioflavonoid that may help keep your airways clear.

wine. Study after study has shown that light to moderate consumption of wine reduces your risk of developing heart disease or of dying from it. The theory is that the pigment in red grape skins contains quercetin, a potent bioflavonoid that has anti-clotting and antioxidant properties. One glass of wine a day is all you need.

■ **Macular degeneration.** Bilberry has a long history of use for eye complaints. High in bioflavonoids, it helps improve circulation to the eyes and protect against macular degeneration. Make a tea using 1 teaspoon of herb per 1 cup of hot water. Steep for 10 to 15 minutes, strain, and drink two or three cups per day.

■ **Heart problems.** Colorful fruits and vegetables, especially dark berries, are rich sources of bioflavonoids, which strengthen your cardiovascular system. Eat ½ to 1 cup of blueberries a day to keep your heart strong.

■ **Hemorrhoids.** If hemorrhoids are cramping your style, load up on crunchy veggies, hearty whole grains and legumes, and oranges and pineapple, all of which are brimming with vein-strengthening bioflavonoids, suggests Anil Minocha, M.D. These foods are also high in fiber, which softens stools and reduces the bathroom straining that can cause hemorrhoids.

Bioflavonoids

Shingles. Studies show that when combined with vitamin C, immunity-boosting bioflavonoids appear to prevent the viral growth and spread of shingles—especially if taken in the early stages of a flare-up. Look for a commercial formulation that includes both, then follow the label directions.

Groin injuries. If you've been laid up by a blow below the belt, keep a bowl of cherries within reach. The bioflavonoids in these tasty treats are custom-made for groin injuries because they help your body repair the delicate blood vessels that were damaged. Try to eat a cup of cherries every day.

Leg pain. If your daily walks are curtailed by intermittent claudication, in which insufficient blood flow during activity causes leg pain, make your tea the green kind. It's a great source of bioflavonoids, which make blood vessels stronger and less vulnerable to blockages.

Stubbed toe. Since bioflavonoids help your body repair and replenish damaged tissue, they're a smart choice when you've stubbed a toe. All fresh produce is good, but berries are tops because they're jammed with these protective chemicals. Treat yourself to a bowl of cherries, blueberries, or raspberries every day.

Soothing Sips

HOLLER FOR HAWTHORN

Hawthorn is a famous heart tonic that's high in bioflavonoids. Known to lower blood pressure, it also enhances circulation, providing the heart with extra blood, oxygen, glucose, and nutrients, and improves heart function and exercise tolerance. To use, add 60 drops of tincture to a glass of water or juice. If you're taking any other medications, check with your doctor before using hawthorn.

Bioflavonoids 59

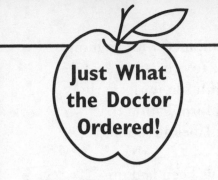

Just What the Doctor Ordered!

Congestion Protection

The bioflavonoids in blueberries, blackberries, and cherries are good for controlling allergies because they keep mast cells from releasing troublemaking histamines, the chemicals that cause stuffiness and other symptoms.

■ **Skin injuries.** Take grapeseed extract for scrapes, cuts, or other skin injuries. The bioflavonoids it contains will help your skin put itself back together. Follow the label directions.

■ **Surgical trauma.** Take advantage of the healing power of black cherries after surgery. Their natural chemicals aid in healing tissue, and they reduce inflammation and strengthen tiny blood vessels that were traumatized by the operation.

■ **Headache.** The next time you have a headache caused by allergies, a cold, or the flu, put some produce on your plate. The bioflavonoids in fruits and vegetables fight off viruses and reduce allergic reactions that can trigger headaches.

■ **Sore throat.** Many over-the-counter sore throat remedies don't work very well, but bioflavonoids can make a real difference because of their anti-inflammatory properties. Two of the best bioflavonoid supplements for sore throats are quercetin and rutin. For a day or two, you'll want to consider taking between 1,000 and 3,000 milligrams a day of one or the other.

Bioflavonoids

Bitters

PUCKER UP

It's natural to avoid bitter foods. For one thing, in nature, they're sometimes poisonous. Nevertheless, there are some good reasons to include more bitter foods and herbs, known collectively as bitters, in your diet. Here are the main ones.

■ **Overweight.** Herbs that tone the digestive system can help normalize eating patterns and prevent overeating. Try a bitters formula taken warm before meals. If you can't find a commercial preparation, mix equal parts of dandelion root, centaury, chamomile, and fennel, then steep 2 teaspoons in 1 cup of hot water for 20 minutes and strain. Drink ¼ to ⅓ cup before meals. People who are taking diuretics or potassium supplements shouldn't use dandelion, and those with ragweed allergies should steer clear of chamomile.

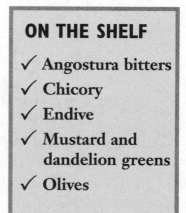

ON THE SHELF

✓ **Angostura bitters**
✓ **Chicory**
✓ **Endive**
✓ **Mustard and dandelion greens**
✓ **Olives**

■ **Hangover.** Bitters may help your liver metabolize alcohol and prevent a hangover. Mix equal parts of dandelion root, gentian, milk thistle, and peppermint. Steep 1 heaping teaspoon of the mixture in 1 cup of hot water for 20 minutes, then strain. Sip it slowly before bed and again first thing in the morning.

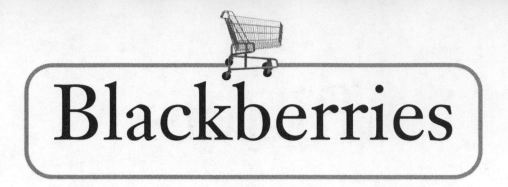

Blackberries

BERRY GOOD FOR YOU

You may think that blackberries are nature's incentive to take long, rambling walks with a berry-picking basket under your arm, but they're actually among the most potent food remedies on the planet. With every bite, you get a burst of intensely flavored juice, along with some impressive benefits. Work $\frac{1}{2}$ cup into your diet each day, and they'll help hold the following aliments at bay.

Soothing Sips

ROOT OUT THE RUNS

If you have irritable bowel syndrome, take advantage of blackberry tea. "The tannins in the blackberry root dry the mucous membranes in your intestine and bind up the bowel," says Michael DiPalma, N.D. Drink several cups a day.

■ **Cancer.** Blackberries are brimming with two recently discovered compounds, catechin and epicatechin. Research has shown that these compounds can prevent cancer by neutralizing free radicals, substances naturally produced by the body that damage cells' genetic material and provoke cancer-causing mutations in DNA. The berries may also inhibit an enzyme associated with the production of free radicals.

Diarrhea. Blackberry is a common diarrhea remedy used by Native Americans, says Gary Null, Ph.D. Squeeze some juice from the berries—fresh or frozen—or make a tea from the leaves. Sip two to four cups a day.

Allergies. Blackberries are bursting with substances called bioflavonoids, which are Mother Nature's answer to allergies. Bioflavonoids inhibit the body's production of histamines, the chemicals that cause runny eyes, a stuffy nose, and other allergy symptoms. Blackberries also boost cell levels of vitamin C, an anti-inflammatory/antihistamine powerhouse that targets the sinus passages.

High cholesterol. One of the chemicals blackberries contain helps lower cholesterol levels, especially levels of low-density lipoprotein (LDL) cholesterol. That's important because LDL is the stuff that clings to artery walls and inhibits the flow of blood to the heart. It also sets the stage for blood clots, the leading cause of heart attacks. Doctors estimate that for every 1 percent reduction in cholesterol, you can reduce your risk of heart disease or heart attack by up to 3 percent.

Fabulous Food Fix

Learn from Our Feathered Friends

Birds sit for hours with their talons wrapped around small branches, but as far as we know, they don't get "carpal claw syndrome." What are they doing that we aren't? It just may be that they fill up on blackberries, nature's remedy for pain and inflammation. The next time you have a flare-up of carpal tunnel syndrome, eat a handful or two of blackberries—and keep it up until you're feeling better.

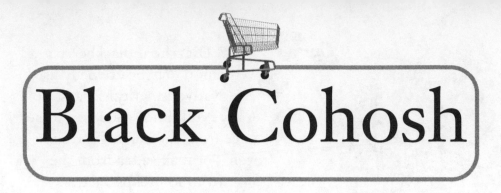

Black Cohosh

A WOMAN'S BEST FRIEND

Native Americans used this powerful herb for literally dozens of conditions, including snakebite. That's probably a bit of stretch, but modern herbalists and even physicians have found that the gnarly roots can play an important role in modern medicine, particularly for "women's problems." Here's how. (Because the herb may have estrogen-like effects, it isn't recommended for use during pregnancy.)

■ **Night sweats.** German studies have found that black cohosh works as well as estrogen for night sweats, sleep disruption, and other types of menopausal discomfort. Follow package directions.

■ **Vaginal dryness.** In studies comparing it with estrogen, this old-time favorite proved to be a worthy remedy for reducing vaginal dryness and boosting tissue tone and elasticity. "Start with two 40-milligram capsules twice a day," says Tori Hudson, N.D.

■ **Back pain.** If you're coping with back pain, look for an herbal formula that contains black cohosh, cramp bark, and oatstraw. These herbs are all excellent antispasmodics and muscle relaxants. Follow the label directions.

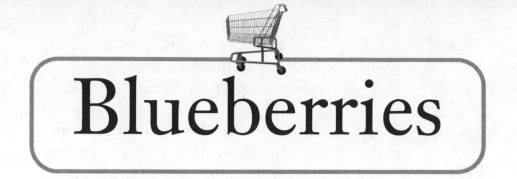

Blueberries

MORE THAN JUST DESSERT

Over the centuries, blueberries have been reputed to cure everything from tonsillitis to loose teeth. Okay, there's probably some historical exaggeration there, but blueberries really do have some remarkable healing powers—and nothing goes better with vanilla ice cream! Here's what they can do.

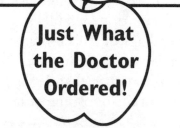

■ **Bruises.** Remember the girl who turned into a giant blueberry in the film *Willy Wonka and the Chocolate Factory*? It wasn't a pretty sight, but the good news is that she probably never bruised again. Blueberries are loaded with vitamin C and chemical compounds called bioflavonoids, which are essential for blood vessel repair. "I advise people to eat a half-cup of blueberries a day," says Sean Sapunar, N.D. The nutrients in the berries will help bruises heal and make your blood vessels stronger and better able to resist future damage.

Just What the Doctor Ordered!

Super Surgery Strategy

Enjoying some tasty blueberries can help you heal after you've had surgery, They help reduce inflammation, mend damaged tissue, and strengthen tiny blood vessels traumatized by the operation.

65

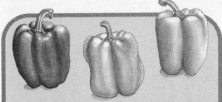

Fabulous Food Fix

Berry Good for the Brain

Eating ½ cup of blueberries a day may clear the sludge from your memory banks and improve your balance and coordination, reports a Tufts University study. Blueberries are reported to have the highest antioxidant content of any fruit or vegetable, so keep bags of frozen blueberries on hand and add them to oatmeal and salads for a brain-boosting treat.

■ **Heart problems.** The bioflavonoids in blueberries work to strengthen your cardiovascular system and help prevent molecular damage that makes cholesterol more likely to form thick sludge on artery walls and prevent heart-nourishing blood from getting through. Eat ½ to 1 cup of blueberries a day to keep your heart strong.

■ **High blood pressure.** The fiber in fruit apparently works even better than the fiber in vegetables and grains to lower systolic blood pressure, studies show. (Fiber is also tops when it comes to preventing constipation.) Blueberries are especially good examples, so top your morning oatmeal or cold cereal with these delicious berries and reach for a fruit snack later in the day, every day.

■ **UTIs.** Blueberries provide the same anti-infection protection as their crimson cousins, cranberries, when it comes to keeping bacteria from binding to the bladder wall and causing urinary tract infections (UTIs). Add them to your diet daily.

■ **Allergies.** Why load your body with antihistamines, which frequently cause side effects, when you can fight allergies with blueberries? They contain chemical compounds that inhibit the release of histamine, the body chemical that causes congestion. So berry up!

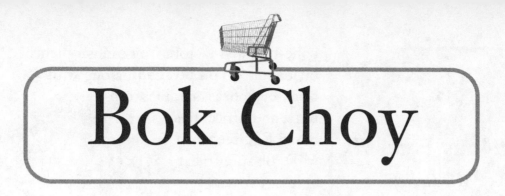

Bok Choy

GO FOR THE GREEN

You can think of bok choy as cabbage without the attitude: It isn't the mildest vegetable on the planet, but during cooking, it doesn't have the same room-clearing smell as its more cantankerous cousin. It isn't meek when it comes to your health, however. Take a look.

■ **Heart disease.** Calcium and magnesium help reduce the tension on artery walls and relax the muscles that control blood vessels so blood flows freely—the keys to lowering blood pressure and reducing the risk of heart disease. Feast on calcium king bok choy as well as magnesium-rich navy, pinto, and kidney beans.

■ **Weak bones.** When you're trying to protect your bones, you need more calcium. Food (as opposed to supplements) is the best source of calcium, possibly because it contains other, still-undiscovered

> ### Just What the Doctor Ordered!
>
> ### *The Vegetarian's Friend*
>
> One cup of bok choy serves up as much calcium as half a glass of milk, an unusually large quantity for a nondairy food. For that reason, bok choy is especially important for vegetarians who don't "do" dairy.

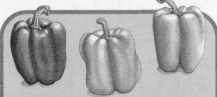

Fabulous Food Fix

PMS Relief

Women with PMS would do well to add bok choy to their menus. One cup of bok choy contains about 200 milligrams of calcium, a nutrient that may be a key to PMS symptoms. In one study, women who boosted their intake of calcium had half the number of symptoms they had before, according to dietitian Nadine Taylor, R.D.

bone-building factors. You can get plenty by loading up on bok choy, along with black-eyed peas, sardines, cabbage, and broccoli, says Susan L. Greenspan, M.D. Be sure to eat at least two servings of calcium-rich foods every day.

■ **Cancer.** Bok choy is packed with flavonoids, organosulfides, coumarins, and terpenes, chemical compounds that protect your cells against cancer-causing agents. It's particularly effective against cancers of the breast, prostate gland, and colon. One of the chemicals in bok choy, sulforaphane, has been shown to boost the body's production of tumor-preventing enzymes. At the same time, it increases levels of glutathione in the colon. This enzyme appears to help remove toxins from the body before they have a chance to damage the cells lining the intestinal wall.

■ **High blood pressure.** If you're taking medications for hypertension, you should eat more bok choy. Eating plenty of fruits and vegetables (8 to 11 servings) each day, along with a couple of dairy foods, can lower blood pressure just as well as medication can.

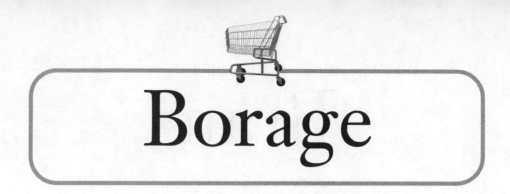

Borage

IT'S ALL IN THE OILS

Its bright blue, star-shaped flowers make borage one of the prettiest herbs in the garden, but its good looks belie the fact that it's a mighty hard worker. Herbalists have endorsed borage for centuries, for some very good reasons.

■ **The blues.** Borage can be just the thing to lift a low mood. Steep 1 teaspoon of the dried herb in 1 cup of boiling water for 10 minutes, then strain. Drink two or three cups a day.

■ **Dry skin.** To combat dry skin as a result of thyroid disease, supplement with 800 to 1,200 milligrams of borage oil a day.

■ **Asthma.** Borage flowers are packed with gamma-linolenic acid (GLA), which helps reduce the airway inflammation that comes with asthma. Check with your doctor about taking 3 grams in supplement form daily.

■ **Raynaud's disease.** When your fingers or toes are icy due to Raynaud's, massage borage oil into them to reduce the discomfort.

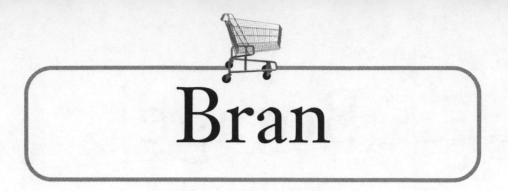

Bran

FIBER OF CHAMPIONS

Pure, unadulterated bran—from oats, wheat, rice, or other grains—isn't exactly a culinary treat, but it goes down well when it's blended into fruit smoothies or used as an ingredient in cereals. More important, it can keep your intestines and arteries in top-notch form. Here's how.

ON THE SHELF

✓ **Whole wheat bread**

✓ **Brown rice**

✓ **All-Bran cereal**

■ **IBS.** Rice bran oil extract, called gamma-orysanol, helps reduce diarrhea, protects the mucous lining of the gastrointestinal tract, and relieves other symptoms of irritable bowel syndrome (IBS) in a jiffy. Take 100 milligrams three times a day.

■ **High blood sugar.** Chewy, high-fiber foods packed with bran not only make you eat more slowly, they also enter your bloodstream in turtle-like fashion, preventing your blood sugar from spiking and then dropping—along with your energy and your resistance to Milky Ways. Choose a bowl of steel-cut oat bran instead of sugary, melt-in-your mouth cereal and have hearty, whole grain bread instead of soft white bread.

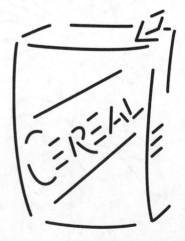

■ **Fatigue.** All of the B vitamins can help improve energy levels, but one of the more important Bs is thiamin pyrophosphate (the activated form of vitamin B_1), which is necessary for the breakdown and release of energy from carbohydrates. To make sure you get enough, take a B-complex supplement, add some wheat germ to yogurt, and choose rice bran cereal for breakfast. Since too much thiamin can cause nerve damage, though, don't take high-dose supplements.

Fabulous Food Fix

Bran Pounds Pressure

Researchers at Texas A&M University tested the effect of barley bran flour (along with barley oil capsules and wheat flour) on men and women. The result? Those who got either kind of barley had significant reductions in blood pressure.

■ **Hemorrhoids.** Most hemorrhoids are caused by straining to pass hard, uncooperative stools. The best way to prevent them is to eat bran or other kinds of fiber, which absorb water in the intestine and make stools softer and easier to pass. This helps in two ways: It makes bowel movements a lot less painful when you have anal irritation, and it reduces the risk that you'll have problems in the first place.

■ **Bowel spasms.** To reduce painful intestinal spasms and promote easier bowel movements, start the day with a bowl of oat bran cereal or sprinkle a tablespoon of oat bran on cereal or yogurt. Because your intestine doesn't have to work very hard to pass high-fiber foods, you'll have fewer painful cramps.

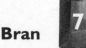

Bran 71

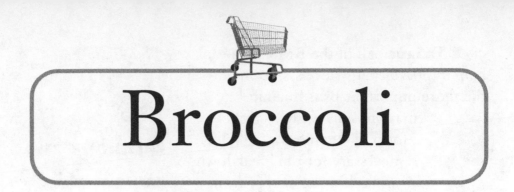

Broccoli

THE KING OF CRUCIFERS

Don't be fooled by the festive green color: Broccoli is serious stuff. A cruciferous vegetable (like cabbage and brussels sprouts), it contains more chemical compounds than most laboratories—and a few weekly servings can protect your body in ways you never thought possible. Here's a sample.

■ **Heart disease.** Studies have found that if you have broccoli just once a week, you could potentially cut your risk of heart disease in half compared with people who don't eat it.

Skin Saver

To help your skin heal from cuts or scrapes, eat five or six daily servings of antioxidant-rich foods such as broccoli.

■ **Stroke.** Researchers at Harvard analyzed the diets of more than 100,000 people for as long as 14 years and found that the more broccoli and other fruits and veggies the participants ate, the lower their risk of stroke was. In fact, broccoli and other crucifers may be as effective for preventing stroke as controlling blood pressure and engaging in physical activity, says Ralph Sacco, M.D.

■ **Alzheimer's.** Broccoli is rich in folate, a B vitamin that lowers levels of homocysteine, an amino acid that's been linked with Alzheimer's disease. Steam up some florets as often as possible!

■ **CFS.** Broccoli, which is rich in vitamin C, aids your body in making glutathione, the powerful antioxidant that helps your body rid itself of toxins and can reduce symptoms of chronic fatigue syndrome (CFS). John Reed, M.D., suggests that you load up on broccoli, red peppers, oranges, and other vitamin C–rich foods and take 750 milligrams of C in supplement form daily.

■ **Endometriosis.** You should definitely eat more broccoli if you have endometriosis. It contains an abundance of phytoestrogens, compounds that are structurally similar to but weaker than the estrogen found in your body. When you eat broccoli and other crucifers, the phytoestrogens compete with natural estrogen to bind to receptors in your body, but when they bind, they have a weaker effect. This means that overall estrogen activity is reduced, which may decrease endometriosis symptoms.

■ **Brain fog.** Broccoli is high in magnesium, potassium, and boron, minerals that are important for mental alertness. Try it in a salad every day!

■ **Lupus.** Doctors often advise women with lupus to eat more broccoli. Each mini-tree is chock-full of powerful anti-inflammatory vitamin C and contains indole-3-carbinol, a

Fabulous Food Fix
Your Brain on Broccoli

People who get high levels of antioxidants from broccoli and other produce tend to score better on memory tests.

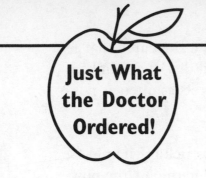

Just What the Doctor Ordered!

Gum It!

To protect your gums, load up on broccoli. It's practically dripping with vitamin C, an antioxidant that toughens gums, reduces swelling, and squelches infection.

chemical that may help rebalance hormones in women with lupus.

■ **Weak bones.** Broccoli is absolutely brimming with calcium, the mineral that you need for strong bones. Blanch it and serve with dip!

■ **Cancer I.** Researchers have found that the more broccoli people eat, the lower their risk of colon cancer.

■ **Cancer II.** Like the Brady Bunch, broccoli is comprised of at least six do-gooders: vitamin A, vitamin C, vitamin K, fiber, and the plant compounds lutein and sulforaphane. Scientists believe that many of these elements work together to provide broccoli's cancer-fighting benefits. A study at the Fred Hutchinson Cancer Research Center found that eating three servings of vegetables daily can lower the risk of prostate cancer by an amazing 45 percent. "If some of those vegetables are the cruciferous kind like broccoli, men could drop their risk even further," says study coauthor Alan Kristal, Dr.P.H.

■ **Cancer III.** A research survey of 50,000 men determined that those who ate a ½-cup serving of broccoli just twice a week reduced their chances of developing bladder cancer—the fourth leading cancer—by half.

■ **Broken hip.** The vitamin K in broccoli may help lower the chance of fracturing a hip when you get older, according to a study at Tufts University.

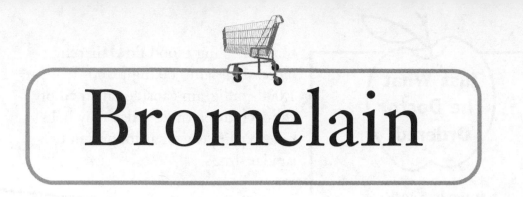

Bromelain

PINEAPPLE IN A PILL

Every now and then, Mother Nature outdoes herself. Take the pineapple. Not only is it the sweetest of tropical fruits, equally delicious in smoothies and upside-down cakes, it's also the source of an enzyme, bromelain, that can ease joint pain, clobber inflammation, and reduce pain after injuries. People with sensitivities to pineapple should avoid bromelain, as should those who use aspirin regularly or take blood thinners. For the rest of us, though, here are all the things this amazing enzyme can help.

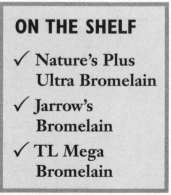

■ **Bursitis.** Has bursitis pain got you down? Take 200 milligrams of bromelain several times a day between meals to reduce inflammation. The enzyme can also help inhibit the formation of scar tissue that can slow your recovery time.

ON THE SHELF

✓ **Nature's Plus Ultra Bromelain**

✓ **Jarrow's Bromelain**

✓ **TL Mega Bromelain**

■ **Lupus.** During lupus flare-ups, bromelain supplements can break down fibrin, the tissue that forms during inflammation and

75

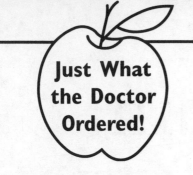

Sneeze Stopper

During hay fever season, pop a combination supplement of bromelain and quercetin. Quercetin may help inhibit the release of histamines, the chemicals that cause allergy symptoms, while bromelain boosts quercetin's effect and may reduce inflammation in its own right. Follow the label directions.

blocks healing blood flow, thereby increasing pain. Taking a 500- to 1,000-milligram capsule on an empty stomach three times a day may help relieve pain as well as ibuprofen or similar drugs.

■ **Sinusitis.** Bromelain reduces inflammation and fluid retention and helps shrink swollen sinuses during attacks of sinusitis.

■ **Surgical trauma.** If you've had surgery, start taking bromelain as soon as you get home. (Check with your doctor first, just to be safe.) It helps in several ways. It promotes circulation so more healing nutrients reach the injured area. It cleans up the cellular debris in inflamed tissue and can usher out pain-causing chemicals. It works so well, in fact, that in some cases, it can help people heal twice as fast. At the very least, you'll probably have less pain, swelling, and bruising.

■ **Pneumonia.** Bromelain can help your body overcome pneumonia. "It's an enzyme that helps break up mucus and reduce inflammation," says Christian Dodge, N.D. Bromelain

The next time carpal tunnel syndrome makes your fingers or wrists feel as if they're clamped in a vise, take some bromelain. It works as a natural anti-inflammatory.

also helps your body absorb antibiotics more efficiently, which is important if you're being treated for bacterial pneumonia.

■ **Digestive problems.** If your stomach doesn't do an effective job of digesting your meals, you're sure to get heartburn or a stomachache. Supplemental digestive enzymes such as bromelain can help, says Andrew Parkinson, N.D. They improve your body's ability to digest proteins and fats, which can help minimize those miserable after-meal flare-ups of pain.

■ **Cancer.** Animal studies suggest that bromelain holds promise for fighting cancer—particularly lung cancer and leukemia—but more tests need to be done. In the meantime, however, ask your doctor whether taking a bromelain supplement is right for you.

■ **Sprains.** Bromelain and the spice turmeric are powerful partners when it comes to reducing the pain and inflammation of a sprain. Take 250 to 500 milligrams of each three times daily between meals.

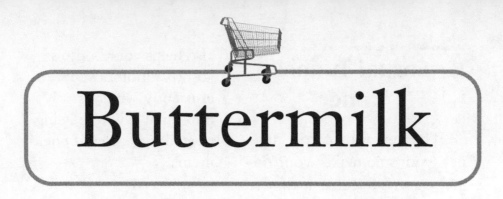

Buttermilk

NATURE'S WHOLESOME SOOTHER

The word *butter* in its name makes it sound as though this thick, creamy drink is loaded with fat. In fact, it's leaner than regular milk, so you can use it as a healthful substitute. As a bonus, it has some healing powers that are all its own. Take a look.

■ **Age spots.** Sick of those big brown spots on your hands? Soak your hands in buttermilk twice a day to keep the spots from enlarging.

■ **Rough skin.** Buttermilk's high lactic acid content means that a buttermilk bath will soothe and soften the skin. Since that's a lot of buttermilk, an easier option is to bathe the parts of you that get roughed up by nasty weather by splashing your face or hands with buttermilk once or twice a day.

■ **Weak bones.** A couple of glasses of buttermilk a day will provide an abundance of bone-building calcium.

■ **Large pores.** To tighten up enlarged pores, mix a little buttermilk and table salt into a paste, then apply it to your face and massage well. Leave it on for about 5 minutes, rinse with warm water, and pat dry.

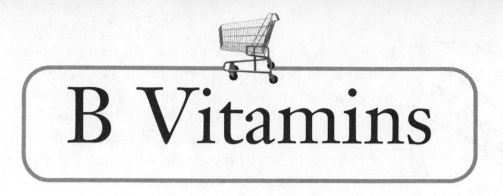

B Vitamins

"B" GOOD TO YOURSELF

If you're like millions of Americans, you take a daily supplement that contains all of the essential B vitamins. That's a smart move (although you should avoid individual B supplements, since large amounts of some Bs—particularly thiamin—can cause nerve damage). The Bs are involved in hundreds of bodily functions, from regulating your mood to ensuring optimal blood flow. It's no exaggeration to say that you need Bs just to, well, be. Here's what we mean.

■ **Mouth sores.** Folic acid (folate) helps the body replace gum cells that are damaged by poorly fitting dentures. Until the sore heals, take at least 400 micrograms daily, along with 1,000 micrograms of B_{12}. Taking folic acid alone can mask a B_{12} deficiency, which can lead to nerve damage.

■ **Heart attack.** In a study of 80,000 healthy professional women, those whose diets included the most vitamin B_6 and folate were

Monthly Skin Saver

The B vitamins—particularly B_6—help regulate those pesky hormones that set the stage for adult acne, especially breakouts triggered by hormonal changes during menstruation and menopause.

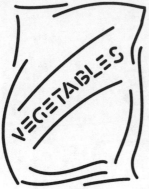

the least likely to have heart attacks. In another study of almost 500 people at high risk for heart disease, increasing their intake of folate and vitamins B_6 and B_{12} helped control their blood levels of homocysteine, a risk factor for heart attack. You can get plenty of Bs from beans, whole grains, and many fruits and veggies, especially orange juice and leafy greens.

■ **Scalp problems.** The B vitamins, particularly biotin, are essential to a healthy scalp. Make sure your multivitamin contains biotin, or find a B-complex vitamin that contains 300 micrograms of biotin.

■ **Mood swings.** It's common for women in the menopausal years to experience mood swings. All of the B vitamins, especially B_6, can help keep your emotions on an even keel.

■ **Gum disease.** Folate helps keep mucous membranes, including your gums, healthy. Be sure to get adequate amounts by eating two or three servings of folate-rich foods every day. Barley, brown rice, dark leafy greens, legumes, oranges, salmon, lamb, and dates are several excellent sources.

■ **Allergies.** Pantothenic acid is a B vitamin that works like an antihistamine. It also lowers levels of cortisol, a stress hormone that can trigger or aggravate allergy attacks. Taking 100 milligrams of pantothenic acid three times a day after meals should help relieve congestion and sneezing.

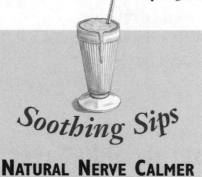

Soothing Sips

NATURAL NERVE CALMER

Sipped as a tea, the herb oatstraw is packed with B vitamins, which soothe jangled nerves. Buy the herb packaged in tea bags and have a cup two to four times a day.

■ **Anemia.** Folate is a red blood cell builder, but since it isn't stored in your body, you need to replenish your supply daily to help prevent anemia. Be sure to eat lots of whole grain products, dark leafy greens, citrus fruits, and beans.

■ **Canker sores.** A deficiency of B vitamins can irritate the tender tissues in your mouth and create the perfect environment for canker sores to develop. If you're prone to these painful sores, make sure your multivitamin contains 100 percent of the Daily Value for all the Bs.

■ **Fatigue.** All of the B vitamins can help boost energy, immune function, and mental sharpness, but a form of thiamin called thiamin pyrophosphate is crucial for the breakdown and release of energy from carbohydrates. In addition to getting thiamin in a B-complex supplement, you can add more to your diet by sprinkling wheat germ on yogurt, having rice bran cereal for breakfast, and snacking on peanuts, pecans, and walnuts.

■ **Raynaud's disease.** If your hands and feet are chilled by Raynaud's, you can increase blood flow to your extremities with inositol hexaniacinate, a form of the B vitamin niacin. Take 600 milligrams a day, but only after checking with your doctor. People with diabetes, low blood pressure, glaucoma, gout, liver disease, ulcers, or bleeding disorders should consult a physician

Fabulous Food Fix

Eggs-cellent for Nails

Eggs are packed with biotin, the B vitamin that helps your body make and use amino acids, the building blocks of protein. Long ago, biotin was found to strengthen horses' hooves, and more recent studies have shown it works similarly for humans' nails—a good reason to eat more eggs.

before taking any form of niacin—as should anyone who's taking any type of medication.

■ **Fibromyalgia.** Some doctors use high-dose B_{12} injections to chase away the fatigue and weakness of fibromyalgia. (B vitamins are crucial for energy production, immune enhancement, and fighting "fibrofog.") You can also battle those symptoms by eating foods rich in B vitamins, such as fortified cereals, eggs, meat, poultry, shellfish, and milk, and taking a B-complex supplement.

■ **Hangover.** The entire B complex—vitamins that are key for nervous system function—tends to be depleted after drinking. To replenish your supply, pop a supplement that contains 50 milligrams of each B vitamin.

■ **Migraines.** The B vitamin riboflavin has been shown to relieve migraines. You may want to try a supplement formula called MigraHealth, which contains riboflavin and other migraine-busting ingredients.

■ **Ear noise.** A deficiency of B vitamins can cause tinnitus, that ringing or other noise in your ears that you hear when no real sounds are present. Taking a B-complex supplement can minimize your symptoms, possibly by improving the function of the nerves in your ears. Look for a formula that includes thiamin, niacin, and vitamin B_{12}.

"B" Happy

When life feels stale, Mother Nature offers refreshment in the form of nutrient-rich foods, especially those abundant in B vitamins, such as whole grains, leafy greens, poultry, and fish. Vitamin B_6, for instance, helps convert the tryptophan found in foods into serotonin, a natural mood booster.

B Vitamins

Cabbage

GET A-HEAD!

Cabbage is one tough vegetable. Long after celery, lettuce, and asparagus have given up the ghost in the produce drawer, cabbage is still fresh and ready to go. But what about that cabbagey smell when it cooks? Open a window—and remind yourself that there's a lot of healing power in those tightly packed leaves. Here's what they can do.

■ **Cancer I.** Harvard researchers studied nearly 48,000 men and found that those who consumed five servings of cruciferous veggies a week—namely, cabbage and its family members—were half as likely to develop bladder cancer as those who ate only one serving or less per week. It didn't matter how many other veggies the men consumed overall.

■ **Cancer II.** At the Fred Hutchinson Cancer Research Center, researchers showed that men who consumed three or more servings of veggies daily—especially the cruciferous

Fabulous Food Fix
Wrap for Relief

Cabbage leaves have been used for centuries to soothe inflammation. A sturdy outer leaf is just the right shape to place over a bent knee or elbow. Blanch a leaf or two and apply warm or cool to your inflamed joint, then secure with a gauze or elastic bandage.

kind—could lower their risk of prostate cancer by nearly 50 percent.

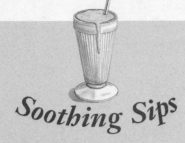

Soothing Sips

LEAF ULCERS BEHIND

Studies show that drinking a quart of freshly made cabbage water daily can heal ulcers in about 10 days. Simply soak a whole head in water overnight, then drink four cups of the soaking water (flavored with carrot juice, if you like) throughout the day.

■ **Brain fog.** Our brains need lecithin, which is found in cabbage as well as beans and egg yolks, to produce chemicals that act as messengers for thoughts and memories. Is your mental alertness slipping? Put a daily helping of coleslaw on the menu!

■ **Endometriosis.** Compounds called phytoestrogens, which are plentiful in cabbage and other cruciferous veggies, are similar to the estrogen found in your body but are weaker. The phytoestrogens you get from cabbage compete with natural estrogen to bind to receptors in your body, and when they bind, their weaker effect reduces overall estrogen activity and may decrease endometriosis symptoms.

■ **Weak bones.** Cabbage is brimming with calcium, a mineral that's crucial for strong bones. It's best to get calcium from foods rather than supplements because foods probably contain other, undiscovered bone-building factors along with their calcium.

■ **Heartburn.** Cabbage is loaded with glutamine, an amino acid that appears to promote healing in the digestive tract. People who eat cabbage several times a week may be less likely to experience heartburn than those who never eat it.

Cabbage

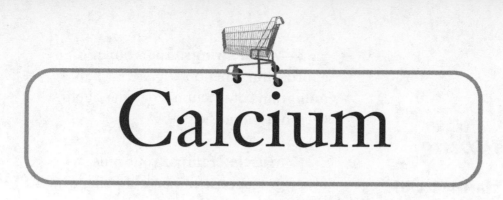

Calcium

THE MAGIC MINERAL

Think calcium is just for strong bones? Think again: Calcium, one of the electrolyte minerals, is responsible for literally dozens, if not hundreds, of your body's normal processes. Take away calcium, and your muscles wouldn't move, your mind wouldn't work, and your bones, of course, would all but collapse. Here are some of the key reasons to load up.

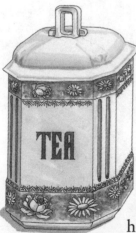

■ **Pregnancy aches.** Leg aches and muscle cramps often worsen in the last half of pregnancy, but eating foods rich in calcium and magnesium will help stave them off. To get both, make your own pregnancy tea by stirring 1 teaspoon of blackstrap molasses into 1 cup of hot water and drinking one cup daily. Other nondairy calcium sources include canned salmon (with the bones), dried beans, and soy milk.

Help for High Blood Pressure

Calcium and magnesium help reduce the tension on artery walls and relax the muscles that control blood vessels so blood flows freely—the keys to lowering blood pressure.

Soothing Sips

HAMMER OUT WEAK NAILS

Calcium and magnesium are essential to nail health. Make your own herbal mineral potion by mixing together equal parts of nettle, horsetail, and oats. Steep 1 heaping teaspoon in 1 cup of hot water for 10 minutes, strain, and drink one or two cups daily. Caution: Be sure to wear gloves when handling fresh nettle to avoid the stinging hairs.

■ **Mood swings.** For women approaching menopause, about 2,000 milligrams of calcium a day may help even out mood swings.

■ **Muscle cramps.** Your muscles move in response to nerve signals, which they receive via electrolytes, the minerals that surround your muscle cells. An imbalance in these minerals can interrupt the flow of signals and cause cramps, so give your body what it needs by including adequate calcium, chloride, sodium, potassium, and magnesium in your diet. Try to get 1,200 milligrams of calcium a day (1,500 milligrams after menopause).

■ **Weak bones.** Although there is a genetic component to osteoporosis, one of the biggest risk factors for the disease is a lack of calcium. Along with weight-bearing exercise such as weight lifting, calcium builds up your bone bank and keeps your skeleton strong.

■ **PMS.** One cup of greens such as broccoli, bok choy, or kale contains about 200 milligrams of calcium, a nutrient that may be a key to the PMS riddle. "A calcium deficiency could be central when you consider that women [in one study] who boosted their intake of this mineral had half the number of symptoms they had before," says Nadine Taylor, R.D. The dose used in the study was 400 milligrams three times a day. To be sure you get enough, supplement with calcium citrate, the most absorbable form.

■ **Migraines.** If you're susceptible to migraines, you may not be getting enough magnesium and calcium. When that dynamic mineral duo is combined with riboflavin (a B vitamin shown to crush head pain) and the herb feverfew, it wards off severe head pain in about half the women who try it. In fact, those who take a formula called MigraHealth, which combines these ingredients, have either fewer headaches or milder episodes.

■ **Sugar cravings.** Calcium and magnesium can help relax a stressed nervous system and nip sugar cravings in the bud. Some doctors suggest taking 750 milligrams of calcium and 375 milligrams of magnesium once a day with food. Magnesium may cause diarrhea in some people. If this occurs, reduce the dose. Capsules tend to work better than tablets because they're easier for the body to break down, doctors say.

■ **Sciatica.** Supplements that contain both calcium and magnesium are like a magic bullet for sciatica because they help tight muscles relax. Check with your doctor first, then look for a combination supplement and take it daily until the pain is gone.

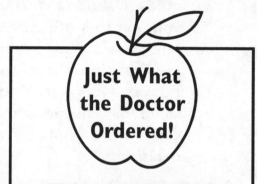

Just What the Doctor Ordered!

Take the Kick Out of Restless Legs

If restless legs syndrome disturbs your sleep, ensure that your nerves and muscles get the nutrients they need to function properly by taking a supplement that contains calcium and magnesium.

Calendula

MARVELOUS MARIGOLD

The next time you're in the garden admiring your marigolds (*Calendula officinalis*), tip your hat to Mother Nature: She packed some powerful medicine into these lovely flowers. Herbalists have used them for centuries for skin care—and a whole lot more. Here's what we mean.

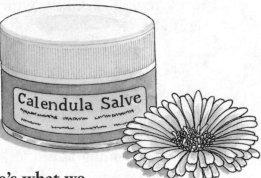

A Friend for Your Feet

Calendula is a gentle antifugal that can prevent athlete's foot fungus from getting a toehold. Dust calendula powder on your feet morning and night.

■ **Sore throat.** For a speedy ending to soreness, paint your throat with fresh calendula juice or tincture. Simply dip a cotton swab in the liquid and apply it generously to the back of your throat, paying particular attention to the sides. Too unpleasant for you? Make a strong infusion of calendula by steeping 1 heaping teaspoon in ½ cup of hot water, then gargle with it as needed.

■ **Chafing.** Calendula has antimicrobial properties that can reduce the risk of infection when you're chafed. After washing and drying the area, apply a layer of calendula cream or oil and cover it with a bandage. Leave it in place for at least 20 minutes and reapply it once a day until your skin is healed.

■ **Dry skin.** Native Americans in the U.S. Southwest and Mexico have long used calendula flowers as skin fresheners because of their mild, pleasing fragrance and soothing oils. A cream made from these flowers absorbs well into the skin, especially during the heat of summer. Combine 1 ounce of dried, crushed calendula petals with glycerin or beeswax, distilled water, and some dried mint or bergamot. Simmer in the top of a double boiler for about 3 hours to create a fine emulsion, then pour it into a clean bowl and whip until it cools and sets. Native Americans also make body talc by mixing crushed calendula leaves with cornstarch.

■ **B.O.** For a fragrant body powder that absorbs odors, mix the powdered flowers of calendula and lavender and add to an equal part of slippery elm powder. Dust it under your arms once or twice daily.

MAGIC MIXES

TONE YOUR PELVIS
Calendula not only soothes skin irritation, it also tones tissues and increases circulation to the pelvic organs. Make a strong infusion of calendula (simply steep 1 cup of fresh flowers in 1 quart of water for 15 minutes, then strain), add it to your bathwater, and slide into the tub for a soak. Better yet, alternate hot and cold water in the bath to increase circulation. After soaking for 5 to 10 minutes, get out of the tub and wrap a cold, wet towel around your lower body like a diaper, leaving it on for 3 to 5 minutes. You can repeat these steps two or three times per session. The greater the contrast between the heat and cold, the greater the toning effect.

Calendula

Sore No More

For ingrown hairs, use calendula in the form of a succus (the juice of the herb preserved with a small amount of alcohol), suggests Heidi Weinhold, N.D. Apply it to sore spots once or twice a day with a cotton swab or a clean cloth.

■ **Irritated skin.** Calendula is noted for its healing properties—especially for skin. According to Native American traditional medicine, ground petals combined with sunflower-seed or corn oil can be rubbed on to soothe minor skin irritations.

■ **Burns.** Calendula is also used to make mild washes for healing burns. To make a wash, steep 1 heaping tablespoon of fresh calendula flowers in a cup of hot water until the water cools. Strain, then pour over the burn.

■ **Skin injuries I.** Use calendula to clean cuts, scrapes, and other skin injuries. This herb is an anti-inflammatory, astringent (cleanser), and antiseptic (germ killer) all rolled into one. Plus, it helps repair tissues and prevent scarring. Some physicians advise applying calendula cream, but you could also add several drops of calendula tincture to a cup of water, dip a cloth in the mixture, and dab it on the wound.

■ **Skin injuries II.** Calendula fights a broad range of bugs, including bacteria and fungi. "I like to use it as a poultice to clean out debris," notes Sharol Tilgner, N.D. To prepare a poultice, saturate a piece of sterile gauze or cloth with calendula extract, place the soaked material on your cut or scrape, and leave it there for about an hour to help soften the skin and make any debris easier to remove. Afterward, pour a drop or two of extract directly on the wound to keep it germ-free and reduce the chance of scarring.

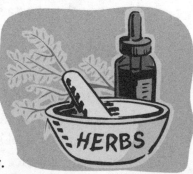

■ **Cold sores.** At the first indication of a cold sore outbreak, add six drops of calendula extract to a tablespoon of hot water, along with six drops each of extracts of tea tree oil, slippery elm, and myrrh—all of which are either excellent astringents or inflammation and infection fighters. Let the solution cool, then dab it directly on your cold sore for instant pain relief.

■ **Pelvic pain.** Many women who have taken mind-numbing narcotics for severe pelvic pain are finding that Menastil, an FDA-registered, roll-on herbal pain reliever made from calendula (which is often used to reduce menstrual pain) brings swift relief for a few hours. Plus, it has no side effects to speak of. Follow the label directions.

Just What the Doctor Ordered!

Cream the Itch

Calendula is one of the best herbs for itch control. After a bath or shower, lock moisture into your skin by smearing calendula cream or lotion on the itchy area. The herb's anti-inflammatory properties will help relieve your discomfort, says Jeanette Jacknin, M.D. You can even keep the emollient in the fridge for instant relief whenever itching flares.

■ **Stubbed toe.** The next time you stub your toe and break the skin, apply calendula. It's a popular choice among herbalists for healing wounds. Buy some calendula cream and use it once or twice a day.

■ **Blisters.** To reduce blister tenderness, try a salve that contains calendula along with skin-protecting vitamins A and E. You can apply it once a day. As an alternative, buy some dried calendula, crumble it between your fingers, and add enough water to make a paste. Cover the blister with the paste and leave it on for about 20 minutes, then rinse it off.

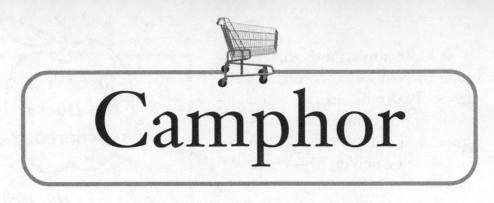

Camphor

AN AROMATIC ANTIDOTE

The penetrating aroma that wafts from the closet when you pull out your cold-weather sweaters comes from camphor, the main ingredient in moth-control products. It's much more than a bug beater, however. In fact, it has a long history of healing. Take a look for yourself.

■ **Queasiness.** The camphor-bearing oil in basil leaves makes them a nice nausea remedy. To make a tea, steep 1 teaspoon of dried leaves or 1 tablespoon fresh in a cup of boiling water for 15 minutes, then strain and sip.

■ **Back pain.** To relieve the muscle aches that accompany disk problems, look for products that contain camphor or menthol, both of which produce a cooling sensation and decrease pain and inflammation in the area. Follow the label directions.

■ **Foot aches.** "Anything that has menthol or camphor in it will stimulate the flow of blood to the feet and wash away the inflammation that causes soreness," says Pamela Taylor, N.D.

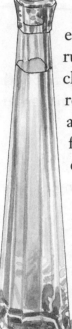

■ **Flu.** Slathering a camphor rub over your chest can help relieve the aches and pains of the flu, along with congestion. Add 6 to 12 drops of oil of camphor to an ounce of olive or almond oil and rub it on.

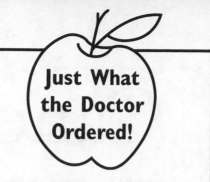

Just What the Doctor Ordered!

Herbal Hair Helper

Here's an easy way to help prevent hair loss: Use a hair-care product that contains camphor. It will dilate blood vessels in the scalp, attract blood to the balding or thinning areas, and perhaps slow hair fallout.

■ **Sprains.** An herbal ice pack is just the thing when you've sprained an ankle. Fill a bowl with ice-cold water and sprinkle in several drops of camphor oil, then soak a clean washcloth and wring it out. Lay the washcloth over the sprained area and cover with an ice pack for about 10 minutes. The pain should begin to ease.

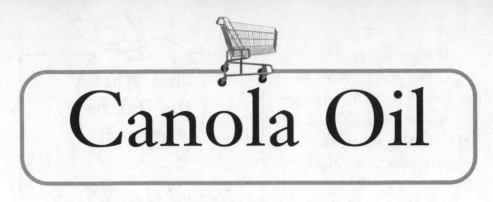

Canola Oil

COOKIN' WITH CLOUT

The next time you're in the mood for sautéed vegetables or scrambled eggs, replace the usual pat of butter with a splash of canola oil. It's good for your brain, arteries, and everything else in between! Here's what we mean.

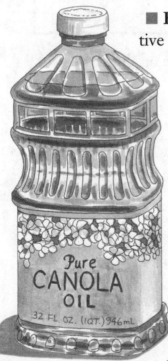

■ **Brain fog.** An Italian study found that cognitive impairment was less common among elderly people who ate a Mediterranean diet, which includes lots of monounsaturated fat, such as canola or olive oil. So when you cook, swap the saturated, brain-fogging fats, such as butter and marbled meats, for healthy monounsaturated fats. Use them not only on pasta but also in salad dressings and hearty soups.

■ **Hay fever.** Soybean, corn, cottonseed, safflower, and sunflower oils all contain omega-6 fatty acids, which can encourage hay fever symptoms such as sneezing and congestion. Canola oil, on the other hand, contains omega-3's, which may help keep your body from erupting into sneezing fits.

■ **Heart attack.** Canola oil reduces the stickiness of blood cells called platelets. That means they're less likely to clump together and get stuck in a coronary artery, setting off a heart attack.

■ **Heart disease.** Canola oil is the only cooking oil rich in heart-healthy alpha-linolenic acid. This substance protects against heart disease by lowering levels of low-density lipoprotein (LDL) cholesterol (the bad kind) and triglycerides (another troublesome component of cholesterol).

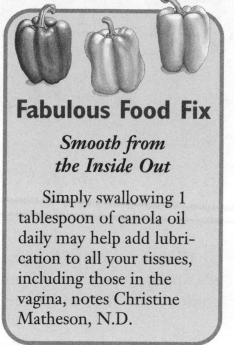

Fabulous Food Fix

Smooth from the Inside Out

Simply swallowing 1 tablespoon of canola oil daily may help add lubrication to all your tissues, including those in the vagina, notes Christine Matheson, N.D.

■ **Vitamin deficiencies.** Adding a little canola oil to your diet can help your body absorb fat-soluble nutrients, such as vitamin E and beta-carotene—the same ones that help reduce damage to cells throughout the body, including those in the heart, arteries, and brain.

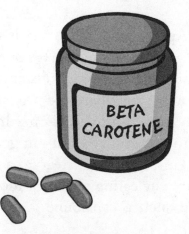

BETA CAROTENE

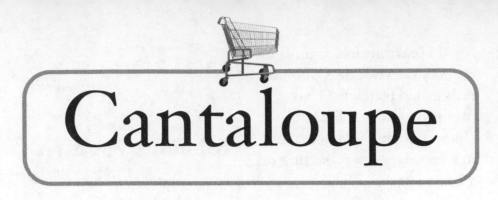

Cantaloupe

START YELLIN' FOR MELON

Forget the 4th of July watermelon. Sure, it's juicy, and it's fun to spit the seeds, but cantaloupe is a much better choice—and not just for the sweet, tangy flavor. Here's why.

■ **Macular degeneration.** Macular degeneration is among the leading causes of vision loss in older adults. One of the best ways to prevent it is to eat more cantaloupe. It's loaded with beta-carotene, a plant chemical that's converted to vitamin A in the body and used every minute of every day by your eyes.

■ **High blood pressure and stroke.** Cantaloupe is a great source of potassium, which can reduce the risk of high blood pressure and stroke.

■ **Aging skin.** Vitamin A is vital for proper skin growth and repair. It's one of a family of natural and synthetic substances known as retinoids, which are the primary ingredients in many prescription skin-care drugs, such as tretinoin (Retin-A). You can get some of the same skin-protecting effect (at a fraction of the cost) simply by eating plenty of foods that are rich in beta-carotene, such as canaloupe.

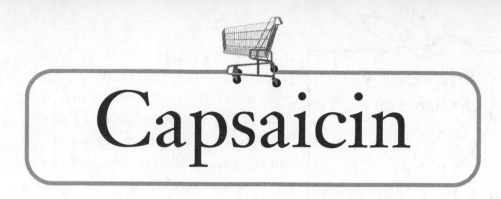

Capsaicin

A RED-HOT HEALER

The next time you bite into a hot pepper and break into a sweat, wipe your brow and thank capsaicin, the chemical that puts the heat into peppers and other spicy foods. Scientists have recently learned that capsaicin does a lot more than make you sweat. As it turns out, it's a hot prospect for dozens of health threats, including arthritis, colds, and even ulcers. See what we mean.

■ **Hangover.** Many people swear by a Bloody Mary— tomato juice seasoned with a splash of vodka and dashes of Tabasco, Worcestershire sauce, and red pepper—to cure a hangover. And the crimson lady may actually work, but probably not for the reason you think. It's not the vodka, which actually delays relief, but the red pepper that does the

MAGIC MIXES

HEAT CREAMS JOINT PAIN
For quick relief from achy joints, apply an over-the-counter capsaicin cream three or four times during the day. It helps deplete nerves of substance P, a pain-causing chemical. You can also make your own salve by adding three or four drops of cayenne pepper tincture to 1 teaspoon of olive oil.

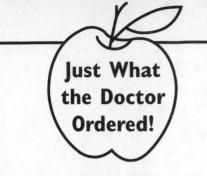

Just What the Doctor Ordered!

Torch Your Worries

The next time you feel that life's stresses are getting to be too much, have some chiles. These little peppers are packed with capsaicin, which pours on the heat. Your body responds to it with a flood of endorphins, the natural painkillers that boost mood and help you forget your worries.

trick. The capsaicin it contains is a potent ingredient that helps stop the production of substance P, which promotes both inflammation and pain. Try a pinch of pepper in a glass of tomato juice (which is loaded with the electrolytes you may have lost if you vomited), suggests Linda White, M.D. Just be sure you make it "virgin" (that is, sans the alcohol).

■ **Itchy skin.** Capsaicin cream, made from the red-hot component in chile peppers, stimulates nerve endings and helps convert a maddening itch to a more tolerable sting. You can think of capsaicin as a form of "chemical scratching"; it causes the same sensation as scratching, but without injury to your skin. Be sure to wash your hands thoroughly after using the cream, and don't use it on areas of broken skin or near your eyes.

■ **Overweight.** Capsaicin-containing red pepper may help raise both your body temperature and your metabolism, so you burn calories for fuel rather than storing them as fat. Plus, it may speed your digestion. People with sluggish digestion tend to gain weight, says Dana Myatt, N.D. In fact, in one small study, dieters who added 1 teaspoon of red pepper sauce and 1 teaspoon of mustard to every meal raised their metabolic rates by 25 percent.

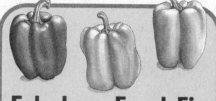

■ **Shingles.** For pain that lingers after shingles blisters heal, try smearing on a paste made by blending a small amount of red pepper with 1 tablespoon of aloe vera gel (if the mixture feels too hot, add more aloe, and use a cotton swab to apply the mixture so you don't burn your fingers). The capsaicin in the pepper helps reduce pain-producing substance P, which your body releases during shingles outbreaks. It may take about six weeks for the treatment to work.

■ **Heel pain.** On your tongue, fiery red pepper makes you want to guzzle a gallon of water, but when you apply capsaicin cream to a painful heel, you'll feel sweet relief. Besides decreasing the concentration of substance P, which transmits pain signals to the brain, it helps warm the muscles surrounding the heel that go into spasm due to an over-stretched arch, says John Hahn, N.D., D.P.M. When these muscles bunch up, they can irritate the nerves in the heel. Applying capsaicin (following the package directions) can help short-circuit the pain-spasm-pain cycle.

■ **Raynaud's disease.** Capsaicin can relieve extremity-chilling symptoms of Raynaud's by dilating

Fabulous Food Fix

Fiery Fat Foe

Capsaicin is one of the chemicals in spicy foods that make them savory, so you need less fat (such as oil) to make recipes palatable, and you can feel satisfied with smaller portions. To start, instead of butter, sprinkle some red pepper on your baked potato or some grated ginger on your veggies. Like the results? Break open a south-of-the-border cookbook, then let 'er rip!

Suck Some Heat

Early studies indicate that red pepper lozenges made with capsaicin may help soothe chemotherapy-related mouth sores. It seems that not only does capsaicin numb inflamed tissue in the same way that benzocaine or other topical anesthetics might, it may also draw white blood cells to the site to heal it. Another plus: Capsaicin has antioxidant properties that may help fight nitrosamine, a cancer-causing agent.

your blood vessels. "If you don't love heavily peppered food, I recommend taking capsaicin capsules at every meal," says Dr. Hahn. You can even sprinkle a little red pepper straight from your spice rack into your shoes or gloves; you'll feel the heat instantly.

■ **Fibromyalgia.** Here's a hot tip for people with fibromyalgia: Over-the-counter capsaicin creams can block the chemical that transmits pain signals to your brain.

■ **Facial pain.** Capsaicin cream can sometimes reduce the frequency or severity of trigeminal neuralgia. The active ingredient appears to block the transmission of pain signals from your face to your brain.

■ **Neck pain.** The next time you have a pain in the neck, try applying some capsaicin cream. Since capsaicin makes your body deplete its normal supply of pain-causing chemicals, your aching neck should soon be a thing of the past.

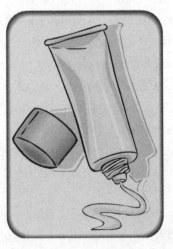

■ **Rotator cuff injuries.** Creams or gels made with capsaicin are good for sore shoulders. Capsaicin is a counterirritant, which means that it helps deplete the area of the substance P that transmits pain signals.

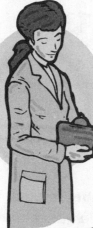

■ **IBS.** While some people with irritable bowel syndrome (IBS) have painful flare-ups when they eat spicy foods, others find that a little culinary heat makes them feel better. The capsaicin in hot foods may make your intestine less sensitive. Ask your doctor to help you work out a careful trial to see if capsaicin can calm your gut.

■ **Stuffy nose.** Hot peppers are just the thing when you have a cold or allergies. They make your nose run, which clears your sinuses and sends germs packing.

■ **Heart attack and stroke.** It turns out that capsaicin is an antioxidant that helps lower bad low-density lipoprotein (LDL) cholesterol and reduce the stickiness of blood platelets so they don't clot and cause a heart attack or stroke. What's more, chile peppers are packed with plenty of other disease-fighting ingredients. One fresh pepper provides 126 percent of the vitamin C and 95 percent of the vitamin A you need daily, creating a powerful antioxidant team that fights the kind of cell damage that sets you up for heart disease, cancer, and premature aging.

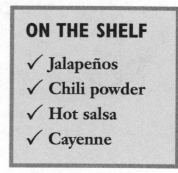

ON THE SHELF
- ✓ Jalapeños
- ✓ Chili powder
- ✓ Hot salsa
- ✓ Cayenne

■ **Ulcers.** For years, part of ulcer treatment was to avoid hot, spicy foods. Now that we know that most ulcers are caused by bacteria, chiles and capsaicin are being explored as a treatment for ulcers because of their bacteria-fighting ability. One caveat: If you suspect that you have an ulcer, check with your doctor before you try any spicy food.

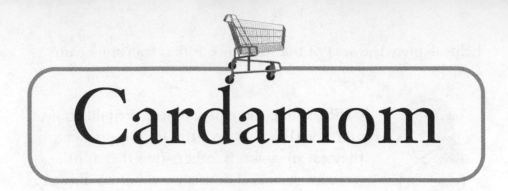

Cardamom

ONE NICE SPICE

Research into the world of spices is still in its infancy, so scientists have just begun to figure out which ones really make a difference. Cardamom, it appears, is right at the top of the list. Here's why.

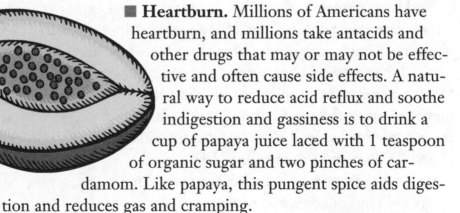

■ **Heartburn.** Millions of Americans have heartburn, and millions take antacids and other drugs that may or may not be effective and often cause side effects. A natural way to reduce acid reflux and soothe indigestion and gassiness is to drink a cup of papaya juice laced with 1 teaspoon of organic sugar and two pinches of cardamom. Like papaya, this pungent spice aids digestion and reduces gas and cramping.

■ **Inflamed gums.** If your gums are red or bleeding, chew on a few cardamom seeds. They're rich in cineole, an antiseptic that fights bacteria and can help reduce the risk of gum disease. Plus, here's a bonus: People who take care

102

of their gums and prevent infection and inflammation have less risk of getting heart disease.

■ **Food poisoning.** Researchers now think that cardamom, cloves, and other spices typically used in Asian cuisine may actually prevent food spoilage. They can't replace proper food handling and refrigeration, but they can sure provide some extra protection when it counts!

■ **High cholesterol.** There's some evidence that spices such as cardamom and cinnamon may help stimulate antioxidant enzymes in the body. That's important because blocking oxidation helps prevent cholesterol from sticking to the walls of arteries and setting the stage for heart disease. So add a pinch to veggies and meats on a daily basis—and your morning tea!

Soothing Sips

CARDAMOM CLOBBERS COLDS

Hot chicken soup is a proven cold chaser—but it's not the only liquid healer out there. Try sipping hot tea that contains a natural decongestant such as cardamom. In addition to the sinus-clearing effects of the steaming tea, this antiviral spice may help open nasal passages in its own right, says David Zeiger, D.O.

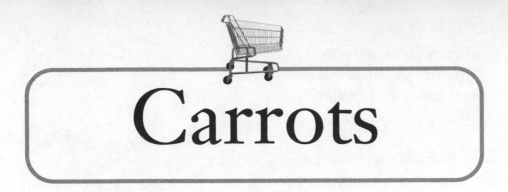

Carrots

THAT WASCALLY WABBIT WAS RIGHT

All your life, you've heard that carrots are good for your eyes. That's true enough, but scientists today see more than better vision in these brash orange vegetables. Turns out, Bugs and all of his bunny friends are going to live a *looong* time, thanks to carrots and the remarkable chemicals hiding under those thin peels. In fact, there's not much a carrot can't do. Here's a sample.

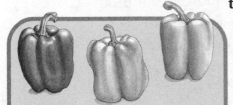

Fabulous Food Fix

Clean Your Choppers

Carrots and other crunchy foods, such as celery and apples, can help sand away tooth stains— and they're a lot cheaper than commercial whiteners. As a bonus, carrots are one of nature's best breath sweeteners!

■ **Heart attack.** Pectin, a type of fiber in carrots, binds up artery-clogging cholesterol, thus helping to prevent heart attacks.

■ **Sore throat.** A carrot neck wrap can help you recover more quickly from a sore throat. To make one, grate a carrot onto a length of cheese-cloth. Fold the cloth in half lengthwise and moisten it with warm water. Wrap it around your neck, wrap a warm towel on top, and keep it on for 20 to 30 minutes.

■ **Blocked milk duct.** If your breast is inflamed because of a blocked milk duct, apply a poultice made by grating a carrot onto some cheesecloth and moistening it. Place it on the breast all the way up to the armpit, cover it with a hot water bottle, and leave it on for 1 hour. Apply a fresh poultice several times daily until the inflammation clears up. If you also have a fever and flu-like symptoms, see your doctor immediately; you may have an infection that could get worse.

■ **High blood sugar.** Chewy, high-fiber foods such as carrots not only slow down your intake of food—and calories—they also enter your bloodstream slowly, preventing your blood sugar from spiking and then dropping.

MAGIC MIXES

MOP UP THE OIL

Here's a facial mask that really works for oily skin. Boil three large carrots until they're soft. Mash them and add 5 tablespoons of honey. Using a circular motion, massage the mixture gently onto your face, then leave it on for 20 minutes. Rinse with warm water and pat dry. (Before you use this on your face, test it on an inconspicuous spot, such as inside the crook of your arm, to make sure it doesn't turn your skin slightly—but temporarily—orange.)

■ **Vision problems.** Yes, carrots really are good for your eyes—and so are other orange and yellow vegetables and fruits. They're all rich sources of beta-carotene, the plant-based building block of vitamin A, a nutrient your eyes suck up like candy. So add some carrots to your menu, along with plenty of greens.

Carrots 105

■ **Weak nails.** Carrot juice contains loads of calcium and phosphorus and is great for strengthening nails.

■ **Aging skin.** Did you know that carrots can promote healthy, younger-looking skin? That's because their beta-carotene is converted in the body to vitamin A, which is vital for proper skin growth and repair.

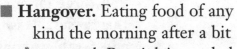

■ **Hangover.** Eating food of any kind the morning after a bit too much Beaujolais can help to ease a hangover, says Stephanie Brooks, R.D. By eating, you'll replace any electrolytes (salts such as sodium and potassium) you lost if you vomited. If your tummy is still tender, chug a sports drink, which packs lots of electrolytes. Or, if you find the citrus in sports drinks irritating, reach for carrot juice. It's loaded with potassium and sodium.

Soothing Sips

MAKE TREATMENTS EASIER

When radiation or other cancer treatments make you too sick to eat, juice a pile of carrots. You'll get a high concentration of antioxidants, which you need to help neutralize toxins from chemotherapy or radiation.

■ **Fading memory.** Estrogen mops up oxygen damage to brain cells caused by free radical molecules, says Claire Warga, Ph.D. When your body's estrogen levels wane during menopause, she suggests turning to plant estrogens that do double duty as natural antioxidants. "People with high levels of antioxidants tend to score better on memory tests," she says. To help keep your memory in tip-top condition, feast on antioxidant-rich fruits and veggies, such as carrots.

Carrots

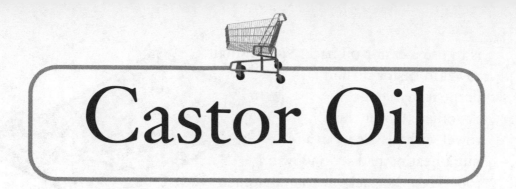

Castor Oil

HEAL FASTER WITH CASTOR

Children aren't punished any more (thank goodness!) with a dose of castor oil. In fact, hardly anyone ever sips this ghastly-tasting oil. It can be applied to the skin, however, and there are some good reasons to keep a bottle in your medicine chest. Here they are.

■ **Bra constriction.** Wearing a tight bra can stall the flow of lymph fluid from the breast and cause congestion in the tissues. If this occurs, rely on the old standard castor oil pack to reduce any inflammation. Saturate a clean cloth with castor oil and completely cover the affected breast with it. Top with plastic wrap (the oil stains clothing) and a hot water bottle or a heating pad set on low. Leave the pack on for 1 hour and repeat daily until the discomfort is gone.

■ **Constipation.** One way to gently encourage things to move along when you're constipated

Soak Away Scaly Skin

To soften psoriasis lesions on your hands or feet, soak in a bath laced with Epsom salts, pat the itchy areas dry, and (unless you have a peanut allergy) massage them with warm peanut oil. Cover with a paste made with baking soda and castor oil, don white cotton gloves or socks, and hop into bed.

107

is to use a castor oil pack. Soak a small towel in castor oil and drape it over your abdomen. Cover the towel with plastic wrap and put a heating pad set on low on top. Keep the pack on your abdomen for about 20 minutes.

MAGIC MIXES

OIL AWAY SCIATICA
A combination of arnica oil, St. John's wort oil, and castor oil can help relieve the pain of an inflamed sciatic nerve. Combine equal parts of the oils and gently massage the mixture onto the nerve track, starting at your buttocks and going down the back of the leg. If your symptoms persist, or if the pain seems unusually severe, see your doctor right away. Sciatica can lead to permanent nerve damage.

■ **Shin pain.** Moist heat is a great treatment for shin pain, and adding castor oil to the mix increases the anti-inflammatory power. Rub the oil onto your sore shin, cover with plastic wrap, and top with a hot, moist towel. Leave everything on for about 20 minutes, then wash off the oil with soap and water.

■ **Muscle pain.** To make a liniment for muscle aches, first fill a 12-ounce glass jar with freshly chopped comfrey leaves. Add enough castor oil to cover the leaves completely, then add the oil from a vitamin E capsule. Put the jar in a sunny window for one week, shaking it once or twice daily. Strain the mixture into a clean glass bottle and add 15 drops of essential oils of juniper and wintergreen. Rub into sore muscles as needed. To prolong the life of the oil, store it in a cool place or in the fridge.

Castor Oil

Wrist pain. A compress made with castor oil is a great way to ease wrist pain. Soak a cloth with castor oil, heat it in the microwave until it's warm but not hot, and place it on your wrist. Cover your wrist with plastic wrap and leave the compress in place for several hours.

Wipe Out Warts

Get rid of unsightly and bothersome warts on your hands by using castor oil once a day as you would hand cream.

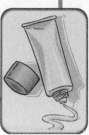

Menstrual pain. Some women swear by hot castor oil packs to ease cramps. Supposedly, the packs increase circulation and decrease inflammation when placed on the lower abdomen. Just soak some folded flannel cloth in castor oil and place it on your abdomen, covering your liver and reaching from your breastbone to your pubic bone. Top it with some plastic wrap, a hot water bottle, and a towel, then relax for 30 to 60 minutes. You can use castor oil packs three to seven days a week, but only when cramping isn't accompanied by heavy bleeding. For best results, though, use this remedy between periods.

Bruises. A castor oil pack is a traditional and powerful way to treat bruises. "Castor oil has excellent anti-inflammatory properties, and it penetrates the skin very well," says Sean Sapunar, N.D. Spread castor oil over the bruise, wrap the area with plastic wrap, and place a heating pad set on low or a washcloth soaked in hot water on top. Leave it in place for about 20 minutes, then wash off the oil. You can repeat the treatment several times a day until the bruise is gone. Don't use heat with deep bruising where bleeding may be a problem.

Rough hands. Soften rough, dry hands with this simple routine: Mix 1 teaspoon of castor oil with 1 drop of lemon or peppermint oil. Massage it into your skin before bed and wear cotton gloves while you sleep.

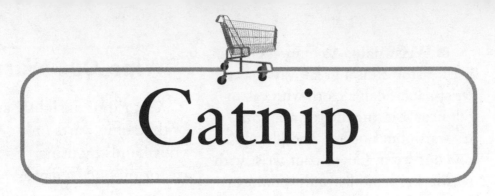

Catnip

A PURR-FECT REMEDY

Have you ever seen cats lolling away the afternoon in a catnip patch? Some folks speculate that the cats get a little buzz from the stuff, while others suspect they just like the smell. But maybe what really makes cats go crazy for catnip is that they know a good thing when they smell it—and catnip really is one of Mother Nature's blessings. Take a look.

Soothing Sips

KITTY'S COUGH CURE

Catnip may make a kitty go crazy, but this herb can also make your cough just go! Fix up some catnip tea by steeping 1 to 2 teaspoons of dried catnip in a cup of boiling water for 10 to 15 minutes, then strain. You can drink up to three cups a day.

■ **Vomiting.** The volatile oil in minty herbs such as catnip helps relieve spasms and may help allay bouts of vomiting—when the flu sneaks up on you, for example, or when you've made a little too merry at holiday feasts. Make a tea by steeping 1 teaspoon of dried leaves in 1 cup of hot water. Strain, then take small sips while it's still warm. If you're pregnant, talk to your doctor or midwife before taking catnip.

110

■ **Gas.** When gas gets trapped in bends in the intestine, it can be really painful, but you can relieve the discomfort with a simple belly rub containing antispasmodic herbs. Add four to six drops each of lobelia and catnip tincture to 2 tablespoons of olive oil, then gently massage it into your abdomen in a clockwise motion.

■ **Insomnia.** Catnip may turn your lazy feline into a rowdy cat, but it has the opposite effect on us humans. In fact, long before pharmacists began dispensing powerful chemicals—with all their side effects—herbalists recommended catnip tea to speed the journey to Dreamland. To make the tea, steep 1 teaspoon of dried catnip in 1 cup of hot water for 10 minutes, then strain and enjoy.

■ **Bug bites.** Sure, you can treat bites and stings naturally, but you can prevent them naturally, too. In fact, catnip oil contains nepetalactone, which, according to studies at the University of Iowa, is 10 times more effective at deterring insects than DEET (short for diethyl-meta-toluamide, a powerful insecticide that does the job but can also cause skin rashes, lethargy, muscle spasms and nausea).

■ **Acid reflux.** Do you take an acid blocker such as famotidine (Pepcid)? You may—with your doctor's okay—be able to wean yourself off the drug with the help of a pair of stomach-settling herbs, says Robert Pyke, M.D., Ph.D. Start by taking a 200- to 300-milligram capsule each of chamomile and catnip after each meal, gradually increasing the interval between doses. "When you reach two days between doses, you're home free," says Dr. Pyke. Don't use chamomile if you're allergic to ragweed.

Catnip

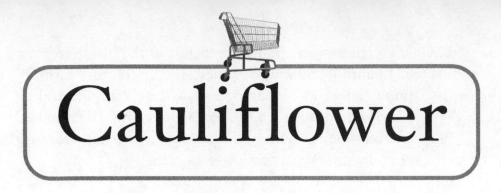

Cauliflower

GET A HEAD FOR HEALTH

When you're in the mood for something a little robust and full-flavored, get the cauliflower steaming—and reap the benefits. There's some powerful medicine in those pale florets. Here's why you should add it to your diet regularly.

■ **Fatigue.** If your life is a little hectic, it's vital to eat more cauliflower. It provides a bushel of pantothenic acid, which is critical for keeping your adrenal glands in good working order when stress puts a strain on them.

■ **Weak nails.** Cauliflower is rich in biotin, a B vitamin that helps your body make and use amino acids, which are the building blocks of protein—and the secret to strong, healthy nails.

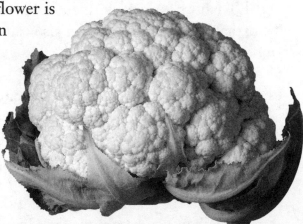

■ **Stroke.** In a study of more than 75,000 women, researchers found that those who ate the most produce, especially cauliflower and other crucifers, had a 30

percent lower risk of having strokes than those who consumed the least.

■ **Heart disease.** Cauliflower offers a big helping of vitamin C, which helps protect your heart by gobbling up free radicals, compounds that play a role in the development of heart disease. Cauliflower is also loaded with folate, a B vitamin that may safeguard your heart by lowering levels of the amino acid homocysteine.

■ **Cancer.** Men who eat three or more servings of vegetables daily—especially the cruciferous kind such as cauliflower—have about half the risk of developing prostate cancer compared with those who don't eat vegetables.

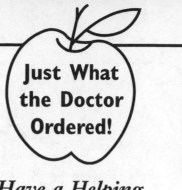

Just What the Doctor Ordered!

Have a Helping of Hormones

If you have endometriosis, put cauliflower on the menu. This hearty vegetable contains an abundance of phytoestrogens, compounds that bind to estrogen receptors in your body. When they do, they have a weaker effect than natural estrogen, thereby reducing overall estrogen activity in your body and perhaps decreasing endometrisis symptoms.

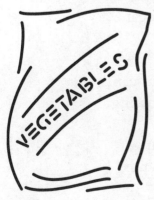

VEGETABLES

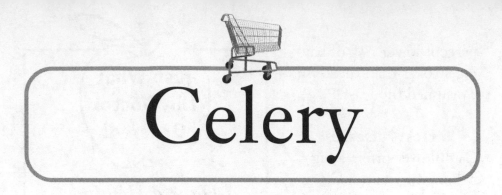

Celery

TAKE STOCK OF STALKS

According to folklore, celery is the perfect diet food because chewing it burns almost more calories than it delivers. That's a bit of a stretch, but celery does have some interesting attributes in addition to that watery crunch. Here's what it can do.

■ **High blood pressure.** Crunching your way through just four stalks a day could ease down your blood pressure. A component in celery (3-n-butyl phthalide) acts as a diuretic and vasodilator and helps relax the muscles lining the blood vessels.

■ **Tooth stains.** Before you spend big bucks on over-the-counter tooth-whitening products, consider stocking up on stalks: Celery acts like gentle sandpaper and can safely abrade away tooth stains.

■ **Bloating.** Celery acts as a gentle diuretic that can remove excess water from the body and reduce bloating.

■ **Dragon breath.** The burst of water that you get with each bite of celery helps flush food particles and odor-causing bacteria from your mouth.

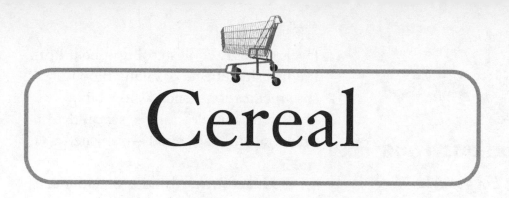

Cereal

MORE THAN JUST BREAKFAST

The cereal aisle is one of the biggest stretches of real estate in the supermarket, and most of those boxes contain basically sugary snacks, with as much sugar per serving as a thick slice of pecan pie. If you shop wisely and avoid the super-sweet kid stuff, though, you can get a tremendous bang for your nutritional buck. Here's why.

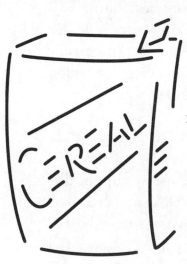

■ **High blood pressure.** In a study of a 500,000-member HMO group, 50 percent of patients on blood pressure medication were able to stop taking it after eating 5 grams of soluble fiber from oatmeal and oatmeal squares every day for four weeks. Another 20 percent were able to cut their medication in half. (Always consult your doctor before making changes in your medication.) In addition, the patients' total and

B Good to Your Gums

Folate is a B vitamin that helps repair and replenish gum cells that have been damaged by gingivitis. Fortunately, most cereals are fortified with plenty of Bs.

levels of LDL cholesterol dropped. Plus, the bad side effects of taking blood pressure medication—such as low blood potassium, muscle cramps, sexual dysfunction, and bad moods—vanished.

■ **Heartburn.** Millions of Americans have heartburn, and a big part of the problem is the super-rich American diet. High-fat meals stay in the stomach longer than low-fat meals, says Lila Wallis, M.D. As a result, they cause more acid to accumulate, slowing digestion and often triggering heartburn. To give your gut a rest, follow a sensible diet that's low in fat, moderate in protein, and high in complex carbohydrates—a recipe for cereal, in other words.

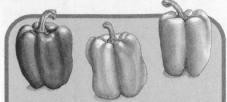

Fabulous Food Fix

Forget Me Not!

Memory loss is often attributed to low blood sugar and fatigue, so be sure to eat nutritious, well-balanced meals—especially a good breakfast of protein and complex carbohydrates such as whole grain cereals. You may find that your spells of forgetfulness come less often.

■ **Diabetes.** A Harvard study published in the *Journal of the American Medical Association* noted that people who eat lots of starches to avoid fats may unwittingly set themselves up for diabetes. Study participants drank a lot of soft drinks and crowded their plates with potatoes, white bread, and white rice—all of which have almost no fiber. The result? They had 2.5 times the rate of diabetes found in people who ate less of these foods and more fiber, specifically from whole grain cereals.

■ **Bladder leaks.** It may sound strange, but chronic constipation can contribute to urinary incontinence. The two body systems aren't directly related, but constipation may increase pressure on the bladder or pelvic floor muscles, in turn causing urine to leak out without warning—when you sneeze or laugh, for example. In some cases, eliminating constipation can clear

Cereal

up the urinary problems. A good way to start is to eat more whole grain cereals, along with breads and at least two servings of juicy fruit, such as prunes, daily.

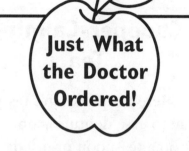

■ **Kidney stones.** If you're prone to kidney stones, eat more cereal. Studies have shown that people who have high-fiber diets are less likely to get stones. You want to get at least 20 grams of fiber a day, but 30 to 35 is even better. A lot of cereals are fiber lightweights, so when you're in the supermarket, check the labels to find those that provide at least 5 or more grams of fiber per serving.

■ **High cholesterol.** An impressive pile of research shows that adding oats to your diet lowers total and bad low-density lipoprotein (LDL) cholesterol without lowering good high-density lipoprotein (HDL) cholesterol. That's important because lowering LDL reduces fatty buildup in the arteries, and maintaining healthy HDL levels makes it easier for the body to eliminate LDL from the blood. These are keys to preventing heart disease.

■ **Folliculitis.** If the itching of folliculitis is making you crazy, a colloidal oatmeal bath can put you at ease. *Colloidal* simply means that the oatmeal has been finely ground so it readily disperses in water. Just add the mix to a warm bath. If the outbreak is on a small area of skin, such as on your arm, you can soak it in the sink or a basin.

Just What the Doctor Ordered!

Energy in a Bowl

The carbohydrates and nutrients in high-fiber foods such as cereal enter your bloodstream slowly, which prevents blood sugar from spiking and then crashing—a common cause of fatigue.

Chamomile

THE HERB THAT KEEPS ON GIVING

Chamomile is one of the country's best-selling herbs. This is due in part to its subtle, apple-like taste and refreshing scent, but mainly it's because chamomile tea can be used inside and out for rapid relief of literally dozens of symptoms and conditions. To make the tea, simply measure 1 teaspoon of dried chamomile flowers (not the weak, store-bought kind in tea bags) into your cup. Fill the cup with hot water and steep, covered, for 10 to 15 minutes, then strain out the herb. As long as you're not allergic to chamomile's cousin ragweed, here's what it can do for you.

■ **Anxiety.** When your troubles start escalating, reach for the chamomile tea. Studies show that it blocks anxiety-promoting brain chemicals triggered by worry. While you wait for the tea to steep, close your eyes and count all the

Chopper-Calming Tea

Here's a quick (and tasty) way to ease denture pain. Drop a teaspoon of dried chamomile into a cup of hot water and steep for 10 to 20 minutes. Strain out the herb, and when the tea is cool, take a mouthful, swish it around for 30 seconds or so, and spit it out. Keep rinsing until you've used all the tea.

118

wonderful things you're grateful for, then sip your tea and feel your worries slip away.

■ **Back pain.** When your back is aching, call on chamomile, ginger, and peppermint. To make a pain-relieving tea, use any of the herbs individually or mix them in equal parts and brew according to the recipe on the opposite page. You can drink a cup three or four times a day.

■ **Scalp irritation.** Herbal rinses add sheen to your hair and relieve scalp irritation at the same time. Traditional herbs include chamomile and calendula for blondes, rosemary and sage for dark hair, and cloves for auburn or red hair. Make a strong tea using 4 tablespoons of herb to 1 quart of boiling water.

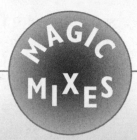

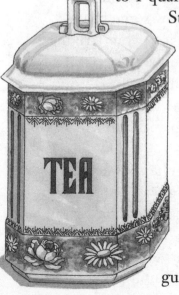

INSTANT EYE RELIEF
Warm compresses made with an infusion of chamomile may help relieve eyestrain from macular degeneration. Steep 1 teaspoon of the herb in 1 cup of hot water, covered, for 10 to 15 minutes. Strain and let cool, then saturate a clean cloth or gauze pads with the solution. Cover your eyes with the cloth or gauze and rest for 20 minutes.

Steep for 15 minutes, then add ¼ cup of apple cider vinegar to restore the scalp's proper pH. Use as a final rinse after shampooing your hair.

■ **Cranky gut.** Chamomile tea has been used as a digestive aid throughout history because its gentle astringent action and antispasmodic effects relax and heal the gut. Drink two or three cups per day.

■ **Gum disease.** You can also keep your gums healthy with chamomile tea. Use 2 tea-

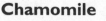

spoons of herb for a slightly stronger tea, then drink a cup after every meal so the herb can do what it does best: kill germs and reduce your risk of gingivitis.

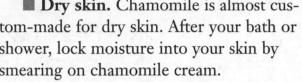

■ **Dry skin.** Chamomile is almost custom-made for dry skin. After your bath or shower, lock moisture into your skin by smearing on chamomile cream.

■ **Athlete's foot.** Tea tree oil is a traditional remedy for athlete's foot, but it may sting. You may want to start out with chamomile, a gentler antifungal herb. Rinse your feet in the tea in the morning, at night, and after showers, then dry them thoroughly.

■ **Calluses.** If you have very thick calluses and want to soak them, try this remedy suggested by Suzanne M. Levine, D.P.M. Brew some chamomile tea and add it to your soaking water. Your skin will soften, but it may also turn slightly yellow. Don't worry, though: The tint is easily removed with soap and water.

■ **Diarrhea.** When Rover has an internal upset, he grazes on grass, but humans should head straight for the chamomile patch. A small handful of these daisy-like flowers can provide a soothing and effective remedy for diarrhea. Simply wash them

Just What the Doctor Ordered!

Ditch the Itch

"A number of cooled herbal teas can calm inflammation and itchy skin, but my favorite is chamomile," says Bradley Bongiovanni, N.D. First, steep a few tea bags in hot water. Let the tea cool, then soak a clean cloth in the solution and apply it to the irritated area several times daily.

Chamomile

and let them dry out for a while, then use them to make your tea. Drink several cups a day until your runs subside.

■ **Sore throat.** Chamomile tea is a traditional remedy for sore throat pain, says Jane Hopson, N.D. And don't forget to add honey. It coats your throat and helps soothe the pain.

■ **Foot aches.** A great way to relax your tired tootsies at the end of the day is to soak them in water spiked with Epsom salts and a few drops of chamomile oil. The oil reduces inflammation as well as muscle spasms.

■ **Dry skin.** If you live in an arid climate or indoor heat dries the air in your home, your skin can get parched. One way to add moisture to the air is to add 10 to 12 drops of chamomile oil to a pot of water and keep it simmering on the stove. (Of course, this only works when you're home to keep an eye on it.)

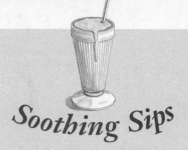

Soothing Sips

HEAD OFF HEAD PAIN

The best teas for tension headaches include chamomile, passionflower, cramp bark, cinnamon, and ginkgo. When using dried herbs, add about 1 tablespoon to a cup of freshly boiled water and steep for 10 to 15 minutes. Strain the tea before drinking.

■ **Stress.** Here's the perfect relaxer: Wrap a few chamomile tea bags in gauze or a leg from a pair of pantyhose. Next, cut an orange into thin slices. Suspend the tea pouch under your bathtub spigot and let warm water flow over it as it fills the tub. Float the orange slices in the water, climb into the tub, and soak your troubles away.

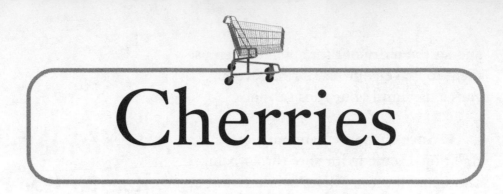

Cherries

A PITTED PLEASURE

When you feel that your life's the pits, turn it into a bowl of cherries with these delicious, shirt-staining little fruits. Cherries are almost like small chemical factories, with dozens of powerful compounds that can help keep you healthy year after year. Here's what we mean.

■ **Bursitis.** Cherries are among the best remedies for bursitis because they help relieve inflammation. Eat about ½ cup every day until you're feeling better.

■ **Surgical trauma.** Take advantage of the healing powers of black cherries after surgery to aid in tissue repair. They contain substances that help reduce inflammation and strengthen tiny blood vessels that were damaged during the operation. Enjoy a cup a day.

■ **Cancer and heart disease.** Dark red cherries, both sweet and sour, are packed with flavonoids called anthocyanins. In nature,

Below-the-Belt Relief

If you've been laid up by a blow to the groin, keep a bowl of cherries within reach. The bioflavonoids in these tasty treats will help your body repair the delicate blood vessels that were damaged. Try to eat a cup of cherries every day.

122

these plant chemicals defend fruits and vegetables against attacks from invading germs and hungry bugs, but in your body, they seem to act as antioxidants that protect against cancer and heart disease. Americans don't consume anywhere near enough of these substances, considering that our record for eating fruits and veggies is the pits. So chomp on cherries and double your pleasure as well as your protection. Just six juicy, dark red cherries a day deliver 200 milligrams of anthocyanins!

■ **Weak bones.** Cherries are a good source of the mineral boron, which seems to be important for bone health.

■ **Arthritis.** Cherries may help relieve joint pain. Laboratory research at Michigan State University has shown that, at least in the test tube, tart cherry juice is 10 times better than aspirin for reducing pain and swelling—and it won't irritate tender tummies as aspirin can. Try 1 to 2 cups a day.

Fabulous Food Fix
Help for the Heart

Cherries are just quivering with quercetin, a flavonoid that fights heart disease. How high are they in quercetin? As high as apples, which are the top bananas when it comes to fruits that deliver the goods. And the best news is that processed cherries, the kind you get in cans and as prepared pie filling, deliver double the quercetin of fresh cherries. That means you can get cherry-good protection all year long.

■ **Allergies.** Cherries are bursting with substances called bioflavonoids that keep mast cells from releasing troublemaking histamines—the culprits that trigger allergy symptoms. Cherries also boost cell levels of vitamin C, an anti-inflammatory/ antihistamine powerhouse that targets the sinus passages. Fresh, frozen, or dried, try working a handful or two into your diet every day during allergy season.

Chicken Soup

Chicken soup has long been a traditional remedy for colds and flu. Studies show that this rich, flavorful broth really does seem to work—and not only for upper-respiratory problems. Here's the lowdown.

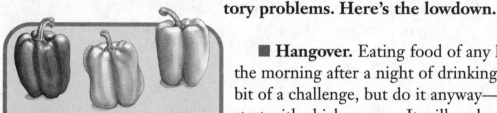

Fabulous Food Fix

Steam and Breathe

Inhaling the steam from a bowl of hot chicken soup will help open your nasal and bronchial passages. Of course, eating the soup is even better. An amino acid in chicken is very similar to a drug that doctors prescribe for patients with bronchitis.

■ **Hangover.** Eating food of any kind the morning after a night of drinking is a bit of a challenge, but do it anyway—and start with chicken soup. It will replace any electrolytes (salts such as sodium and potassium) you lost if your overindulgence resulted in vomiting. Besides, it's warm and soothing and easy to get down.

■ **Surgical trauma.** Chicken soup has a little bit of everything you need when you're on the mend after surgery, says Cristopher Bosted, N.D. "It has lots of vegetables in it, and some protein, and you can put in garlic and onions, which are helpful for healing and immunity," he says. If you know someone who makes fresh chicken soup—or you can make it yourself—freeze several serving-size batches before your surgery, then thaw some every day to enjoy.

■ **Colds.** Scientists have studied chicken soup for years trying to figure out how it works. They're still looking for the answer, but one thing is certain: It does seem to help colds. Most doctors theorize that the steam from the hot soup promotes drainage and thus makes you feel better.

■ **Nighttime congestion.** Chicken soup made with spicy red pepper can clear out congestion and make it easier to sleep at night.

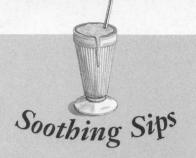

Soothing Sips

INFECTION PROTECTION

Slurp lots of chicken soup if you have pneumonia. For one thing, it helps make coughs more productive. It also provides an abundance of healing nutrients, and it's easy to eat when you're sick and your appetite is low.

■ **Viruses.** Adding mushrooms to chicken soup makes it downright therapeutic. Smoky-tasting shiitakes amp up production of interferon, a protein that girds the body to defend against viral invaders, while reishi mushrooms may help ease respiratory tract inflammation. Add both to your soup, advises John Hahn, N.D., D.P.M.

■ **Earache.** There's some evidence that chicken soup may relieve ear pain. Studies have shown that it stimulates immune cells and helps ease symptoms of infection. For a healing boost, chop a few cloves of garlic, which has antimicrobial effects, and leave it on the cutting board for 10 minutes before you toss it into the soup. This little "rest" allows its healing agents to form.

Chicken Soup

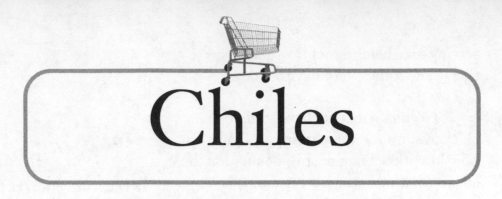

Chiles

TONGUE-TORCHING HEALERS

Chile lovers swear that hot peppers make them feel better. You would think that anything hot enough to blow off the top of your head would have the opposite effect, but researchers say there really is something to it. Here's what chiles can do.

■ **Itchy skin.** Because capsaicin, the heat-producing chemical in chiles, stimulates nerve endings, it can help turn a maddening itch into a minor stinging sensation. Just buy some capsaicin cream and follow the package directions. Wash your hands thoroughly after using it, and don't use it near your eyes or on areas of broken skin.

■ **Heart attack and stroke.** Capsaicin is an antioxidant that helps lower levels of bad low-density lipoprotein (LDL) cholesterol and makes blood platelets less likely to clot and cause a heart attack or stroke. Chiles are also packed with plenty of other heart-smart ingredients, including vitamins C and A.

■ **Ulcers.** Go ahead and dig into chiles if you have an ulcer. Since a type of bacteria called *Helicobacter pylori* causes most ulcers, researchers believe hot peppers may help because of their bacteria-fighting ability. Check with your doctor to determine whether your ulcer is caused by bacteria, though, before you start chowing down.

■ **Tendinitis.** The next time you have tendinitis, load up on red peppers. They're rich in vitamin C, an antioxidant nutrient that may help reduce the swelling in your tendons that's causing your pain, says Andrew Lucking, N.D.

■ **Stuffy nose.** Is your nose so clogged you can't sleep? There's no need to drive to your local drugstore in the middle of the night. Instead, keep your pajamas on and dig into a pita stuffed with lettuce, tomato, and a heap of chopped onions and chile peppers. Your nose will start running almost instantly.

Just What the Doctor Ordered!

Feel-Good Painkillers

The ribs and seeds of chiles are packed with capsaicin, a heat-producing chemical that causes the brain to chill out with a flood of endorphins—high-flying, mood-lifting natural painkillers that create a sense of well-being. Just eat enough to feel the heat, and relief is on the way!

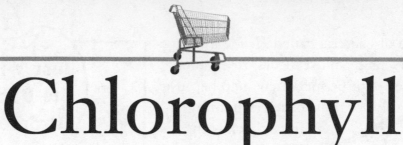

Chlorophyll

IT'S GOOD TO BE GREEN

Chlorophyll, the stuff that makes plants green, can also put you in the pink of health. You'll even *smell* better when you get enough!

■ **Chemo and radiation side effects.** Fruit and vegetable juices deliver a high concentration of antioxidants and chlorophyll, both of which may help protect against the side effects of chemotherapy or radiation during cancer therapy. Have five or six servings a day before, during, and after treatment.

■ **Dragon breath.** The chlorophyll in fruits and vegetables is a natural deodorant that sweetens your breath. It's especially helpful when you've been eating garlic, onions, or other pungent foods. Just munch on a little parsley at the end of a meal.

■ **B.O.** To deodorize your body along with your breath, drink up to three cups of alfalfa tea daily or take alfalfa tablets. Alfalfa is one of the best sources of chlorophyll, and as a bonus, it helps clear up constipation.

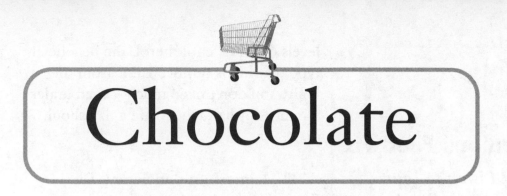

Chocolate

GET YOUR JUST DESSERTS

Chocolate is probably the one sweet that most women (and men!) can't do without. You obviously don't want to eat too much—it's not exactly light on fat or calories—but a little taste now and then can do wonders for your health. Check it out.

■ **Brain fog.** If you have trouble focusing—and have a hankering for chocolate—chances are that your brain really needs it. Chocolate contains phenylethylamine, methylxanthines, and caffeine, which together improve mood, energy, and concentration. A 1.75-ounce bar of dark chocolate will do the trick.

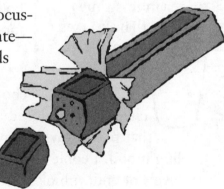

■ **High cholesterol.** Drinking a frothy cup of hot chocolate made with pure cocoa powder (or eating an ounce of dark chocolate with a high cocoa content) does more than stave off winter's chill: Cocoa is rich in flavonoids, which have been shown to prevent oxidation of LDL cholesterol. When LDL is oxidized, it clings to arteries and increases the risk of heart disease and stroke. Studies also show that chocolate helps raise

129

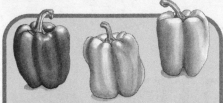

Fabulous Food Fix

Listen to Your Sweet Tooth

When PMS gets you down, give in to your chocolate cravings. Create a cocktail to fight the symptoms by adding 1 tablespoon of fat-free chocolate syrup to a glass of calcium-rich fat-free milk. You'll feel better in less time than it takes to wash the glass.

levels of HDL cholesterol, the beneficial type that helps remove LDL from the body. You don't need much—a tad under 3 ounces of dark chocolate a day should do it.

■ **Magnesium deficiency.** *The Journal of the American Dietetic Association* reports that some people may crave chocolate to compensate for a magnesium deficiency. When you're stressed, your body uses more magnesium than it would normally, depleting your supply. So go ahead, have a little chocolate and replenish your magnesium. A 2-ounce serving of dark chocolate contains about 50 of the 200 to 400 milligrams your body needs every day for muscles to function properly.

■ **Stress.** Research has shown that chocolate helps release endorphins, chemicals produced in the brain that play a key role in controlling mood. People with higher levels of endorphins feel less stressed and more relaxed and confident.

Chocolate

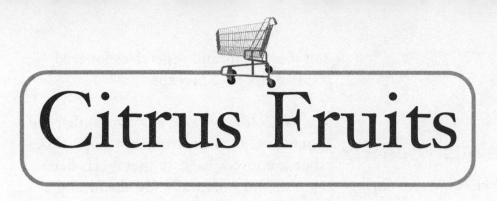

Citrus Fruits

GET THE BEST WITH THE ZEST

The acidic blast that fills your mouth when you eat citrus fruits does more than just make your mouth pucker. It unleashes a flood of chemical compounds that affect just about every system in your body and can improve your ability to fight infection, resist digestive problems, and even stave off cancer. Take a look.

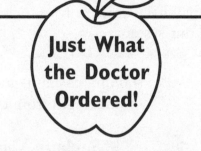

■ **Queasiness.** If your stomach's doing flip-flops, head for the fridge. Grab an uncut lemon, scratch into the peel, and sniff the clean, fresh citrus scent. That's what they do in India to handle nausea.

■ **Stroke.** A Harvard study found that men and women who ate citrus fruits, along with cruciferous vegetables and green leafy vegetables, were less likely to have ischemic strokes, the kind caused by a blood clot in the brain. Each daily serving

> ### Just What the Doctor Ordered!
>
> ### *Turn Down the Heat*
>
> For quick relief from hot flashes, carry a small spray bottle filled with water and "seasoned" with a dash of lemon or lime juice. You'll get a cooling citrus sensation when you spritz your skin.

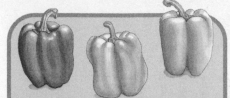

Fabulous Food Fix

Citrus Smoke-Out

Are you trying to quit smoking? This trick will help: Whenever you get the urge to indulge, suck on a lime. Besides curbing your desire for tobacco, it will replace some of the vitamins, phosphates, and calcium that smoking may have drained from your system.

of these fruits and vegetables lowered stroke risk by 6 percent.

■ **Colds.** No one has proven that the vitamin C in citrus fruits can stop colds, but scientists speculate that it acts like interferon, a natural body chemical that stops virus growth. Even if it can't prevent colds entirely, though, there's some evidence that getting enough C can decrease their duration and intensity, so eat plenty of citrus at the first sign of the sniffles.

■ **Muscle cramps.** An imbalance in electrolytes, the minerals that surround your muscle cells and transmit nerve signals, can cause muscle cramps. You can make sure your body has what it needs by including potassium (along with chloride, sodium, calcium, and magnesium) in your diet. You'll get plenty of potassium from citrus fruits. All you need is one serving a day.

■ **Sunburn.** Citrus fruits are among the best sources of antioxidants, which can help your skin heal from sunburn and protect you from the free radical damage that can cause skin cancer. One of the main antioxidants in citrus, vitamin C, helps strengthen collagen, the protein that supports the skin, and helps quell the flood of free radicals that are produced when you get burned. Doctors recommend eating five or six servings of antioxidant-rich foods daily.

■ **Cancer.** The pulpy white membrane on orange and tangerine wedges provides pectin, a form of fiber that may help reduce the spread of cancer—which is important if you're undergoing radiation or chemotherapy treatments. Pectin also lowers cholesterol and can reduce the risk of heart disease.

■ **Iron-deficiency anemia.** When you eat foods high in vitamin C, such as citrus fruits, the vitamin helps your body absorb iron from other foods. Basically, it moves the iron through the gastrointestinal system and into your bloodstream so it doesn't pass through to be eliminated. This is particularly important if you have iron-deficiency anemia, which can sap your strength and energy in a hurry. Women tend to get this type of anemia due to menstrual bleeding, so protect yourself ahead of time and load up on citrus all month long.

■ **Folate-deficiency anemia.** A condition called folate-deficiency anemia tends to affect moms-to-be and women who are breastfeeding. The B vitamin folate (folic acid) is a red cell builder that comes from citrus fruits as well as whole grain foods, dark leafy greens, and beans. Unlike iron, it isn't stored in your body, so you need to eat folate-rich foods every day.

■ **Bruises.** Your body uses vitamin C to repair damaged capillaries. When you have a bruise, you've injured dozens or even hundreds of them,

Soothing Sips

SLOW THE RUNS

Here's a diarrhea remedy that's a bit more palatable than drugstore products: In a blender, puree a peeled and cored apple with about a teaspoon of lime juice, a few drops of honey, and a pinch of cinnamon. Drink it down and relax.

Citrus Fruits 133

Citrus Stops Stones

Anyone who's concerned about kidney stones will want to start the day with an orange or a tall glass of juice, then continue to eat oranges or quaff orange juice throughout the day. The fruit raises your body's level of citrates, natural chemicals that keep new stones from forming and existing ones from getting worse. Discuss this with your doctor before you try it, though, because not all types of stones are affected by citrates.

so you need as much of this important nutrient as you can get. While the bruise is healing, eat plenty of fruits (especially citrus fruits) and vegetables, which are loaded with vitamin C.

■ **Dragon breath.** If your breath tends to be, well, less than sweet, and there's no medical or dental problem, try this remedy. At bedtime and between meals, drink the juice of one lime and a teaspoon or so of honey mixed into a glass of water.

■ **Gum disease.** For healthy gums and whiter teeth, mix lime juice and salt into a paste and rub the mixture onto your gums and teeth several times a day.

■ **Stings.** A drop of lime juice will ease the pain of a bee or fire-ant sting. (But it's not a substitute for medical attention. If you suspect you're allergic to stings, or if you notice swelling or start to have trouble breathing, call 911!)

■ **Drab hair.** Want to lighten your hair without chemicals—or a beauty-salon price tag? Just mix 1 ounce of mild shampoo with the juice of two limes and one lemon. Pour the solution onto your hair and massage it in. Sit in the sun or under a helmet-type hair dryer for 15 to 20 minutes, then rinse.

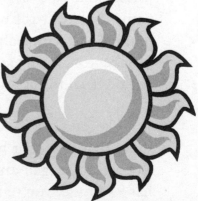

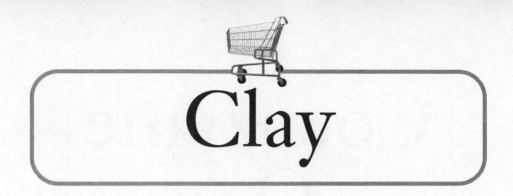

Clay

THE MAGIC OF MUD

Forget fancy-schmancy high-tech medicine; one of the oldest, most effective remedies comes straight from Mother Earth. Here's the scoop.

■ **Smelly feet.** If even the dog runs for cover when you take off your shoes, sprinkle some green clay in them, and your feet will be sweet.

■ **Oily skin.** Clay soaks up excess oil and sloughs off dead skin cells without irritation. Simply add a little water to a teaspoon of green clay, then mix a few drops of lavender oil into the paste. Apply it to your face and rinse off after 15 minutes.

■ **Breast pain.** To reduce monthly breast discomfort, try a poultice made from green clay and cabbage. Mix 4 parts shredded cabbage with 1 part clay and apply it to your breasts. Cover the poultice with a moist cloth, then wear a loose, soft cotton bra to keep it in place overnight.

■ **Ingrown toenail.** A clay pack will help keep swelling and infection from an ingrown nail under control. Apply the clay and leave it on until it dries, then rinse it off and dry your foot thoroughly. Repeat the treatment once or twice a day.

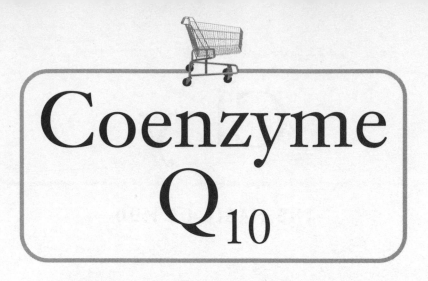

Coenzyme Q_{10}

A JUMP-START FOR THE HEART

If you haven't heard about coenzyme Q_{10} (CoQ$_{10}$) yet, you probably will soon. It's a high-powered supplement (and a chemical in foods) with a lot of science behind it—and good evidence that it really works. Here's how.

■ **Heart problems.** CoQ$_{10}$ is an antioxidant that appears to bring oxygen to the heart and may even help curb the damage caused by a lack of oxygen. For heart health, take 100 milligrams a day. Look for capsules or tablets in an oil base, which your body absorbs better than powder-based forms.

■ **Muscle/organ fatigue.** Tuna, salmon, and other cold-water fish provide the CoQ$_{10}$ needed by your heart, liver, muscles, and brain to produce the energy they need to keep going.

■ **Pain.** CoQ_{10} provides the spark that fires up the ATP in your cells—a chemical that can mean less pain and more energy.

■ **Headache.** Studies have shown that when people took CoQ_{10} daily, they experienced 60 percent fewer headaches than when they weren't taking it. The dose was 150 milligrams a day.

■ **High blood pressure.** CoQ_{10} makes arteries less vulnerable to constriction. Researchers report that people who took 100 milligrams a day were able to cut their doses of blood pressure medications in half. Don't, however, make any changes to your medication regimen without checking with your doctor.

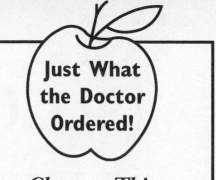

Just What the Doctor Ordered!

Chew on This

"Coenzyme Q_{10} helps tighten gum tissue so plaque can't become trapped in it," says Darin Ingels, N.D. Your best bet is to take a 30-milligram capsule with food twice daily. Alternatively, you can break open a capsule and dip your toothbrush in it, then press it lightly on tender gums.

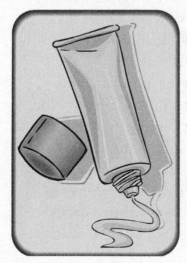

■ **Dry skin.** Try a facial cleansing cream containing CoQ_{10}. It's a natural substance that helps skin stay strong and elastic. Buy the brand that contains the least alcohol and the fewest artificial colors or other ingredients.

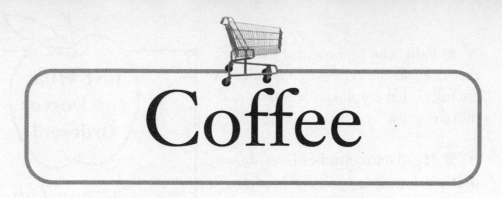

Coffee

BREW SOME RELIEF

A hot, steaming cup of coffee does more than help open your eyes in the morning. It can also stimulate specific parts of your body just when you need it most. Take a look!

■ **Constipation.** The next time you're a little constipated, knock back a cup of strong coffee. It stimulates the intestine and will help you stay regular.

■ **Bloating.** If you don't drink coffee often and have trouble with fluid retention now and then, try a cup—black. It's a natural diuretic that can wash fluids from your body, which is especially helpful for premenstrual bloating.

■ **Headache.** If your head is pounding and you're not too queasy, down some coffee—the high-test kind with plenty of caffeine. Taking 130 milligrams of caffeine (the amount in about 1½ cups of coffee) and two aspirin tablets relieves a headache 40 percent better than aspirin alone, according to the National Headache Foundation.

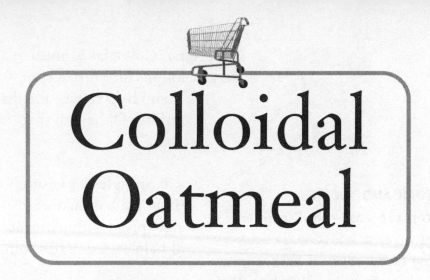

Colloidal Oatmeal

NATURE'S SKIN SOOTHER

The same gel-like substance in oats that lowers cholesterol and soothes your digestive tract can also do wonders for your skin. Haven't had a "cereal bath" lately? Here are some reasons to give it a try.

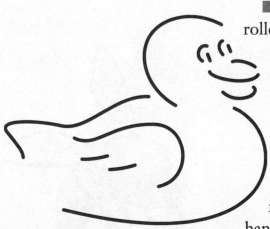

■ **Itchy skin.** Save the rolled oats for breakfast, but try a commercial brand of finely milled or "colloidal" oatmeal, such as Aveeno, when you're itching. It relieves various types of contact dermatitis, such as poison ivy. Just throw a few handfuls into a tepid bath to make your bathwater instantly silky and comforting, then soak for at least 20 minutes to let the tiny particles thoroughly penetrate your pores.

139

■ **Eczema.** Colloidal oatmeal baths and lotions moisturize your skin and help reduce the discomfort of "the itch that rashes."

■ **Shingles.** A leisurely soak in a tub of lukewarm water spiked with oatmeal will help ease shingles pain.

■ **Sunburn.** When your skin is scorched and sore, fill your tub with cool to lukewarm water. Add some oatmeal and soak long enough to soothe the burn.

■ **Folliculitis.** If the itching of folliculitis is making you crazy, a colloidal oatmeal bath can put you at ease.

■ **Bug bites.** Some insect bites really itch while they're healing, but an oatmeal bath provides quick relief.

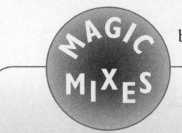

SOAK AND SOOTHE
You can ease the discomfort of a yeast infection by soaking in an oatmeal bath, says Jana Nalbandian, N.D. Just fill an old sock with a cup or two of oatmeal, fasten the open end to the faucet with a rubber band, and let the water run through it as the tub fills up.

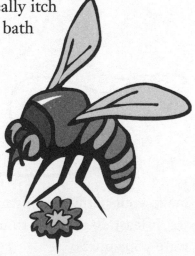

Colloidal Oatmeal

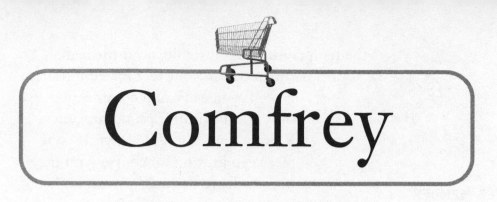

Comfrey

LEAVES OF PROTECTION

Comfrey is like a complete medicine chest jammed into one compact little package. It's been used for thousands of years to treat injuries, relieve rashes, and banish bruises—and that's just the beginning. Here's what else it can do.

■ **Sprained ankle.** A sprained ankle hurts like the dickens and can take weeks or even months to heal completely. A natural way to help it back to health is with a comfrey wrap—and it won't cause the side effects of aspirin or similar drugs. Buy three or four whole leaves of this traditional trauma-treating herb and blanch them by dipping them briefly in boiling water. Let them cool a bit, then drape them over the injured area and cover with an elastic bandage. Replace the leaves daily until the sprain heals.

■ **Bunions.** A comfrey footbath soothes painful bunions fast because the herb contains chemical compounds that reduce discomfort and help sore areas heal. To make a footbath, steep an ounce of dried comfrey leaves in a few cups of simmering water for 10 minutes. Add enough cool water to make

Blister Beater

Been wearing those tight shoes again? Ointments containing comfrey root promote speedy healing of blisters.

the temperature comfortable, pour the water into a basin, and soak your feet for 20 minutes or so. If you can't find comfrey, it's okay to substitute Epsom salts, says Rowan Hamilton, Dip.Phyt. If your feet keep hurting, of course, you may need to leave the pointy-toed high heels in the closet. They're a common cause of bunions.

■ **Hemorrhoids.** Warm sitz baths using an infusion of comfrey and horsetail can help soothe inflamed anal tissues and, over time, make them less susceptible to irritation. Make a strong infusion by simmering 1 cup of comfrey root in 1 pint of water for 20 minutes. Remove from the heat, add 1 heaping tablespoon of horsetail, and steep for an additional 10 minutes. Strain the solution, pour it into the bathtub, and fill the tub with enough warm water to come up to the top of your pelvic bone. Soak for 20 minutes three times weekly.

MAGIC MIXES

MUSCLE MENDER
Prone to sore muscles? Fill a 12-ounce glass jar with freshly chopped comfrey leaves, then cover completely with a mixture of olive oil and the oil from a vitamin E capsule. Put the jar in a sunny indoor spot for a week, shaking it a couple of times a day. Strain the oil and put it into a clean glass bottle, then add 15 drops of juniper and wintergreen oils. You can rub the liniment into sore muscles whenever you feel the need. Store in a cool place or in the fridge.

■ **Irritated skin.** Here's a pleasant way to moisturize your skin and reduce lingering irritation from rashes or other skin conditions. After a bath or shower, lock in moisture by smearing comfrey ointment, chamomile cream, or calendula lotion directly onto the affected area. These herbs have anti-inflammatory properties that will help relieve your discomfort. You can even keep these emollients in the fridge for instant relief whenever itching flares.

Comfrey

■ **Vaginal pain.** Just about any kind of vaginal pain can be helped by a sitz bath—a shallow bath that allows you to soak the vaginal area, says Annette Fuglsang Owens, M.D., Ph.D. Soaking in lukewarm water for 15 minutes before or after intercourse can prevent or relieve pain, she explains. Add 10 to 15 drops of comfrey oil to the bathwater to soothe any inflammation or irritation.

■ **Itchy skin.** The leaves and roots of the comfrey plant contain the healing agent allantoin, which stimulates healthy tissue growth and can help relieve itchy rashes caused by allergies or other conditions. To make a cooling, cell-growth-encouraging poultice, simply mash 1 cup of fresh leaves or soak 1 cup of dried leaves in enough water to cover them. Then wrap the mash in a thin cloth and apply it to the affected area.

■ **Shiners.** Comfrey is among the best treatments for a black eye, says Priscilla Natanson, N.D. If you're using fresh leaves, mash them into a paste and apply it directly to the bruise, being careful not to get any in your eye. If you're using the dried form, crush the leaves between your fingers and add just enough water to moisten. Wrap the powder in a piece of cheesecloth, then hold it on the area. Apply either form of the herb for about 20 minutes twice a day.

Just What the Doctor Ordered!

A Soothing Solution

To clean minor cuts and scrapes, use a healing infusion. Combine equal parts of calendula, echinacea, and comfrey, then steep 1 heaping tablespoon of the mixture in 1 pint of hot water for 20 minutes. Strain out the herbs and wash the wound with the solution.

Cornstarch

SILKY-SMOOTH RELIEF

Cornstarch is one of those household products that just keep on giving. Apart from its use as a kitchen ingredient, it's almost custom-made for skin problems, thanks to its absorbent qualities and super-smooth texture. Here's what we mean.

■ **Itchy skin.** Cornstarch is a reliable itch reliever. Dust this satiny powder right onto your body or add it to your bathwater for soothing itch relief.

■ **Blisters.** Blisters are most likely to develop if your feet are too sweaty. Try sprinkling a little cornstarch into your socks before you put them on, and dust some between your toes, too.

■ **B.O.** Native Americans in the U.S. Southwest and Mexico make body talc by mixing crushed calendula leaves with cornstarch.

■ **Anal itching.** Moisture is the enemy when you have anal itching. After you shower or bathe, towel off and dust on a little cornstarch powder to absorb moisture.

■ **Hemorrhoids.** A cornstarch enema can help ease painful hemorrhoids. To make it, mix 1 tablespoon of cornstarch with a pint of water. Boil the mixture for a few minutes, let it cool, and pour it into an enema bag.

■ **Sunburn.** To relieve sunburn pain, add enough water to cornstarch to make a paste, then apply it directly to the affected area.

■ **Athlete's foot.** Prevent or cure athlete's foot by sprinkling cornstarch on your feet and in your shoes to absorb moisture and reduce friction.

Just What the Doctor Ordered!

Ditchin' Friction

Cornstarch reduces painful friction in places where skin rubs against skin. After bathing and before dressing, use a cotton ball to apply enough powder to lightly cover the chafed area. Check several times a day and apply more cornstarch if the skin looks red or irritated.

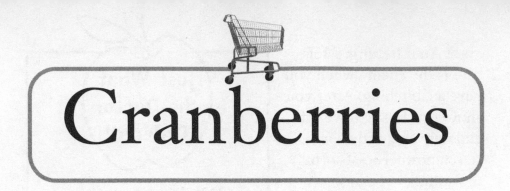

Cranberries

A SAUCE FOR ALL SEASONS

If your only experience with cranberries is the canned, gelatinous glop that makes an appearance on holidays, you're in for a surprise if you ever eat fresh berries or drink the juice. Apart from their deliciously tangy taste, cranberries are jammed with protective chemicals that can keep you healthy all year. Here's the scoop.

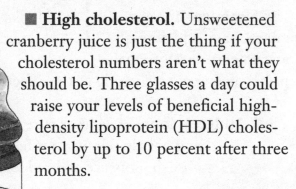

■ **High cholesterol.** Unsweetened cranberry juice is just the thing if your cholesterol numbers aren't what they should be. Three glasses a day could raise your levels of beneficial high-density lipoprotein (HDL) cholesterol by up to 10 percent after three months.

■ **UTIs I.** Turkey Day's star fruit harbors bacteria-fighting weapons called proanthocyanidins. These condensed tannins have been shown to keep the bacteria that cause urinary tract infections (UTIs) from sticking around—even in people who have strains that resist standard antibiotics. Drink 2 cups of unsweetened cranberry juice every hour at the first hint of burning or pop one 400-milligram capsule of cranberry extract four times a day.

■ **UTIs II.** In addition to their role in treating UTIs, cranberries also seem to prevent them. Research done at Harvard Medical School showed that elderly women who drank 1¼ cups of cranberry juice every day for a month were more than 60 percent less likely to have infections than those who did not. And if they continued drinking the tangy thirst quencher, their chances dropped even more.

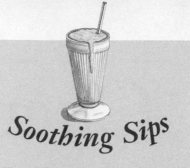

Soothing Sips

THE CRANBERRY CURE

The next time hemorrhoids—and the bleeding that often accompanies them—flare up, simply mix a few ounces of cranberry juice with an equal amount of pomegranate juice and drink it between meals. Both fruits are hemostatics, which help stanch bleeding.

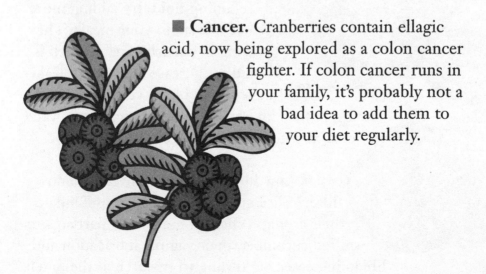

■ **Cancer.** Cranberries contain ellagic acid, now being explored as a colon cancer fighter. If colon cancer runs in your family, it's probably not a bad idea to add them to your diet regularly.

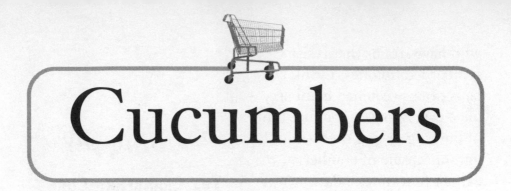

Cucumbers

MORE THAN A SALAD STAPLE

Nothing's tastier on a hot summer day than a cool cucumber salad doused with a little vinegar and salt. In fact, this crisp veggie can cool off all sorts of health problems—and not just when you eat it. Here's how.

■ **Puffy eyes.** To diminish eyelid swelling, place a 1-inch-thick slice of chilled cucumber over each eye and relax for 15 to 20 minutes.

■ **Bloating.** When you're retaining fluid, try adding more cucumbers to your meals. They contain cucurbocitrin, which is said to increase the natural leakiness of tiny blood vessels, or capillaries, in the kidneys. This means that more water escapes into the kidneys for elimination.

■ **Low libido.** Need an instant libido lifter? Slice up some cucumbers and inhale their aroma. When women study participants sniffed cucumber, their vaginal lubrication and libido increased, according to research at the Smell and Taste Treatment and Research Foundation.

■ **Dark circles.** To lighten undereye circles, cut two cucumber slices, lie down in a comfortable place, and put one slice over each eye for about 10 minutes.

■ **Eczema.** Cucumber juice reduces the inflammation caused by eczema. Just moisten a cotton pad with the juice and gently dab the trouble spots.

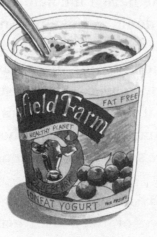

Fabulous Food Fix

Cool as a Cucumber

You can soothe sunburn by placing chilled slices of cucumber on your simmering skin. A dab of cold yogurt or a splash of vinegar will do the job, too.

■ **Irritated skin.** Here's how to make a soothing facial for all skin types: Puree half a cucumber in a blender. Mix in 1 tablespoon of plain yogurt, apply the mixture to your face, and leave it on for about 30 minutes, then rinse with warm water and pat dry.

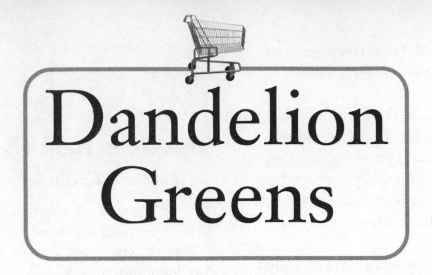

Dandelion Greens

THE "LAWN CURE"

Americans in search of the perfect lawn go after dandelions with everything short of nuclear bombs—and the tenacious weeds just keep coming back. It's a good thing, too, because dandelion greens are among the most potent remedies in the herbal medicine chest. If you don't feel like picking your own, you can check the gourmet section of your supermarket's produce aisle. (Don't use dandelion if you take diuretics or potassium supplements, however.) Here's what these greens can do.

■ **Anemia.** Dandelions are super sources of iron and are gentle to the liver, points out Ryan Drum, Ph.D. Plus, they taste great—a

Weed Out Migraines

Because dandelion helps support the liver, which metabolizes estrogen, it can also ease migraine pain associated with fluctuating hormone levels. Plus, it's rich in magnesium, which is often deficient in people with migraines. Take 400 to 500 milligrams of dandelion leaf capsules a day throughout your cycle.

little like arugula, a nutty, spiky-leaved salad green. It's the leaves at the crown of the dandelion plant that you want. Just be sure to pick them from an area that you're sure is free of pesticides and lawn chemicals—then rinse them thoroughly and toss 'em into salads.

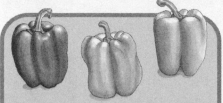

Fabulous Food Fix

Bitter Stomach Saver

Dandelion greens are a traditional remedy for stomach problems of all kinds. Eaten before a meal, the pleasantly bitter greens stimulate digestive secretions and reduce cramping. The leaves are most tender when they're picked just before the flowers bloom.

■ **Bloating.** The fresh, young leaves of the dandelion (which the French call *pissenlit*, or "urinate in bed") act as a natural diuretic. In fact, in head-to-head tests, dandelion leaf tea was shown to be as effective as the prescription diuretic furosemide (Lasix). Drink two to four cups of tea a day to deflate swollen tissues, suggests Michael DiPalma, N.D., or take up to two standard capsules of dried dandelion leaf daily. You can even toss fresh leaves into your summer salads to benefit from their cleansing effect. If you have fluid retention due to heart problems, talk to your doctor about using dandelion; don't, under any circumstances, do it on your own.

■ **Endometriosis.** If you have endometriosis, search your supermarket for "lipotropic" supplements that contain dandelion, milk thistle, and choline, all of which help support the liver, which metabolizes estrogen. That's important because estrogen is what fuels the growth of endometrial tissue, which is overproduced and grows on other tissues or organs in women with endometriosis. Without the estrogen stimulus, the endometrial tissue grows more slowly, which helps reduce cramping and other symptoms.

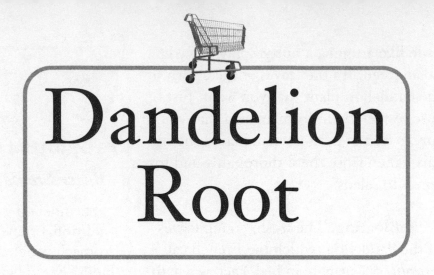

Dandelion Root

A SUPER HEALER

If you spend a lot of summer hours digging dandelions out of your lawn, you may find it hard to think of them as your friends. Believe it or not, though, they're some of nature's best medicine (except for people who take diuretics or potassium supplements). Here's what we mean.

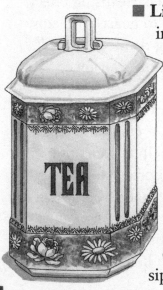

■ **Liver problems.** To tone your liver, relieve inflammation, and relax spasms, try dandelion root. Add 1 teaspoon of dried root to 1 cup of hot water. Steep for 15 minutes, strain, and drink between meals.

■ **Anal itching.** Anal itching is often a sign of poor digestion. Boost your digestive power by drinking ½ cup of dandelion tea before meals. To make your own, steep 1 teaspoon of dandelion root in ½ cup of hot water for 20 minutes. Strain and sip warm before meals.

■ **Hormone imbalance.** If your hair has suddenly become extremely oily or startlingly dry, it probably means that your levels of androgen hormones, which have an effect on sweating and oil production, have either soared or taken a nosedive. One way to help your liver rebalance the hormones is to take 150 milligrams of dandelion root in capsule form twice daily.

■ **Hangover.** The next time you've stayed out a little too late dancing on tables (or sleeping under them), reach for dandelion root tincture. It may be the perfect little hangover helper. It not only stimulates the liver, which may speed alcohol metabolism, it's also a gentle diuretic that can reduce excess fluid buildup that leads to puffiness. Unlike more powerful diuretics, it won't flush out all-important electrolytes—minerals that are essential for normal muscle movement, nerve function, and just about everything else that happens in your body. Take 30 to 60 drops of tincture three times a day.

Soothing Sips

HEMORRHOID HELPER

Most hemorrhoids are caused by nothing more than constipation. You can make an anti-constipation/anti-hemorrhoid decoction by simmering 1 teaspoon each of dandelion root and burdock root in 2 cups of boiling water for 20 minutes. Remove from the heat and add 1 teaspoon of peppermint, then cover and steep for another 10 minutes. Strain and sip ½ cup first thing in the morning and before each meal.

Dandelion Root 153

Decongestants

STOP THE STUFFINESS

Hay fever, colds and flu, and even sinusitis can leave you feeling so stuffed up that you almost feel as if you need to use a jackhammer on your nasal passages just to breathe. Here's how supermarket decongestants can help.

■ **Earache.** The next time you have an earache, you might have to start out by fixing your nose. Over-the-counter decongestants or nasal sprays may help decrease nasal secretions, shrink the mucous membranes, and open the Eustachian tubes in your ears, reducing pressure and pain. Be sure to follow package directions, and don't use them longer than the recommended period. One caution: If you have high blood pressure, check with your doctor or pharmacist before using decongestants.

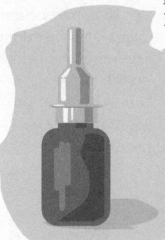

■ **Sinus headache.** Sinusitis, which is basically infection and inflammation of the sinus cavities in your head or face, can often cause headaches. Antibiotics are frequently needed to clear up the infection, but decongestants—saline sprays, nose gels with eucalyptus, and eating spicy foods—are the only thing that will unstuff your sinuses.

■ **Stuffy nose I.** Is your nose so clogged up you can't sleep? Head to the produce aisle. It's probably well stocked with natural decongestants, such as garlic, onions, chile peppers, and horseradish. Eat as much hot stuff as you can comfortably handle. Your nose will probably start running within seconds.

■ **Stuffy nose II.** Hot chicken soup is a proven cold chaser. The steam acts as a natural decongestant, and it appears that there are substances in chicken that are chemically similar to those in commercial decongestants.

Soothing Sips

SPICY HEAD CLEARER

When you're so congested that you feel as though your nose and sinuses are packed with cotton balls, sip hot tea that contains natural decongestants such as ginger or cardamom. "In addition to the steam of the hot tea, these antiviral spices may help open nasal passages in their own right," says David Zeiger, D.O.

Decongestants

155

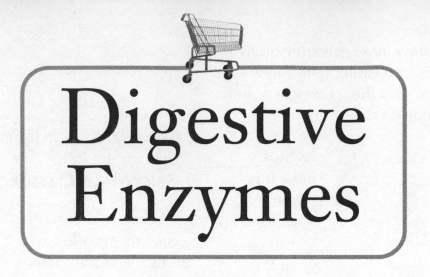

Digestive Enzymes

THE ACID TEST

The acid in your stomach is just about as strong as battery acid, but even that isn't always enough for proper digestion or the absorption of nutrients—and that in turn can lead to all sorts of health problems. The solution? For some people, digestive enzymes can make all the difference. Here's why.

■ **Brittle hair.** "Hair that's brittle and breaks when you brush it could indicate that you're not absorbing the minerals you need from your diet," says Kathleen Flewelling, N.D. Try taking digestive enzyme supplements to aid absorption. Check for formulas that include hydrochloric acid to help break down fats and proteins, plus papain and bromelain for better carbohydrate

ON THE SHELF
✓ Pineapple
✓ Papaya

156

absorption. Follow the package directions, and don't use hydrochloric acid if you're prone to ulcers.

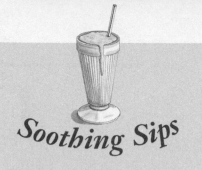

■ **Heartburn.** If your stomach doesn't digest food efficiently, you're sure to get heartburn or a stomachache. Supplemental digestive enzymes can help. Many different types are available, including bromelain and papain, but it doesn't really matter what kind you get; they're all helpful.

Soothing Sips

TROPICAL FUME FIGHTER

To soothe indigestion and gassiness, drink a cup of papaya juice laced with 1 teaspoon of organic sugar and two pinches of cardamom.

■ **Laryngitis.** Clear-Ease tablets contain papaya and pineapple enzymes, which help reduce inflammation and swelling of the vocal cords when you have laryngitis.

■ **Gas.** When you don't thoroughly chew your food, you produce less saliva, which contains digestive enzymes that help break down food before it hits your digestive tract. The undigested food then ferments, and the result can be painful gas and bloating. The answer? Eat papaya. Its natural digestive enzymes may help relieve your distress.

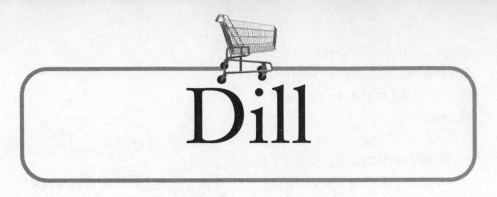

Dill

A DILLY OF A SEED

If all you know about dill is that it's a type of pickle, you're in for a few surprises. This fresh-tasting herb is a traditional remedy that will help you get out of a pickle. Here's how.

■ **Queasiness.** A homemade infusion of dill seeds can help calm an upset stomach. Steep 1 teaspoon of seeds in 1 cup of hot water, covered, for 15 minutes, then strain and sip.

■ **Dragon breath.** You've probably seen fennel seeds next to the cash register at Indian or Asian restaurants. It's not because the proprietors want to save money on candy mints; it's because chewing dill or fennel seeds after meals will help freshen breath and promote healthy digestion.

■ **Gas.** If beans and other starchy foods make you gassy—as they do to nearly everyone from time to time—simply sprinkle your food with tasty carminative (gas-reducing) seeds, such as dill, fennel, or caraway. For more oomph, stir in some basil, rosemary, oregano, or sage, all of which are carminative. You can buy over-the-counter products that reduce gas, but the herbal approach may work just as well—and cost a lot less.

Echinacea

POWER UP IMMUNITY

The next time you have any kind of infection, reach for echinacea. As with most herbal medicines, some pretty grandiose claims have been about its healing benefits, but echinacea is unique because, unlike some of its herbal counterparts, it truly deserves the accolades. It fires up your immune system and increases your body's ability to repel viral as well as bacterial invaders. One caveat: People with autoimmune conditions, such as lupus or rheumatoid arthritis, shouldn't use this herb.

■ **Sore throat.** Is your throat so sore that you can hardly swallow? Echinacea—a renowned mucous membrane healer—numbs on contact and may kill off any virus that may be causing sore throat misery. You can put 60 drops of tincture and some water in a small

A Sex Rx

For pain that occurs after intercourse, use a vaginal wash made with soothing antimicrobial herbs. Combine equal parts of echinacea, goldenseal, and lavender and steep 1 heaping teaspoon of the mixture in 1 cup of hot water for 20 minutes. Strain and pour into a peribottle. Keep the bottle by the toilet, and after intercourse, wash your labia and vaginal opening with the solution. If the irritation persists, see your doctor to rule out an infection.

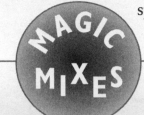

MAGIC MIXES

spray bottle and spritz your throat several times a day, or take echinacea in capsule form (check the label for dosage directions) until your symptoms disappear.

A SUPER SKIN HEALER
The healing herbs echinacea and goldenseal spell double trouble for the bacteria that cause folliculitis, says Heidi Weinhold, N.D. They kill some germs on contact, and they create an unfavorable environment for future populations. The easiest approach is to buy an ointment that contains both herbs and apply it several times a day until the outbreak is over.

■ **Cold sores.** Echinacea isn't just a plain old cold fighter; it battles cold sores, too, perhaps by boosting the antiviral immune fighters in mucous membranes. Mix ¼ teaspoon of extract in water or juice and drink it three times a day for as long as your symptoms last.

■ **Athlete's foot.** You can kick athlete's foot with a tea made with equal parts of echinacea, oregano, calendula, and cleavers, which have immune-boosting effects that fight the fungus from the inside. Add 1 heaping teaspoon of the mixture to 1 cup of boiling water and steep, covered, for 15 minutes. Strain and drink up to three cups a day. For mild cases of athlete's foot, you can make an external wash with the same herbs, using ½ cup per 1 quart of water. Let the mixture cool to a comfortable temperature, soak your feet for 15 to 20 minutes, and dry them well.

■ **STDs I.** People with sexually transmitted diseases (STDs) need to strengthen their immune systems even while using medical treatment. To make an immunity-boosting tea, combine equal parts of echinacea, goldenseal, and licorice root and steep 1 heaping teaspoon in a cup of hot water for 15 minutes.

160

Echinacea

Strain and drink two or three cups daily. If you have high blood pressure or kidney disease, skip the licorice root.

■ **STDs II.** Echinacea boosts production of T cells that fight viruses and of phagocytes that battle bacteria, says Tori Hudson, N.D. That's especially important if you have chlamydia, an STD that's becoming increasingly common. In addition to antibiotics, Dr. Hudson suggests taking ½ teaspoon of liquid extract every 2 hours for two days, then taking ¹/₂ teaspoon three times daily for the next two weeks.

■ **Colds.** Echinacea has a strong reputation as an herbal cold fighter. At the first sign of a cold, start taking it according to the package directions. This immune stimulant battles cold germs after they enter your body. In fact, studies show that it will decrease the duration of your cold and cut the severity of your symptoms in half.

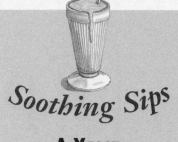

Soothing Sips

A YEAST PREVENTION PLAN

Studies in Germany have shown that echinacea tea can prevent yeast infections if you drink it regularly. Make a cup of tea by steeping ½ teaspoon of dried herb in 1 cup of boiling water for about 10 minutes, then strain out the herb. Researchers found that the tea loses its effect after eight weeks, so stop for a month, then start drinking it again.

■ **Pneumonia.** All liquids are helpful when you have pneumonia, but warm echinacea tea is in a class by itself. It reduces chest congestion and soothes your throat and lungs while boosting the ability of your immune system to fight the infection. Steep a teaspoon of dried herb in a cup of hot water for about 10 minutes, then strain and sip. Plan on drinking two or three cups of tea a day until the infection is gone and you're feeling better.

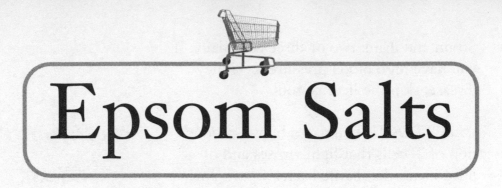

Epsom Salts

MAKE YOUR BATH BETTER

You already know how soothing a long, hot soak can be at the end of the day, but you can make it heck of a lot better by adding Epsom salts. Not only do the salts soften bathwater and soothe your muscles and joints, they also knock out skin problems in the time in takes to lie back and say "Ahh!" Take a look.

Natural Bruise Beater

A body bruise is a good excuse to use that box of Epsom salts that's been sitting in the back of your bathroom cabinet all these years. Add a cup or two of the salts to a warm bath (or a smaller amount to a basin of water), then soak the bruised area for about 20 minutes. The magnesium in the salts is very soothing for bumps and bruises.

■ **Muscle pain.** The mineral magnesium is a must for muscle pain. Epsom salts are just the ticket because they're a form of magnesium that's easily absorbed through the skin. The next time you're stuck in bed staring at the ceiling because your back's in spasm, gently move yourself to the bathroom, run a hot bath, and add 2 cups of Epsom salts, then relax and feel the relief. In some cases, in fact, you'll notice the pain fading even before the water cools.

■ **Kidney stones.** Your doctor will probably advise you to take an over-the-counter or prescription painkiller during kidney stone attacks. While you're waiting for it to work, add a cup or two of Epsom salts to a warm bath and soak for a while.

■ **Aches and pains.** For general pain—from a cold, the flu, or simply accumulated stress—treat yourself to a fragrant remedy. First, scoop ⅓ cup each of chamomile, lavender, and lemon balm into a muslin bag. Toss the bag into the tub while you run warm water, then add 2 cups of Epsom salts and agitate the water to dissolve them. Soak for 10 to 15 minutes.

■ **Bunions.** To soothe painful bunions fast, try an Epsom salts footbath. First, add a cup or two of the salts to a few cups of simmering water, then add enough cool water to make the temperature comfortable. Pour the water into a basin and soak your feet for 20 minutes or so.

■ **Ingrown toenail.** The next time you have an ingrown nail, take advantage of Epsom salts. "An Epsom salts bath will help draw out pain and infection," says Pamela Taylor, N.D. Fill a basin with warm water, add a cup of Epsom salts, and soak your foot for 20 to 30 minutes.

MAGIC MIXES

CALM A COLD
When you're congested, climb into steamy bathwater laced with 2 drops each of eucalyptus, thyme, and rosemary oil, plus a cup or so of Epsom salts. The steam will increase the flow of nasal mucus; the molecules from the oils will dilate your small airways, easing your breathing; and the magnesium in the Epsom salts will be absorbed through your skin and may help relax your bronchial passages.

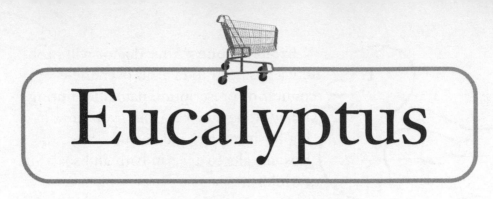

Eucalyptus

A SNIFFER SOOTHER

The penetrating scent of eucalyptus is unmistakable in products such as Listerine mouthwash and Vicks VapoRub. This fast-growing herb contains a chemical compound, eucalyptol, that clears congestion in a jiffy—but that's not all.

■ **Stuffy nose.** The next time you have a cold, pick up a bar of eucalyptus soap and use it in the shower. The scent will permeate your nose and help open the nasal passages. As a bonus, laboratory studies show that eucalyptol kills the flu virus!

■ **Allergies.** When those headachy, runny-nose, sneezy allergies hit, try placing a dab of soothing salve on your temples. Choose one that contains an essential oil, such as eucalyptus or peppermint. The scent will soothe and relax you while the oils open your respiratory passages and ease the headache-causing congestion.

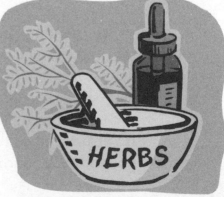

ON THE SHELF

✓ Listerine

✓ Vicks VapoRub

✓ Eucalyptus Chest Rub

✓ Eucalyptus essential oil

■ **Sinus headache.** Sinusitis, an infection and inflammation of the sinus cavities in your head or face, often causes headaches because the openings through which fluids drain out of your sinuses become clogged and create a vacuum. It's exquisitely painful. If you're prone to sinus headaches, check with your doctor. You may need an antibiotic for the infection, but decongestants, such as nose gels with eucalyptus, will open your sinuses quickly.

■ **Earache.** Eucalyptus may help ease the pressure in your Eustachian tubes and encourage drainage of fluid that's been dammed up in the middle ear—a common cause of earaches. Fill a bowl with boiling water, add several (up to 10) drops of eucalyptus oil, and lean over the bowl (but not so close that you could burn your face). Drape a towel over your head and the bowl to capture the steam, then inhale the mist for at least 5 minutes. You can also place a few drops of eucalyptus oil in your bathwater, but don't put it directly into your ears.

■ **Thinning hair.** If you comb the hair-care aisle at your local supermarket, you'll find lots of pricey hair-thickening products (such as "volumizer" shampoos) that contain chemicals called polymers. These chemicals carry a positive electrical charge, and since hair has a negative charge, polymers stick to hair shafts, actually coating them to make them look thicker,

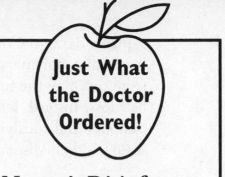

Just What the Doctor Ordered!

Nature's Disinfectant

To prevent passing the flu bug by hand contact, be sure to clean high-touch household surfaces, such as telephones, countertops, and toilet handles. You can disinfect them with a few drops of eucalyptus oil mixed into a pint spray bottle of water. It smells a lot better than commercial cleaners and is better for you, too.

explains Bernard Cohen, M.D. The trouble is, by coating the hair shafts, polymers also suffocate them, preventing oxygen from reaching the follicles—and ironically, perhaps encouraging hair loss. Instead, look for herbal hair products that contain camphor and eucalyptus, which dilate the blood vessels in your scalp and help discourage hair loss.

■ **Sore throat.** Treating a sore throat with a saltwater gargle is like rubbing your eyes when they're inflamed, says Murray Grossan, M.D. Instead, boil some water in a pot, remove it from the stove, and lean over it so your face is close enough to inhale the rising steam but not close enough to be burned. Then stick out your tongue and breathe in the vapors. Adding a few drops of eucalyptus oil to the water will help thin mucus and increase healing blood flow to your inflamed larynx.

Soothing Lung Sauna

When asthma has you so congested that you can hardly breathe, treat your lungs to a sauna. Fill a teapot with water and bring it to a boil, then remove it from the stove and add a few drops of eucalyptus oil. Hold a towel over your head and the pot and breathe deeply. Be careful not to lean close enough to scald your face. The combination of eucalyptus and steam will thin the sticky mucus that's clogging your airways.

■ **Sprained ankle.** The usual advice for a sprained ankle is to apply ice, and that certainly works, but *brrr*—it's cold! Instead of using ice cubes, fill a bowl with ice water and sprinkle in several drops of eucalyptus oil. Soak a washcloth in the herbal water, wring it out, and lay it on your ankle. Surround it with an ice pack for extra cooling power and leave it in place for about 20 minutes. Repeat the treatment once or twice a day until your ankle's healed.

Eucalyptus

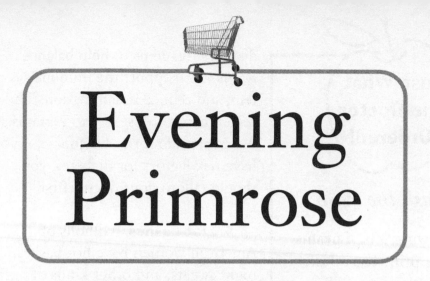

Evening Primrose

AN ALL-AROUND HEALER

Evening primrose is a beautiful, night-flowering blossom that adds a touch of exotic romance to any garden, but it's the seeds—or specifically, the oil extracted from them, called gamma-linolenic acid (GLA)—that makes it one of the most popular healers in nature's medicine chest.

■ **Breast pain.** Evening primrose oil is one of the best-known Native American remedies for fibrocystic breasts, and it does seem to relieve breast pain in some women, although no one's found a medical explanation. The oil is available in capsules; follow the package directions.

Oily Fatigue Fighter

According to one study, 85 percent of a group of people with chronic fatigue syndrome reported some improvement after 15 weeks of taking a combination of evening primrose oil and fish oil supplements. Start with 1,500 milligrams twice a day.

■ **Diabetes.** Evening primrose oil can be used to help prevent a range of ailments, including

167

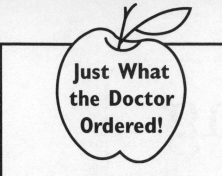

Just What the Doctor Ordered!

Thrash the Rash

Swallowing 3 to 6 grams of evening primrose oil daily may correct a fatty acid imbalance and reduce any itching and redness associated with eczema.

diabetes. It seems to help balance hormones, support the immune system, and reduce inflammation. The recommended dose is 1 to 2 grams a day in capsule form. Of course, if you have risk factors for diabetes, you should talk to your doctor first.

■ **Hot flashes.** Millions of American women have hot flashes, night sweats, and other kinds of menopausal discomforts. Vitamin E and primrose oil can be very effective at reducing hot flashes, according to Orli Etigen, M.D. Before you resort to powerful (and possibly dangerous) hormone replacement, ask your doctor about these natural alternatives and the amount that's right for you.

■ **Dry skin.** Essential fatty acids are crucial for healthy skin, and a deficiency can leave skin looking dried out and wrinkled. Take 1 gram of evening primrose oil once or twice daily, or be sure to eat one serving of foods containing omega-3 oils every day (salmon, almonds, and sesame seeds are good sources).

■ **Inflammation.** Whether you've twisted an ankle, wrenched your back, or are recovering from an infection, much of the discomfort you experience is due to inflammation. The GLA in evening primrose seeds helps the body make prostaglandin E, which has anti-inflammatory properties. Check for

Evening Primrose

capsules whose label says "standardized to 8 percent gamma-linolenic acid," which means they contain an adequate amount of the active ingredient, and take 2 to 3 grams a day.

■ **Raynaud's disease.** The GLA in evening primrose oil can help relieve moderate pain in people with Raynaud's disease. Studies indicate that massaging some of the oil into your chilled fingertips and toes can not only help them feel better but also help thaw them out.

■ **Lupus.** Protein from land-based animals may encourage inflammation, which can be a real problem if you have lupus. Trout, salmon, and other cold-water fish, however, contain beneficial omega-3 essential fatty acids that squelch it. If a fishy diet isn't to your taste, and you're not taking blood thinners, try 1 to 2 grams of evening primrose oil, which has an anti-inflammatory effect. Be patient, however, since you may not see benefits for two months or more.

■ **Rashes.** If your skin has erupted in a red, bumpy rash on your forearms and thighs, it could be a telltale sign that you're lacking essential fatty acids—the kind found in fish oil, flaxseed oil, and evening primrose oil—which help keep skin lubricated, supple, and smooth. Jeanette Jacknin, M.D., suggests taking 1 teaspoon or 500 milligrams of flaxseed oil, evening primrose oil, or fish oil three times a day. You can also apply evening primrose oil directly to your rash. If the irritation has progressed to the point where the skin is cracking, you should see healing within a week or two.

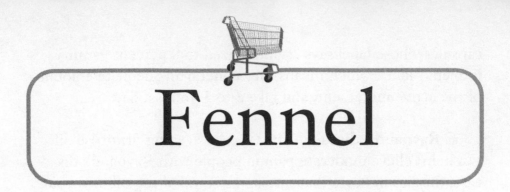

Fennel

A FRIEND FOR DIGESTION

Sweet-tasting fennel seeds do more than liven up sauces. They've been used for centuries to relieve digestive problems, freshen the breath, and make coughs a little less troublesome. Not bad for something that's smaller than a grain of rice!

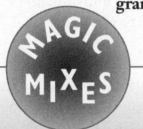

MAGIC MIXES

TAME A REBELLIOUS TUMMY If you're nauseated, try dipping a cloth into a brew made with fennel and placing it on your stomach. The warmth will settle tense digestive muscles, while simply inhaling the aroma of fennel may have a calming effect on your roiling belly.

■ **Dragon breath.** Fennel tea is a sweet postmeal drink—especially if you've had garlic or other smelly foods that not only cause bad breath but may also make odor pour from your pores. In fact, fennel is such an excellent natural deodorizer that Indian restaurants often offer fennel seeds instead of after-dinner mints.

■ **IBS.** The antispasmodic properties of fennel make it one of the best weapons against the symptoms of irritable bowel syndrome (IBS), says Anil Minocha, M.D. The intestinal contractions that often accompany IBS can be excruciatingly painful—and may also lead to emergency pit stops due to diarrhea. Dr. Minocha recommends munching 1 teaspoon of fennel seeds or sipping fennel tea three times a day after meals. For the tea, boil 1 teaspoon of seeds and a ½-inch slice of fresh ginger in a cup of water for 5 to 10 minutes, then strain before drinking.

■ **Chest congestion.** You don't have to buy over-the-counter products when your chest is so tight you can hardly draw a breath. Essential oil of fennel works wonders as a chest rub to clear up congestion. Just dissolve 10 drops of fennel oil, 10 drops of thyme oil, and 10 drops of eucalyptus oil in 4 ounces of sunflower oil and massage your chest gently with the mixture. You'll probably start breathing better within minutes, with less chest pain.

■ **Gas.** It's amazing how painful even a little gas can be—especially when it's accompanied by after-meal intestinal contractions. Fennel seeds contain 8 percent volatile oil, which relieves gas and is an antispasmodic, so they're a tasty way to settle your stomach and sidestep gas after rich meals. Try chewing ½ teaspoon any time you feel bloated with gas.

■ **Puffy eyes.** A cold compress made with fennel tea can reduce eyelid puffiness. Just pour 1 cup of boiling water over 2 teaspoons of fennel seeds, cover, and steep for 10 minutes. Store it in the refrigerator overnight, and in the morning, strain

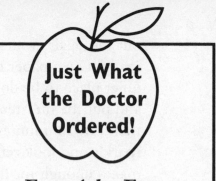

Just What the Doctor Ordered!

Ease Achy Eyes

A warm compress of eyebright and fennel seeds can refresh your eyes when they're dry and tired. Make a tea using 1 teaspoon of eyebright and 1 teaspoon of fennel seeds in 1 cup of hot water. Add a clean cloth and steep for 10 minutes. Wring out the cloth, make sure it's not too hot, and apply it to your eyes for 20 minutes once or twice daily.

Fennel 171

out the seeds. Your eye-pleasing medicine is ready! Dip a paper towel into the tea, find a quiet place to lie down, shut your eyes, and put the moistened paper towel over them. In 10 minutes or so, your eyes will sparkle and look refreshed. This recipe makes enough for five daily treatments.

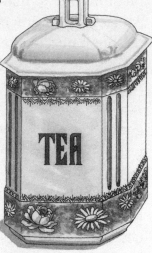

■ **Oily skin.** Here's a great cleanser for oily skin: Combine ½ cup of buttermilk with 2 tablespoons of fennel seeds and heat them in the top part of a double boiler for 30 minutes. Turn off the heat and let the mixture steep for 3 hours. Then strain, cool, and pour into a bottle. Keep it refrigerated between uses.

■ **Heart disease and cancer.** Fennel seeds contain a chemical compound called anethole, which has been shown to block inflammation and prevent the development of cancer. They provide modest amounts of cancer-fighting flavonols, including quercetin, as well. These plant chemicals can also prevent harmful oxygen molecules called free radicals from damaging cells and setting the stage for heart disease. Try a few after meals.

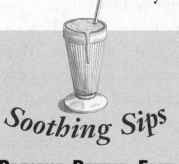

Soothing Sips

BREATHE BETTER FAST

If you're having trouble breathing because of asthma, allergies, or simply a cold, sip some fennel tea. It's a traditional remedy for opening the bronchial passages, says Jamison Starbuck, N.D. And because fennel helps thin mucus, it's especially helpful when you have a dry, unproductive, wracking cough.

Fennel

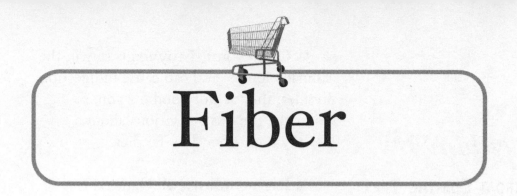

Fiber

More than a century ago, food manufacturers began stripping away the outer coatings of grains to make pure white flour—and guess what? Serious conditions such as heart disease, diabetes, and even cancer shot through the roof. So did not-so-serious but annoying problems such as constipation and hemorrhoids. Was this sudden deterioration in American health due to a lack of fiber? Yep. To put it simply, the fiber in plant foods keeps you healthy in more ways than you ever thought possible. Here's a sample.

■ Heart disease. Researchers believe that both the protein and fiber in legumes may help hearts stay healthy, and one study of 12,000 Americans ages 25 to 75 provided evidence that it's true. In the study, people who ate different types of legumes several times a week had a 19 percent lower risk of heart disease than those who ate them less than once a week. Beans, peas, and peanuts all qualify as heart-healthy legumes.

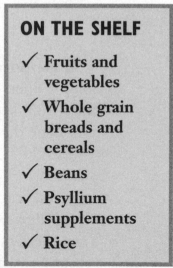

ON THE SHELF
✓ Fruits and vegetables
✓ Whole grain breads and cereals
✓ Beans
✓ Psyllium supplements
✓ Rice

■ **Cranky gut.** Fatty foods stay in the stomach longer and can cause indigestion. Besides, they're not good for you, so now's the time to get serious about a healthy high-fiber, low-fat diet.

■ **High cholesterol.** Oatmeal is a great source of soluble fiber. Savor a bowl every day, and you'll lower your cholesterol, according to more than 40 scientific studies. Not only is it rich in a type of fiber called beta-glucan, oatmeal also fills you up so you may eat less of other foods that aren't as good for you, according to Joseph Keenan, M.D.

■ **Stiff arteries.** The soluble fiber in beans not only lowers cholesterol but also may make your arteries more flexible, according to one study.

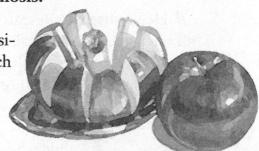

Soothing Sips

THROAT-COATING TEAS

The herbs marshmallow and mullein contain gel-like fiber that helps coat mucous membranes to ease irritation when you have a sore throat. Sip either of these teas throughout the day.

TEA

■ **Hemorrhoids and diverticulosis.** Soluble fiber, found in apples and other fruit, keeps stools soft for easier passage through the colon, which reduces the risk of hemorrhoids as well as diverticulosis, a potentially dangerous condition that occurs when bulges form in the intestine. Then there's the insoluble fiber found in whole grains and vegetables, which adds bulk to stools and decreases pressure on the colon walls. Bulk up your diet with these good-for-you foods, and as a bonus, you may find that your hips lose some bulk, too.

■ **Insulin resistance.** Getting 50 grams of fiber daily—almost double the amount normally recommended—may lower insulin resistance, studies show. Those fiber-rich psyllium powders sold in supermarkets could help you meet that quota, but select brands without sugars or laxatives, follow the package directions, and consult your doctor before using them.

■ **Leg pain.** You can't walk away from intermittent claudication, leg pain caused by poor circulation, without making lifestyle adjustments. One of the most important steps is to eat a high-fiber, low-fat diet.

■ **Chemo side effects.** The fiber in flaxseed turns into a soothing, protective gel in your digestive tract, which helps promote intestinal function with none of the harshness of bran or other types of insoluble fiber. This makes it a great addition to your diet when you're undergoing chemo-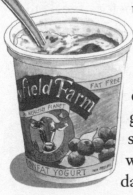therapy. Plus, flax contains omega-3 essential fatty acids to help squelch the inflammation that results from chemotherapy. Stir a few teaspoons of ground flaxseed into your morning smoothie or yogurt, and your taste buds won't have a clue that you're getting your daily quota of roughage.

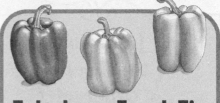

Fabulous Food Fix

Knock Down the Pressure

The fiber in fruit apparently works even better than the fiber from vegetables and grains to lower systolic blood pressure, studies show. Strawberries, blueberries, and peaches are especially good examples, and in some studies, strawberries lowered diastolic pressure, too. So top your morning oatmeal or cold cereal with these fruits and have a fruit snack every day.

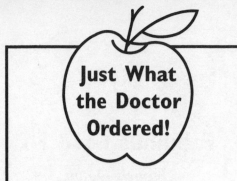

Just What the Doctor Ordered!

Eat Away Stones

People with high-fiber diets are less likely to get kidney stones. You can get loads of fiber by filling up on fresh fruit and vegetables as well as legumes, whole grains, and high-fiber cereals. You should get at least 20 grams of fiber a day, but 30 to 35 grams is even better.

■ **IBS.** Few things are more painful than the colon spasms caused by irritable bowel syndrome (IBS), but bulking up stools with fiber supplements such as psyllium or flaxseed can reduce their severity. Each morning, add a heaping tablespoon of the powdered form of either fiber to a full glass of water, stir to thicken, and down the mixture on the spot. Chase it with another glass of water, then be sure to drink 8 to 10 more glasses throughout the day.

■ **PMS.** A high-fiber, low-fat, vegan (no meat, no dairy) diet significantly limits water retention, pain, and other kinds of discomfort caused by premenstrual syndrome.

■ **Ulcers.** Eat plenty of fiber-rich foods if you're prone to ulcers. It appears that people with high-fiber diets get them less often.

■ **Overweight.** When you're trying to control your weight, taking a fiber supplement such as psyllium before meals may help reduce the number of calories absorbed by your body. Plus, psyllium helps you feel full and stabilizes blood sugar levels, which may help control food cravings, notes Glen Rothfeld, M.D. Take 1 to 3 tablespoons of psyllium powder mixed in water or juice three times a day before eating, he suggests. Be sure to swallow another full glass of water with the supplement and drink 8 to 10 additional glasses throughout the day.

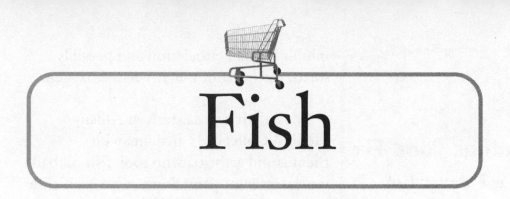

Fish

A BOATLOAD OF HEALTH

Have you ever wondered how fish stay warm in their frigid, watery homes? They don't mind the cold because they're bundled up in the equivalent of insulated, fatty sweaters—and the same fat that keeps them toasty has special properties that would warm any doctor's heart. Folks who want the benefits can eat more fish or take fish oil supplements (unless they're taking aspirin or blood-thinning medication).

■ **Heart attack.** Fish, especially cold-water varieties such as tuna and salmon, are loaded with omega-3 fatty acids. When you eat fish a few times a week, the omega-3's are incorporated into blood platelets, which are responsible for clotting, and make them less sticky and less likely to clump. This is important because most heart attacks are caused by clots that form in the arteries that carry blood to the heart, and even a small clot can

The Perfect Brain Food

Cold-water fish are the richest sources of docosahexaenoic acid (DHA), a type of omega-3 fatty acid that helps to promote cell-to-cell communication in the brain, improve focus, and possibly reverse memory loss.

inhibit normal circulation and possibly starve the heart of much-needed oxygen.

■ **Arthritis.** In a study at Albany Medical College, 33 patients with rheumatoid arthritis who took fish oil had much less joint pain. Some were even able to stop taking nonsteroidal anti-inflammatory drugs, such as ibuprofen and naproxen sodium. Since these drugs often cause stomach upset and other side effects, anything you can do to take less of them is sure to pay off in the long run. Follow package directions.

■ **Depression.** Finnish research suggests that people with low levels of omega-3's in their neural membranes are more likely to have depression. Adding 1 to 3 grams of fish oil a day to your diet may help prevent the problem. Remember, though, that depression needs a doctor's diagnosis.

■ **Allergies.** Much of the discomfort caused by allergies is due to inflammation in the airways and other parts of the body. The omega-3 fatty acids in cold-water fish inhibit inflammation, notes Richard N. Firshein, D.O. Fish also provide vitamin A, which boosts IgA, a "good guy" antibody that's released in saliva and attaches to allergens to keep them from invading your system. For allergy relief, some doctors recommend taking 1 to 3 grams of fish oil daily if you don't regularly eat fish.

■ **Heart disease.** According to the American Heart Association, people with heart disease should take at least

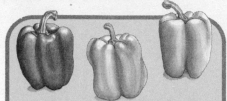

Fabulous Food Fix

Look Better Fast

To keep your skin and hair healthy, eat fish two or three times a week. The omega-3 fatty acids in fish can help your skin retain water, which will keep it plump, supple, and smooth. And since thin, brittle hair may indicate a deficiency of these fats, adding more fish to your diet should strengthen your tresses as well.

1 gram of fish oil a day, for two reasons. First, the oil that comes from cold-water fish can make red blood cells more slippery and improve their flow, even in tiny capillaries. Second, fish oil helps lower triglycerides—blood fats that can clog arteries—and stabilize insulin resistance, a major factor in heart disease. If you'd like to try fish oil, talk to your doctor.

■ **The blues.** The oils in fish can powerfully improve your mood, says Hyla Cass, M.D. In order to see any effect, however, you'll need to eat fish three times a week.

■ **Joint stiffness.** Fish oils can ease swollen, stiff joints by reducing both inflammation and cartilage destruction, says Michael E. Weinblatt, M.D. Try 1 to 3 grams a day.

■ **Asthma.** The omega-3's in fish do more than battle inflammation. They also may repair airway damage, which is good news if you have asthma. There's some evidence that people with asthma who eat fish regularly have a reduction in symptoms.

■ **CFS.** The beneficial oils in fish that inhibit inflammation can help minimize pain caused by chronic fatigue syndrome (CFS).

■ **Raynaud's disease.** People with Raynaud's and other circulatory problems may experience

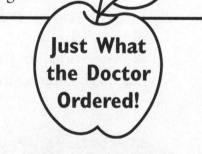

Just What the Doctor Ordered!

Call a Sturgeon!

You should definitely eat more fish if you've been in an accident and your neck paid the price. Fish oils help reduce the inflammation caused by whiplash.

cold, painful hands. If this symptom is caused by underlying inflammation of the blood vessels that pinches off blood flow to your extremities, eating lots of fish could increase your tolerance to cold by inhibiting the inflammation.

■ **High blood pressure.** Omega-3's can help lower blood pressure, but you need about 5 grams a day for the best effect. That's a lot of oil. To reach your quota, Darin Ingels, N.D., suggests that you check with your doctor about taking fish oil capsules.

■ **Lupus.** People with lupus, an autoimmune disease, often experience intense inflammation. The omega-3's in fish naturally reduce inflammation and can help reduce symptoms. Check with your doctor first, then consider taking 3 grams of fish oil a day.

■ **Menstrual pain.** A diet rich in fish can help lower levels of prostaglandin E2, which contributes to menstrual cramps. At the same time, fish boosts levels of prostaglandin E3, which relaxes the uterine muscle.

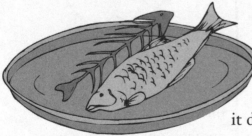

■ **IBS.** Some foods can help quell the intestinal inflammation that contributes to irritable bowel syndrome (IBS). Try three or four servings of fish a week and see what it does for you.

■ **Vaginal dryness.** Believe it or not, the oils in your diet can play a direct role in how comfortable intercourse feels. For example, the abundant fatty acids in fish can help reduce vaginal dryness, so plan on having a few servings a week. As a bonus, the oils in fish will also help normalize vaginal tone.

Flaxseed

FABULOUS FLAX FACTS

Until recently, flaxseed was used for just about everything except eating. Manufacturers used it to make cloth, paints, and livestock feed. Now, though, the ground seeds are almost a kitchen staple, and for the best possible reason—flaxseed is remarkably good for your health. Here's the lowdown.

■ **Dry skin.** Fatty acid deficiency can leave skin looking dried out and wrinkled, but the omega-3 oils in flaxseed can prevent it. Unless you're taking aspirin or prescription blood thinners, take 1 gram once or twice daily.

■ **Depression.** Low levels of omega-3's have been linked to depression and the risk of Alzheimer's disease. Fortunately, flaxseed is overflowing with these fats. To benefit your mind and your whole body, add a handful of nuts, a serving of fish, or 2 table-

Turn Down the Heat

Women in Asia get far fewer hot flashes than Western women, possibly because they eat a plant-based diet brimming with phytoestrogens, plant chemicals that bind to estrogen receptors in the body and may reduce overall estrogen activity. Flaxseed oil (try 1 tablespoon a day) packs plenty of these beneficial compounds.

181

spoons of freshly ground flaxseed to your diet every day.

■ **Sunburn.** For mild sunburn, mix some soothing oil by adding the contents of six capsules each of vitamin A and vitamin E to ¼ cup of flaxseed oil. Apply frequently to the sunburned areas. You can also add this combination to ¼ cup of aloe vera juice and smooth it over your skin.

■ **SAD.** Take 1 tablespoon of flaxseed oil once or twice daily during the winter to head off the cold-weather blues—a.k.a. seasonal affective disorder (SAD).

■ **Allergies.** During allergy season, take 3 tablespoons of flaxseed oil daily to combat symptom-causing inflammation.

■ **Brain fog.** If you notice that your memory and concentration aren't what they used to be, add more flaxseed to your diet or take about 2 grams of flaxseed oil daily. It may reduce the inflammation that can impair focus and memory.

■ **Chemo side effects.** In the digestive tract, flaxseed turns into a soothing, protective gel that helps promote intestinal function

MAGIC MIXES

STOP THE HACK ATTACKS
A flaxseed poultice retains heat for a long time and is ideal for soothing irritating, spastic coughs. Add ½ cup of ground flaxseed to ¾ cup of boiling water, then simmer, stirring, until it makes a thick paste. Spread the paste on a piece of cheesecloth and apply it to your chest (it should be as hot as is tolerable). For deep penetration, you can add five or six drops of an essential oil such as thyme or eucalyptus. Leave the poultice on for 1 to 2 hours.

Flaxseed

and is much gentler than bran or other insoluble fibers. This makes it a helpful addition to your diet if you're undergoing chemotherapy.

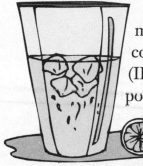

■ **IBS.** Bulking up the stools with fiber supplements such as flaxseed can reduce the severity of colon spasms caused by irritable bowel syndrome (IBS). Each morning, add a heaping tablespoon of powdered flaxseed to a full glass of water, stir, and drink it immediately. Have another glass of water, then be sure to drink 8 to 10 more throughout the day.

■ **Brittle hair.** If your hair is thin and brittle, you may be deficient in omega-3 fatty acids. You can increase levels of these essential fats by eating flaxseed. Andrew Weil, M.D., suggests buying whole flaxseed (keep it refrigerated), grinding it, and sprinkling 2 tablespoons a day on cereal or a salad.

■ **High blood pressure.** Flaxseed may help inhibit inflammatory reactions that can cause arteries to narrow and increase blood pressure. Take 1 to 3 tablespoons of flaxseed oil daily to help bring your numbers down.

■ **Irregular periods.** Studies show that a tablespoon of flaxseed daily can help regulate the menstrual cycle if you're skipping periods.

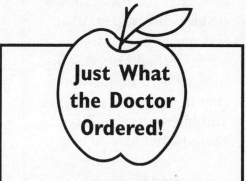

Just What the Doctor Ordered!

Save Your Skin

To help correct a fatty acid imbalance and reduce any itching and redness associated with eczema, take 3 to 6 grams of flaxseed oil, which is rich in omega-3 fatty acids, daily. Even better, apply the oil to the affected areas once or twice a day.

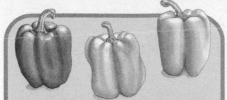

Fabulous Food Fix

Banish Breast Pain

In one study, women with severe cyclical breast tenderness who ate muffins containing 25 grams of ground flaxseed every day for four months had less breast pain than those who ate muffins without the flaxseed. This may be because flaxseed is rich in essential fatty acids and phytoestrogenic compounds that may reduce the impact of estradiol, a form of estrogen. Be patient, though: The pain may not ease for two months. Not up to baking? Some experts suggest taking 3 1/2 tablespoons of flaxseed oil daily.

■ **Dry skin.** If you have dry skin as a result of thyroid disease, taking 800 to 1,200 milligrams of flaxseed oil a day may help.

■ **High cholesterol.** A University of Toronto study of nine healthy women found that their total cholesterol dropped by 9 percent and their bad low-density lipoprotein (LDL) cholesterol dipped by 18 percent when they ate 2 ounces of flaxseed daily for just four weeks. That's a great way to protect your heart.

■ **Brain development.** Omega-3 fatty acids are critical to brain and vision development both before and just after babies are born. Mothers who eat plenty of fish, flaxseed, and walnuts deliver these brain builders through the placenta and breast milk.

■ **Cancer.** Flaxseed contains up to 800 times more lignans than any other plant food. Lignans? They're plant compounds that act like weak estrogens. They've been shown to tie up the body's estrogen receptors and, some scientists suspect that may help prevent hormone-related cancers from getting started.

■ **Constipation.** If you're not as regular as you'd like, eat more flaxseed. It's rich in insoluble fiber, the roughage that keeps you on schedule.

Flaxseed

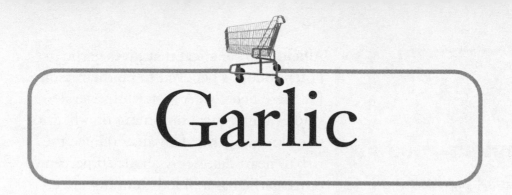

Garlic

You'd have to have a tongue made of asbestos to eat more than a few cloves of raw garlic at one time. Fortunately, you don't have to eat a lot to get impressive results. The oils in garlic—the same ones that give it that room-clearing smell—are intensely concentrated. Research has shown that even small amounts of garlic can fight infection, lower cholesterol, and a zillion other things. See what we mean.

■ **Athlete's foot.** If you're tired of athlete's foot, put your foot down—in a tub of garlic water! Crush several garlic cloves and drop them into a tub of warm water with a little rubbing alcohol added, then gently place both feet in the tub and soak for about 10 minutes once a day.

■ **Heart disease.** Raw garlic inhibits blood clots that can cause a heart attack. It also reduces blood pressure and may even make your blood vessels more flexible.

Blast Away Blemishes

To make blemishes vanish, peel and mash six cloves of garlic and apply the mash to the affected areas (avoiding your eyes). Leave it in place for about 10 minutes, rinse with warm water, and pat dry.

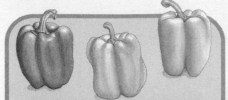

Fabulous Food Fix

Good for Your Gut

Fresh, raw garlic is Mother Nature's antibiotic—and it can help knock ulcer-causing bacteria dead, says Skye Weintraub, N.D. You can take two garlic capsules daily or simply mash two whole, peeled cloves and eat the paste every day, smeared on a cracker.

Allicin, the chemical that gives garlic its potent odor, is believed to be the reason for these benefits. A review of several studies found that consuming one-half to one clove of garlic daily may reduce the risk of heart disease by about 20 percent. Since garlic has a blood-thinning effect, however, don't eat it on a regular basis without your doctor's okay.

■ **Stuffy nose.** Spicy foods such as garlic contain chemical compounds that can help reduce nasal and sinus congestion. Some cold sufferers add garlic to chicken soup to promote drainage.

■ **Stroke and heart attack.** Garlic decreases the stickiness of platelets, cell-like structures in the blood that tend to clump together and form clots, thus helping to reduce the risk of stroke and heart attack. Chop some garlic, let it sit for 10 minutes, then sprinkle it onto your favorite foods. For best results, eat one to three raw cloves a day.

■ **Sore throat.** Garlic is one of the best remedies for sore throats because of its anti-inflammatory, antiviral, and antibacterial properties. The problem, of course, is that you'd have to eat a few cloves a day to take advantage of its healing power—and that much garlic can give you a powerful aroma. To get the benefits without the odor, consider taking garlic capsules that have had the "stink" removed. Look for a supplement that provides about 10 milligrams of allicin, the active ingredient.

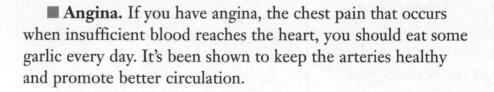

■ **Colds.** The next time you have a cold or any other infection, be sure to eat more garlic. Add a few cloves to pasta sauce, stir-fries, and your favorite chicken soup to take advantage of its powerful antimicrobial effects.

■ **Angina.** If you have angina, the chest pain that occurs when insufficient blood reaches the heart, you should eat some garlic every day. It's been shown to keep the arteries healthy and promote better circulation.

■ **Yeast infections.** "Garlic, garlic, and more garlic." That's yeast-fighting advice from Jana Nalbandian, N.D., who explains that garlic is a powerful antifungal. Raw or lightly cooked garlic delivers the biggest kick. "I tell people to toss the garlic in after the food's off the stove," says Dr. Nalbandian. "Just chop it up and throw it in."

■ **Flu.** As powerful as it is pungent, garlic is great for spurring your immune system to fight off a flu virus. Since raw garlic has the highest concentration of immune-boosting components, chop up a few cloves, let them rest on

Make Nice with Spice

Do you feel better when you eat garlic? There's a reason for that. One study found that when garlic is served at a meal, families are more likely to be nice to each other. A possible explanation is that garlic evokes positive childhood memories, making people chill out.

Garlic **187**

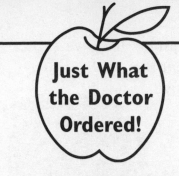

Just What the Doctor Ordered!

Better Digestion in a Flash

Many pungent spices, including garlic, can help relieve stomach problems and improve digestion. You don't have to eat tons of garlic to get the benefits; just look for recipes that already include it.

the cutting board for a few minutes, and toss them into your favorite hot soup. By the time the soup's cool enough to eat, the garlic will have softened and added its flavor to the meal.

■ **Itchy feet.** Garlic is such a potent topical antifungal that Daniel DeLapp, N.D., recommends it for itchy feet caused by fungal infections. Apply a generous film of olive oil to each foot, then place a clove of raw, peeled garlic between all of your toes every night for a week. Be careful not to bruise or break open the cloves, because garlic juice can burn the skin. You'll need to wear a pair of all-cotton socks to bed, then wash and dry your feet each morning. Although you may need to sleep in the guest bedroom (the garlic will stink up your room, your skin, and even your breath!), this treatment should stop the itch in its tracks. Don't use this remedy on broken skin, and discontinue it if irritation occurs.

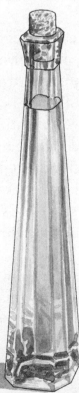

■ **Diarrhea.** Garlic is one of the best ways to fight diarrhea-causing infections. Pick up some garlic capsules at the store and take 200 to 400 milligrams three times a day until your diarrhea subsides.

■ **Earache.** Here's a natural remedy for earaches that really works. Mash a garlic clove with a fork and saturate it with several drops of olive oil. Let the mash absorb the oil overnight, strain out the garlic, and warm the oil so it's pleasantly tepid, not hot. Tilt your head so your sore ear is facing up and plop in two or three drops of the oil. Lie down—again, with your sore ear up—and let the oil settle for 2 or 3 minutes before you raise your head. Do this a few times a day, and your discomfort should disappear within a day or two.

■ **Cancer.** In an analysis of medical studies, researchers from the University of North Carolina found that people who consumed six or more garlic cloves per week had a 30 percent lower risk of colon cancer and a 50 percent lower risk of stomach cancer than those who ate a clove or less weekly. Other studies have hinted that garlic staves off breast and prostate cancers, too, but the evidence is still preliminary. Garlic supplements don't seem to have an effect on cancer, however, because they have only trace amounts of allicin.

■ **High cholesterol.** Garlic is the real deal for lowering cholesterol; according to many studies, it can drop levels by up to 15 percent. To keep your arteries free and clear, regularly peel and chop a clove or two, let it rest on the cutting board for at least 10 minutes, then slip it into everything from soups and stews to salads and poultry dishes. Letting the garlic rest allows the cholesterol-lowering compounds to form.

Geranium

ONE POWERFUL FLOWER

Geraniums probably decorate more windowsills than any other houseplant. Apart from their lush greenery and beautiful flowers, they're a snap to grow. For herbalists, though, beauty is beside the point. A type of oil extracted from geraniums has a long history of healing—and is still widely used today. Here's how.

■ **Dry skin.** An herbal facial steam can deep-six dryness—especially if you use an oil such as geranium that encourages oil production in your skin. Simply bring 3 cups of water to a boil, then remove the pot from the stove. Add one drop each of rose, geranium, rosemary, fennel, and peppermint herbal oil. Drape a towel over your head to capture the steam and create a kind of mini-sauna. Be careful not to get close enough for the steam to burn your face, and limit your steam sessions to about 5 minutes once a week.

■ **Menstrual pain.** For menstrual discomfort, try a geranium-oil massage. It stimulates blood and

Stop Sweat at the Source

For excessively sweaty hands, coat your palms with astringent oils to close the pores and stop the sweating. Margaret Stearn, M.D., recommends using fragrant cypress and geranium oils.

190

lymph circulation and reduces bloating and annoying aching in the small of your back around the time of your period.

■ **Varicose veins.** These unsightly, bulging veins occur when blood that flows down into the legs is unable to entirely overcome gravity on the trip back up, so it accumulates in the veins and causes them to swell. Using hot and then cold compresses soaked in a circulation-boosting herbal solution expands and then contracts the veins, providing a soothing pumping action, says Jeanette Jacknin, M.D. To give it a try, soak a cloth in a mixture of 10 drops each of cypress, geranium, ginger, juniper, lavender, and rosemary oil and 1 quart of hot water. Press the cloth to your leg for 15 minutes, then soak another cloth in a second batch of solution made with the same oils and cold water and apply it for 15 minutes. Follow up with a gentle leg massage (aided by a few of those aromatic, circulation-boosting oils), stroking upward toward your heart.

■ **Corns.** Any oil softens the skin, but herb-infused oil blends stimulate circulation and help keep your feet healthy and ache-free. Here's a blend that can help. Add two drops each of peppermint oil and carrot seed oil to an ounce of calendula oil, then mix in five drops each of lavender oil and geranium oil. Store the mixture in a small bottle and massage it into your feet once a day—more often when your corns are aching.

MAGIC MIXES

SPRAY AWAY STRESS
To help reduce daily stress, put 1 teaspoon of salt mixed with five drops each of oil of lavender, chamomile, bergamot, rose, geranium, lemon balm, and clary sage in a spray bottle, top it off with water, and mist the air. Inhaling the aroma of these calming and stimulating herbs will ease your troubles.

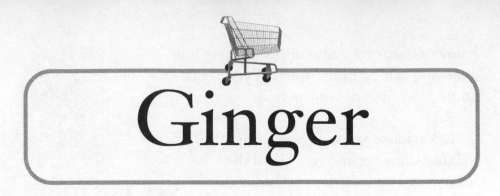

Ginger

IT'S A SNAP!

You wouldn't think that this gnarled, ugly little root would be good for much of anything, but inside that grungy skin is an entire medicine chest of chemical compounds that have been shown to help digestion, reduce nausea, and even protect the heart.

■ **Cranky gut.** Ginger is a jack-of-all-trades for stomach ailments, but it's especially good at relieving pain, since the gingerol it contains helps stop intestinal contractions. You can take ginger in capsule form or drink it as a tea, but chewing a slice of raw ginger also works.

Powerful Germ Killer

Ginger appears to have mild antibacterial properties that may help prevent infection. The next time you get a cut or scrape that may become infected, start loading your recipes with ginger for a little extra protection.

■ **Cluster headaches.** If you have episodes of the excruciating head pain known as cluster headaches, you can make an analgesic tea by adding 1 teaspoon each of dried feverfew, lemon balm, and ginger to a cup of hot water. Steep for 10 minutes, strain out the herbs, and sip. Feverfew may cause mouth irritation in sensitive people, and since it's a uterine stimulant, pregnant women shouldn't use it.

■ **Migraines.** Keep migraines at bay by spicing up your diet with ginger. This pungent root appears to help keep blood vessels from dilating and pressing against sensitive nerves, says Terri Dallas-Prunskis, M.D. Even small amounts of ginger seem to be effective, she adds. You can start by adding fresh or powdered ginger to stews, rice dishes, soups, and even fresh green salads.

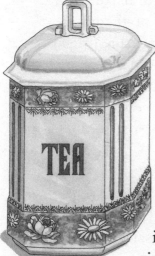

■ **Sinusitis.** The pungent aroma of ginger comes from dozens of powerful chemicals that strengthen immunity, increase healing circulation, and kill germs that can cause sinus infections. Try a cup of ginger tea one to three times a day.

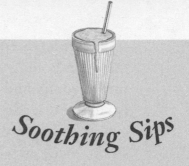

Soothing Sips

EASE A BAD BACK

To relieve back pain, mix equal parts of ginger, chamomile, and peppermint. Use 1 teaspoon of the mixture per 1 cup of boiling water and steep, covered, for 10 minutes. Strain and drink a cup three or four times a day.

■ **Queasiness.** Ginger in any form—including ginger tea, ginger candy, and fresh ginger—dampens the vestibular impulses in the brain that make you nauseated, says William Warnock, N.D. In fact, studies have shown that ginger is superior to dimenhydrinate (Dramamine) when it comes to relieving nausea related to motion sickness. To brew a stomach-soothing tea, either buy some ginger tea and follow the package directions or grate 2 teaspoons of fresh ginger into a cup of boiling water, steep for 10 minutes, strain, and sip. If you're pregnant, ask your doctor before trying this remedy.

■ **Athlete's foot.** "Tea made from fresh ginger simmered in boiling water provides more than 20 antifungal compounds," says Jeanette Jacknin, M.D. To make the tea, add 1 teaspoon of grated ginger to a cup of boiling water, steep for 10 to 15 minutes, and strain. Sweeten with honey and drink a cup three times daily. Swab your hot, itchy feet with a cotton ball soaked in any leftover tea.

■ **Aches and pains.** Anti-inflammatory herbs help relieve pain throughout the body and may be combined with antispasmodic herbs to increase relaxation. To make a tea, combine equal parts of ginger, meadowsweet, lemon balm, prickly ash, and calendula. Add 1 heaping teaspoon of the mixture to 1 cup of hot water and steep, covered, for 15 minutes. Strain and drink two or three cups daily.

Aspirin-Free Arthritis Relief

It's unlikely that the Gingerbread Man ever had arthritis. Yes, he was just a cookie, and a fictional one at that, but all of that ginger must have helped. Ginger is a powerful anti-inflammatory herb that can take the edge off arthritis pain, says Grace Ornstein, M.D. To make a healing tea, grate about an inch of fresh ginger and steep it in hot water for 10 minutes, then strain. Drink it once or twice a day.

■ **Vomiting.** When you've been vomiting, avoid drinking water or other fluids without salt or sugar, because they'll usually come back up. Instead, sip clear, sweetened liquids, such as real ginger ale. Clear beverages and broths will stay down better than juices and cola-based sodas.

■ **Stuffy nose.** The oil in ginger is similar to the capsaicin in peppers because it's slightly irritat-

Ginger

ing and thins out mucus. You can clear your nose with ginger in several ways. Cut the root into pieces, brew a tea, and inhale the vapors as you sip; grate it and toss it into salad dressing; or chop it into a super supper stir-fry.

■ **Gas.** Add ginger to "gassy" vegetables such as brussels sprouts, broccoli, and cabbage. Along with enhancing flavor, it will offset the gassy effects of these healthy foods.

■ **Overweight.** Certain common kitchen spices, such as ginger, red pepper, mustard, and cinnamon, may help raise both your body temperature and your metabolism, so you burn calories for fuel rather than store them as fat. Plus, spices may speed your digestion, which is important because people with sluggish digestion tend to gain weight, says Dana Myatt, N.D. Perhaps what these tasty spices do best, though, is make food savory, so you need less fat (such as oil) to make it palatable, and you can feel satisfied with smaller portions.

■ **Frosty fingers.** When your hands are almost frozen stiff, simply wiggle your fingers and either run warm water over them or order a warm beverage and lace your fingers around the cup. Just steer clear of Irish coffee, since both caffeine and alcohol are blood vessel constrictors. A better choice may be ginger tea, since it has a warming effect and boosts blood flow, says David Zeiger, D.O.

Fabulous Food Fix

The Cookie Cure

When you've overindulged at the dinner table, munch two or three ginger snaps to soothe your stomach.

■ **Heavy periods.** This tangy root dampens production of troublemaking prostaglandin E2 and lightens menstrual flow. To take advantage of this effect, stir ¼ to ½ teaspoon of powdered ginger into a cup of hot water and drink it daily.

■ **Heart disease.** One of the chemicals in ginger, called zingerone, keeps low-density lipoprotein (LDL) cholesterol from being oxidized—the process that makes it more likely to cling to arteries and form blood-blocking deposits that can lead to heart problems.

■ **Cancer.** The gingerol in ginger fights cancer by preventing cancer cells from multiplying—and even by encouraging them to just drop dead.

■ **Heart attack and stroke.** Gingerol also inhibits clotting of platelets in your blood, which reduces your risk of a heart attack or stroke.

Take Down Muscle Pain

The painful muscle inflammation of fibromyalgia should be treated, well, gingerly. A cup of ginger tea contains an inflammation-fighting compound called gingerol—and it tastes good, too! Just steep a few slices of fresh ginger in a cup of boiling water for about 10 minutes, strain, and sip the tea until it's gone.

■ **Angina.** Keep some pungent ginger in the first row of your spice cabinet if you have angina (chest pain caused by impaired circulation to the heart). It contains chemical compounds that lower cholesterol and inhibit the formation of blood clots. Along with other spices, such as turmeric and red pepper, ginger also inhibits arterial inflammation that may lead to or worsen angina. Use it generously when you cook.

Ginger

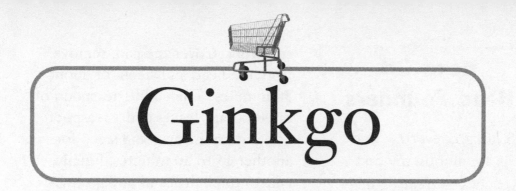

Ginkgo

MORE BLOOD, MORE ENERGY, MORE LIFE

The ginkgo tree was introduced into Europe in the 1700s, but herbalists of the time didn't take it seriously at first. They should have gone back to their books to learn what Asian healers had to say. They had extensive experience with ginkgo and were so impressed that they used it for dozens of common and often serious health threats. Although people taking aspirin or prescription blood thinners should avoid it, here's what it can do for the rest of us.

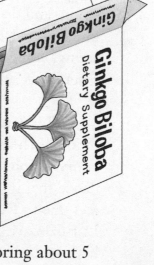

■ **Hangover.** A tiny vial of standardized ginkgo extract may be the perfect party favor because the seeds of this Asian herb contain an enzyme that may help speed the body's metabolism of alcohol. In fact, the Japanese are so convinced of the herb's protective powers that they serve ginkgo seeds at cocktail parties to help guests prevent hangovers, says James A. Duke, Ph.D.

■ **Low energy.** To add a spring to your step, bring about 5 cups of water to a simmer, then add 1 teaspoon of ground gin-

Head Off
Head Pounders

"Ginkgo, feverfew, and coleus are among my first approaches to treating migraines," says Chris Meletis, N.D. Ginkgo "thins" the blood and may inhibit the release of pain-causing chemicals. Take 60 milligrams in capsule form twice daily to relieve your pain. It's also good for preventing migraines, so you may want to take it daily to avert attacks.

seng root. Cover the pan, remove from the heat, and steep for about 30 minutes. Then add 1 teaspoon of dried borage leaves and 1 teaspoon of dried mint leaves and steep for another 15 to 20 minutes. Finally, add 10 to 20 drops of ginkgo tincture. Strain out the herbs and sweeten to taste. You can drink up to three cups a day. Since ginseng can raise blood pressure, it may not be for folks taking blood pressure medication. Check with your doctor before using it.

■ **Erection problems.** Ginkgo is used to increase circulation and may be helpful for some men who have erection problems.

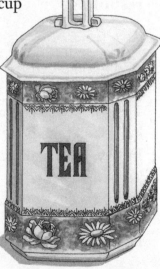

Make a tea using 1 heaping teaspoon per 1 cup of boiling water. Steep for 10 minutes, strain, and drink one or two cups daily. Since tonic herbs such as ginkgo are slow acting, you may need to take the tea for several weeks before seeing improvement.

■ **Raynaud's disease.** Ginkgo has traditionally been used for all sorts of circulatory problems, and there's some evidence that it may help with icy hands and feet due to Raynaud's, says Magdalena Dziadzio, M.D. Add a teaspoon of dried herb to a cup of hot water and steep for about 10 minutes, then strain and drink.

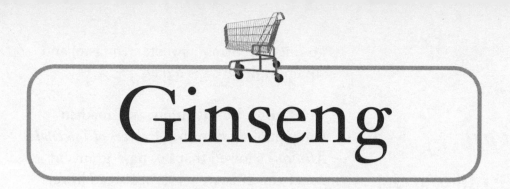

Ginseng

THE ULTIMATE TONIC

The root of an ivy-like groundcover, ginseng has been the subject of more than 1,000 books and scientific papers—and still, no one's entirely sure how it works. One thing is certain: It's been used in Asia for thousands of years (at one time it was more valuable than gold!), and new research into its bevy of powerful chemical compounds suggests that it really can make a difference. Although people with high blood pressure should avoid it, here's what the rest of us will find.

■ **Fatigue.** If you're feeling a little tired, ginseng can help. To make a reenergizing tea, first bring about 5 cups of water to a simmer and add 1 teaspoon of ground ginseng root. Remove from the heat, cover, and steep for about 30 minutes. Next, add 1 teaspoon each of dried borage leaves and dried mint leaves and steep for 15 to 20 minutes. Finally, add 10 to 20 drops of gink-

Good News for Men

Ginseng improves blood flow to the penis and may increase testosterone levels to encourage erections. What's more, the herb is an adaptogen, which means it helps defuse the effects of stress on the body. If stress is at the root of your erection problems, ginseng may be just the sparkplug you need. Give it a few weeks to work.

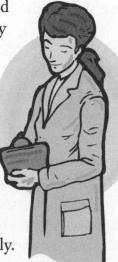

Soothing Sips

GET UP AND GO!

Ginseng is a whole-system tonic that helps increase endurance and improve mental performance. For a revitalizing tea, steep 1 teaspoon of the herb in 1 cup of hot water for 15 minutes, then strain. Drink one or two cups daily.

go tincture. Strain, sweeten to taste, and sip up to three cups a day.

■ **High blood sugar.** A Canadian study published in the *Archives of Internal Medicine* showed that taking 3 grams of American ginseng with meals can lower blood sugar by 20 percent! This was a breakthrough study because it was the first to test an herbal product using accepted scientific criteria, according to Andrew Weil, M.D. The theory is that ginseng may slow digestion, decreasing the rate at which carbohydrates are absorbed into the bloodstream. Researchers also believe American ginseng may modulate insulin secretion, but they don't yet know whether Asian ginseng will give the same result. If you have diabetes, talk to your doctor before using ginseng.

■ **Hot flashes.** This root has been used for centuries to relieve hot flashes, possibly because it is a potent source of phyto-estrogens, or plant estrogens. Phyto-estrogens attach to the same receptors that your body's estrogen and estrogen replacement drugs do, but they have a modulating effect and promote milder estrogen activity. Despite its stellar reputation, don't take ginseng without talking with your doctor first—particularly if you have breast or ovarian cancer in your family.

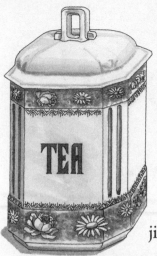

■ **Low libido.** Ginseng has had a reputation as an aphrodisiac throughout the history of folk medicine. It may not be justified, but research has only begun to scratch the surface of this potent herb. If you'd like to try it as a libido tonic, make a tea by steeping 1 heaping teaspoon in a cup of hot water for 15 to 20 minutes, then strain. Drink one cup a day. Be aware, however, that ginseng makes some people jittery.

■ **Heart disease.** According to several studies, ginseng may protect your arteries and heart by improving your cholesterol levels. Unlike most approaches, which lower levels of harmful low-density lipoprotein (LDL) cholesterol, ginseng may actually raise levels of beneficial high-density lipoprotein (HDL) cholesterol. Since HDL basically sucks up LDL cholesterol and sticks it in your body's dumpster, more HDL means that the risk of heart disease declines.

■ **Poor appetite.** Millions of older adults don't get all the nutrition they need because their senses of smell and taste have declined, so they don't eat as well as they should. Ginseng may help because it appears to stimulate appetite while improving the ability of the intestine to absorb vital nutrients.

Get Ease with Zzz's

If you don't get ample or restful sleep, you can feel both drowsy and edgy at the same time. Siberian ginseng—a restorative and stimulating tonic—can help you fight fatigue without making you feel wired, says Victoria Franks, N.D. As long as you don't have high blood pressure, she recommends taking 30 to 60 drops of ginseng tincture daily.

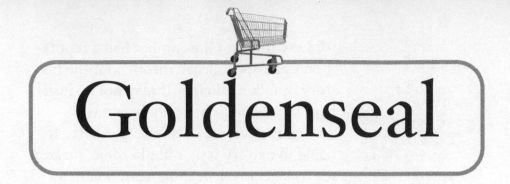

Goldenseal

NATURE'S BUG BEATER

The herb goldenseal gets its name from its rich yellow roots, which were once used to make a dye. For traditional healers and even some modern doctors, it's still as good as gold—for improving immunity, fighting pain and infection, and even improving women's health. Here's what we mean.

■ **Gum disease.** You should definitely stock up on goldenseal if your gums bleed or become sore or infected. Apart from protecting against infection, goldenseal strengthens the tissues of the gums and mouth. Use a clean, new paintbrush and paint your gums with goldenseal tincture once or twice daily. Since the herb can irritate gums, test first by dabbing just one spot with the brush. If no irritation shows the next day, go ahead and paint away!

■ **Vaginal pain.** For pain after intercourse, try a soothing, antibacterial herbal wash. Mix equal parts of echinacea, goldenseal, and lavender,

Soothing Sips

INTIMATE PROTECTION

If you have vaginitis, make goldenseal tea. It's the plant world's leading antibiotic, and drinking two or three cups daily will help flush out bacteria. Don't use during pregnancy.

then steep 1 heaping teaspoon of the mixture in a cup of hot water for 20 minutes. Strain out the herbs and pour the solution into a peribottle. Keep it near the toilet and wash your labia and vaginal opening with the solution after intercourse. If the problem persists, see a doctor to rule out an infection.

■ **Wet rashes.** If you have a rash that's wet and oozing, here's some help: Wash your skin, then dry up the rash and prevent secondary infections by dusting it with an herbal powder. Combine equal parts of slippery elm powder and goldenseal powder and gently dust the mixture on the rash for soothing relief and quick healing.

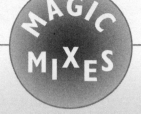

ERASE BLEMISHES FAST
Powdered goldenseal root is a mild but effective disinfectant for acne. Add ½ teaspoon to 12 drops of tea tree oil, dab the resulting paste onto your blemishes, and rinse it off after about 20 minutes. Apply the paste twice a day, and your pimples will vanish, says Jeanette Jacknin, M.D.

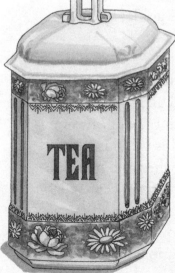

■ **STDs.** If you're getting medical care for a sexually transmitted disease (STD), an herbal tea can help strengthen your body's immune system from the inside out. Combine equal parts of echinacea, goldenseal, and licorice root and steep 1 heaping teaspoon in 1 cup of hot water for 15 minutes. Strain and drink two or three cups daily. Don't use licorice root if you have high blood pressure or kidney disease.

■ **Loose tooth.** To try to save a tooth that's being imperiled by gum disease, pack it with a mixture of powdered myrrh and goldenseal. Add enough hydrogen peroxide to the powders to make a paste and apply it around the tooth one to three times daily. If you also have pain, add a pinch of powdered cloves. See your dentist as soon as possible.

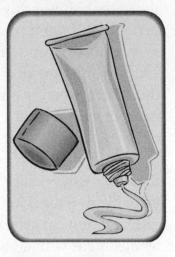

■ **Athlete's foot I.** Goldenseal is an effective treatment for athlete's foot. Look for it in over-the-counter antifungal creams.

■ **Athlete's foot II.** Here's a Native American remedy: First, to relieve the itching and burning, soak your feet in hot water to which you've added a few drops of oil of thyme. Then dust your feet with a mixture of myrrh and goldenseal powder in any proportion and put on a pair of heavy cotton socks. Repeat daily for several days.

■ **Blisters.** You can help open, inflamed blisters heal more quickly by applying an ointment that includes goldenseal and comfrey root.

Dust Off Germs

The next time you remove a splinter, you can reduce the risk of infection by washing the wound thoroughly and, when it's dry, dusting it with goldenseal powder.

■ **Bites and stings.** A mixture of bentonite clay and goldenseal is just the thing for painful insect bites or stings. Goldenseal is well known for healing skin, and when the powder is mixed with a bit of the clay and enough water to make a paste, it makes a perfect poultice for easing pain and inflammation.

■ **Cold sores.** Goldenseal is an antiviral herb that can treat cold sores. Mix ¼ teaspoon each of goldenseal and echinacea extracts in water or juice and drink it three times a day until the sore heals.

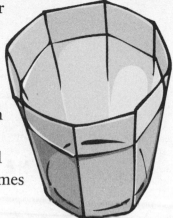

■ **Canker sores.** To relieve the pain of canker sores, make an antiseptic mouth rinse by dissolving ½ teaspoon of goldenseal powder and ¼ teaspoon of salt in 1 cup of warm water. Swish and spit four times a day.

■ **Sinus headache.** Humans have been getting sinus headaches for eons, and they've been easing them with herbal medicines for almost as long. Goldenseal can help because it reduces congestion and inflammation. Try 125 milligrams in capsule form twice a day.

■ **Folliculitis.** The combination of echinacea and goldenseal kills the bacteria that cause folliculitis, an infection of the hair follicles, says Heidi Weinhold, N.D., and keeps the infection from returning. Buy an ointment that contains both herbs and apply it several times a day until the irritation disappears.

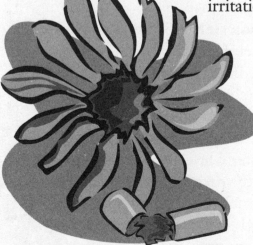

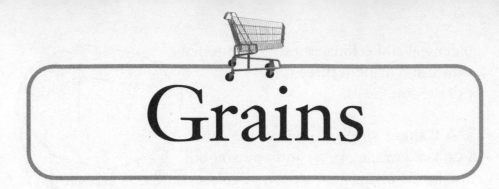

Grains

THE BEST FIBER FIND

You already know that the U.S. government's Food Guide Pyramid calls for eating up to 11 servings of grains a day, but you may wonder why pasta, rice, whole wheat, and other grains are so important. For one thing, they're absolutely jammed with fiber. They're nutritional power-houses that provide key vitamins, minerals, and other chemical compounds that you need for good health. Best of all, grains do all this without overloading your body (including your hips) with excess calories. See for yourself.

■ **High cholesterol.** Scores of studies have shown that the heart-healthiest diet is the one people in Mediterranean areas enjoy. Made up of mostly vegetables and fruit, beans, fish, nuts, grains, and plenty of olive oil, Mediterranean meals have a positive effect on both cholesterol levels and blood pressure. Add generous amounts of vegetables, peas, beans, fish, and whole grains to your low-fat diet, and you'll lower both your total and LDL cholesterol levels by twice as much as people who eat ordinary low-fat

ON THE SHELF

✓ Rice
✓ Quinoa
✓ Wheatberries
✓ Whole grain breads and pasta
✓ Oatmeal

meals, according to results of a study presented to a meeting of the American Heart Association.

■ **Weak nails.** Healthy nails are strong, smooth, and pale pink. To stay that way, they need lots of oxygen and nutrients. If you're not eating a well-balanced diet, the nutrients you do get will rush to meet your body's most important needs, and your nails will be short-changed. Be sure to include high-quality protein, whole grains, and plenty of fresh fruits and veggies in your diet. Your nails will thank you.

■ **Stroke.** Homocysteine, an amino acid your body makes as it digests protein, has been linked to stroke and heart attacks for a long time, but new evidence is coming to light. At a meeting of the American Stroke Association, it was revealed that homocysteine is involved in actually causing strokes, not just increasing vulnerability to them. One way to lower homocysteine is to increase your intake of foods high in B vitamins, specifically folate, B_6, and B_{12}, which you can get from whole grains. Researchers are now trying to find out if these vitamins ward off new strokes in people who have

Just What the Doctor Ordered!

Quench the Flames with Grains

To help your skin heal after a burn, eat five or six servings of antioxidant-rich foods daily. You need antioxidants to minimize the harmful effects of free radicals, oxygen molecules that are produced in profusion after burns and cause additional damage to skin cells. Whole grains are one of the best sources of antioxidants.

already had them, but regardless of whether or not you've had a stroke, it can't hurt to get some more of those big B's.

■ **CFS.** "Good nutrition may be the single most important strategy for whipping chronic fatigue syndrome," says Ralph Ofcarcik, Ph.D. "Since the immune system is functioning at less than an optimum level, it makes good sense to focus on 'nutrient-dense,' or unprocessed, foods,"—and that includes whole grains!

■ **High blood sugar.** Studies have shown that a natural, whole-foods diet heavy on grains is far more likely to help stabilize blood sugar than one that includes fast food and refined sugar.

A Recipe for Better Breathing

The magnesium in whole grains and other foods acts like "a sedative for your bronchial tubes," says Anna Szpindor, M.D. Studies show that if your diet is deficient in magnesium, your asthma may be more severe and flare up more frequently than it otherwise would.

■ **Constipation and diverticulosis.** The insoluble fiber in whole gains and vegetables adds bulk to stools, which helps prevent constipation. At the same time, a diet rich in grains decreases pressure on the colon and reduces the risk of diverticulosis—high-pressure "blowouts" in the colon wall.

■ **Queasiness.** If eating too much of the wrong kinds of foods gives you an upset stomach, sipping barley water is the ideal remedy, since compounds in barley, called catechins, can help quell nausea. Boil a small handful of pearl barley in 1 quart of water for an hour.

Strain out the barley, then add ½ cup of the cooking water to ½ cup of warm milk. Eat the cooked barley, too, if you can, since it may help prevent indigestion and diarrhea.

■ **Rashes.** Forget the fancy bubble baths when you have a rash or hives. Instead, sink into a cool, slimy colloidal oatmeal bath for 5 to 30 minutes, suggests Sharol Tilgner, N.D. When this finely ground grain hits the tub, the water turns milky and coats your erupted skin, moisturizing and reducing the itch. You can also mix colloidal oatmeal with a bit of water to form a paste and apply it directly to the rash.

■ **Ear noise.** If you have tinnitus, those sounds in your ears that you hear when no real noise is present, start eating more grains. They're high in magnesium, a mineral that helps maintain optimal ear circulation.

■ **Stress.** Grains can help you deal with the stresses of a life in overdrive. They're packed with pantothenic acid, a B vitamin that's necessary to keep your adrenal glands working well when your body is stressed, says Jamison Starbuck, N.D.

■ **Folate-deficiency anemia.** Folate (folic acid) is a B vitamin that builds red blood cells and comes from foods such as whole grains, dark leafy greens, citrus fruits, and beans. Women who are pregnant or breastfeeding are most likely to come up short on folate, which isn't stored in the body and needs to be replenished daily.

Fabulous Food Fix

Think Zinc

Men need plenty of zinc to maintain healthy sexual function. This mineral, which the prostate needs to produce seminal fluid, is found in whole grains, shellfish, and poultry, says Marcus Loo, M.D.

Grains 209

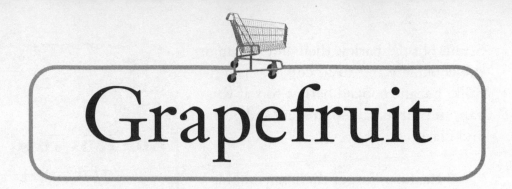

Grapefruit

THE KING OF CITRUS

The sheer size of grapefruit can be a little daunting, and this may explain why it isn't as popular as its more petite—and admittedly sweeter—citrus kin. But if the pucker potential doesn't totally put you off, there are plenty of good reasons to eat grapefruit more often. Here's a sample. If you take any prescription medications, though, check with your doctor before eating grapefruit regularly.

■ **Diarrhea.** Made from the seeds and pulp of grapefruit, grapefruit seed extract may knock out any bacterium, parasite, or virus that may be behind your diarrhea. Add two drops to a glass of water and take it twice a day until you've killed whatever you picked up, but never take it straight, or it may wipe out beneficial bacteria along with the troublemakers. Also, if you're taking cholesterol-lowering medication, you should avoid grapefruit seed extract.

Soothing Sips

JUICE UP STROKE PROTECTION

The antioxidants and potassium in grapefruit may team up to stave off strokes. A Harvard study found that drinking a glass of grapefruit juice or orange juice daily lowered the risk of a common type of stroke by 25 percent.

■ **Heart attack and stroke.** Grapefruit is loaded with pectin, a type of fiber that essentially attaches to cholesterol molecules in your intestine and drags them out of your body in stools. This means that the cholesterol never gets into the bloodstream, so it can't form the fatty deposits that greatly increase the risk of heart attack and stroke. Try one serving a day of the fresh fruit.

■ **Nail fungus.** Fungal infections on or beneath a nail can be difficult to get rid of. Before trying more toxic therapies—many of which are only marginally effective—begin a regimen of nail painting with grapefruit seed extract. Paint only the affected nail once or twice a day, being careful not to apply the extract to the surrounding skin, which may become irritated. Continue the treatment for six weeks for best results.

MAGIC MIXES

SAVE YOUR THIGHS
Troubled by cellulite? Try this copycat version of those herbal wraps the fancy spas use: Mix ½ cup of grapefruit juice, 1 cup of corn oil, and 2 teaspoons of dried thyme. Massage the mixture into your thighs, hips, and buttocks, then cover the area with plastic wrap. Hold a heating pad over each body area for 5 minutes.

■ **Heart disease.** The compound lycopene is known to protect the heart, and grapefruit, along with tomatoes and guavas, is one of the richest sources. Lycopene is a carotenoid, a plant pigment that is believed to have powerful antioxidant properties, and that seems to be one of the main keys to preventing heart disease.

■ **Cancer.** The lycopene in grapefruit is especially important for men. There's good evi-

Grapefruit 211

dence that this brightly colored plant pigment can greatly reduce the risk of prostate cancer.

■ **Infections.** If an infection has taken hold, fight back with a trio of powerful weapons: grapefruit seed extract (100 milligrams three times a day), echinacea (200 milligrams twice daily), and gold-enseal (200 milligrams three times a day), suggests Robert Ivker, D.O. Skip the grapefruit seed extract if you're taking cholesterol-lowering medication, though, and don't take echinacea if you have an autoimmune disease such as lupus, rheumatoid arthritis, or multiple sclerosis, or if you're pregnant or nursing.

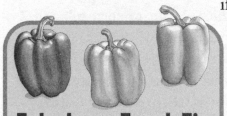

Fabulous Food Fix

Wrinkle Remover

To help relax wrinkles, mix 1½ tablespoons of unflavored gelatin and ½ cup of grapefruit juice in a microwaveable container and heat it until the gelatin is completely dissolved. Put the mixture in the refrigerator until it's almost set (about 25 minutes), then spread it on your face, let it dry, and peel it off.

■ **Gum disease.** Have a few daily servings of grapefruit or other vitamin C–rich citrus fruits when your gums are sore or bleeding. Vitamin C will help keep your gums in the pink, especially if they're recovering from gingivitis. As a bonus, vitamin C helps squelch the inflammatory effects of free radicals, those harmful molecules that damage healthy cells throughout the body.

■ **Injuries.** In addition to clobbering free radicals, vitamin C helps maintain collagen, which repairs your body's tissues after injuries. Eating just half a grapefruit guarantees you all the vitamin C you need for the entire day!

Grapefruit

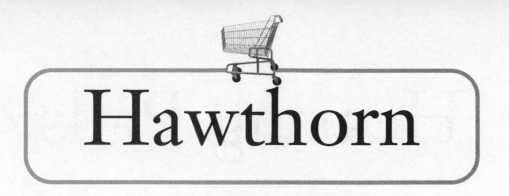

Hawthorn

HELP FOR THE HEART

Hawthorn comes from flowers and berries that have been used for centuries as a heart and circulatory tonic—and it really does seem to help. Take a look below, then check with your doctor about whether it's right for you. Avoid hawthorn if you take medication.

■ **Weak heart.** Hawthorn dilates the blood vessels and helps the heart squeeze harder. People who take it can exercise for longer periods without chest pain. One caution: If you take digoxin for irregular heart rhythm, hawthorn may increase its effects, so check with your doctor.

■ **Leg pain.** Hawthorn can help relieve the pain of intermittent claudication. Add 1 heaping teaspoon to 1 cup of hot water and steep for 15 to 20 minutes, then strain. You can drink two or three cups of this tea per day.

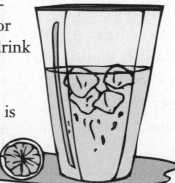

■ **High blood pressure.** Hawthorn is known to lower blood pressure. To use it, add 60 drops of tincture to a glass of water or juice and drink it once a day.

Heating Pads

HOT HEALERS

Mmm…nothing feels better than gentle heat, and few things are better for you when you're hurting. Whether you've sprained an ankle, have an earache, or are simply dealing with a headache at the end of the day, applying heat eases pain, removes harmful toxins, and brings in healing nutrients. Here's how it works.

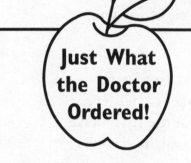

Just What the Doctor Ordered!

Relief for Gym Rats

If joint pain tends to flare after you exercise, a heat treatment can help. Apply a heating pad set on low or a hot, moist towel to aching joints after your workouts. It can cut down swelling and pain.

■ **Earache.** Gentle heat is probably the most soothing home treatment for an adult's aching ear, says John W. House, M.D. The easiest approach is to use a heating pad. Set it on low, cover it with a towel or pillowcase, and lie down for a while with your ear resting against the pad. As long as the pad doesn't get too hot, it's fine to lie there for 20 to 30 minutes or until the pain subsides. Remember to set a timer or alarm clock so you don't fall asleep.

214

■ **Headache.** You've probably seen movies or television shows that portray headache sufferers holding comically large ice bags on their heads. Ice can certainly help in some cases, but heat is usually better for tension headaches because it makes muscles relax instead of contract, says Terri Dallas-Prunskis, M.D. She recommends putting a heating pad or a washcloth soaked in warm water on the areas that hurt. You can also hang out in a warm bath or shower for 10 to 15 minutes.

■ **Shoulder pain.** The next time you have a sore shoulder, apply heat to the area. It will relax the muscle, loosen the joint, and help prevent painful spasms. Hold a heating pad set on low or a warm compress against your shoulder for 15 to 20 minutes at a time whenever it starts feeling stiff. Just this short heat treatment can leave your shoulder feeling loose and relaxed for hours.

Hot Oil for Quick Relief

A castor oil pack is a traditional remedy to soothe and heal injured muscles, and it's easy to use. Just apply some castor oil to the area and cover it with plastic wrap, then top with a heating pad set on low. The heat will help the oil penetrate the skin, where it will ease pain as well as stiffness. Leave the pack on for 20 to 30 minutes, then wash off the oil. Repeat the treatment several times a day.

■ **Finger pain.** Nothing hurts worse than clobbering a finger or thumb with a hammer. If you don't take care of it right away, the throbbing can seem to last forever. Apply ice until the swelling goes down, usually about 24 to 48 hours. After that, apply heat. You can rest your hand on a heating pad set on low or wrap

215

Heating Pads

Protect Your Peeper

Forget about raw meat when you have a black eye. Instead, start a warming trend. Immediately after the injury, apply ice cubes wrapped in a towel to the sore area to help keep swelling from getting started. A day or two after using ice, switch to heat by applying a towel moistened with warm water, for example, or a heating pad set on low and swaddled in a soft towel. The heat will soothe the injured area and boost circulation, which will help your eye heal more quickly.

the digit in a washcloth moistened with warm water. Heat increases circulation, speeds the flow of healing nutrients to the area, and helps flush away pain-causing toxins. This also works for wrist pain.

■ **Back pain I.** It seems that the only time hot water bottles or heating pads come out of the closet is when back pain makes an appearance. There's nothing wrong with using heat after the first few days, but don't use it right away, because it increases inflammation. As soon as your back starts hurting, apply a cold pack or ice cubes wrapped in a towel to your sore muscles. Cool the area for about 20 minutes every few hours for the first 24 hours. Cold constricts, or narrows, blood vessels and reduces blood flow, in turn reducing pain in the first day or two after an injury. After a couple of days of using cold, switch to the heating pad for quick relief.

■ **Back pain II.** Here's another good remedy for back pain. Add some castor oil to equal parts of St. John's wort oil and arnica oil, then have someone apply the whole slick mess to the painful area of your back. Cover it with plastic wrap and a warm compress or a heating pad set

Heating Pads

on low and leave it on for about 20 minutes. The heat will penetrate deeply into the muscles and help them relax.

■ **Constipation.** Millions of Americans suffer from constipation, and way too many of us depend on laxatives. There's nothing wrong with using them occasionally, but they're really too strong for regular use, and they can actually increase the risk that you'll get constipated. A better, alternative way to gently encourage things to move along is to put a castor oil pack on your abdomen. First, soak a small towel in castor oil and lay it over your midsection. Cover it with plastic wrap and then a heating pad set on low. Leave the pack on for about 20 minutes.

■ **Labor pain.** A time-tested way to ease the pain of childbirth is to put a heating pad or hot water bottle on your abdomen or waist. Stores that carry massage and relaxation products sell long, rice-filled pads that you heat in the microwave and wrap around your body under your belly. Check with your doctor to see if it's advisable for you to use one.

■ **Leg cramps.** For calf cramps, drape a heating pad over your leg and set the heat on low. Warm your calf for about 20 minutes at a time.

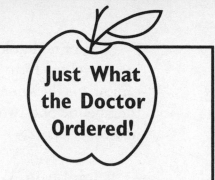

Just What the Doctor Ordered!

Warm Your Rear

You won't know the meaning of pain until you've had an anal fissure, a small tear in the tissue surrounding the anus. The darned things can take forever to heal! A little gentle heat makes everything feel better, and your rear end is no exception, so if you're unlucky enough to get a fissure, try this remedy: Cover a heating pad with a towel, set the heat on low, and sit and relax for as long as it feels comfortable.

Heating Pads   **217**

■ **Sprained ankle.** Apply a cold pack or ice cubes wrapped in a towel for 15 to 20 minutes, followed by a heating pad set on low for the same amount of time. Hit your ankle with this therapeutic one-two punch two or three times a day for a day or two.

■ **Joint pain.** When your joints hurt but there's no swelling, heat works better than cold. Twenty minutes of warmth will promote the flow of healing nutrients to the joint.

■ **Lyme disease.** Lyme disease is notorious for causing symptoms that wax and wane; you may feel fine one day and miserable the next. When you're feeling achy or tired, you may want to experiment with cold or heat treatments. Neither is best; different people respond in different ways. For example, apply a cold pack or ice cubes wrapped in a small towel to an achy joint or muscle. Hold it in place for about 20 minutes, then repeat the treatment throughout the day. If that doesn't seem to help, use a heating pad set on low instead. Once you figure out which approach works for you, use it for soothing relief whenever symptoms threaten to lay you low.

■ **Chest congestion.** Here's a good way to ease a tight chest. Add a few drops of water to a small amount of dry mustard to create a thin paste, then apply the paste to your chest and cover it with a layer of flannel and a hot water bottle or a heating pad set on low. The oils in mustard can easily burn the skin, though, so lift a corner of the flannel every 5 minutes to check for redness, and don't leave the poultice on for more than a total of 15 minutes. After several minutes, the congestion should start to loosen, possibly because mustard helps bring blood to the skin's surface and get fluids moving, says Mary Hardy, M.D.

Heating Pads

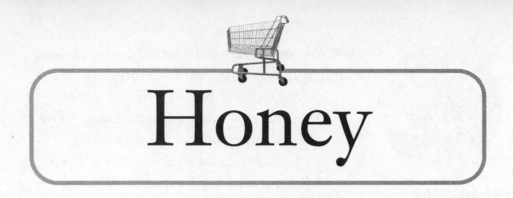

Honey

A SWEET CURE

Winnie the Pooh was always getting caught with his hand in the honey pot. Sure, his hankering for honey had more to do with his insatiable sweet tooth than anything else, but it's safe to assume that all that honey made Pooh one healthy bear! See what it can do for you.

■ **Allergies.** Bee pollen and locally made honey have long been touted as allergy preventives. If you eat bee pollen and honey before allergy season hits, you ingest minute parts of the plants, grasses, and trees that may trigger symptoms. By thus stimulating your immune system, you can build up resistance and lessen the severity of your allergies when the season arrives. A typical dose is 1 teaspoon of honey per day. Caution: Never give raw honey to children under age 1, and avoid bee pollen if you have insect allergies.

Honey for 'heads

Is your face dotted with blackheads? Make a paste of egg white, dry oatmeal, and honey. Apply it to your skin and wait 10 minutes or so, then rinse with warm water and pat dry. The blackheads will disappear!

MAGIC MIXES

A SWEET SOOTHER

You can make your own moisturizer without leaving the kitchen by mixing equal parts of honey and milk. Use this combo as a head-to-toe body lotion, then rinse off the excess. If you're feeling ambitious, toss the mix into a blender and add some apricots, avocado, or coconut oil. The blend feels wonderful, and you can keep it in the refrigerator and massage it into your skin whenever you want.

■ **Cuts and scrapes.** In a study, when crude, undiluted honey was applied to infected wounds, they healed twice as fast as wounds treated with antiseptics. "The thick honey covers the wound and may serve as an antibacterial to keep infection at bay," explains Manfred Kroger, Ph.D. Plus, honey appears to reduce swelling and pain. Just be sure to thoroughly wash your cut, use pasteurized honey (which won't harbor bacteria of its own), and watch for signs of infection.

■ **Cough.** Honey mixed with onion juice was widely used as a cough suppressant during the Great Depression, when few folks could afford store-bought remedies. Honey or sugar is used to draw the juice from an onion, forming an effective cough syrup because the onion, it's said, stimulates saliva flow, which clears the throat, and perhaps

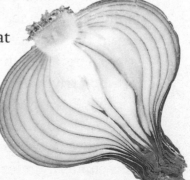

reduces inflammation. Here's what to do: Slice an onion into rings and place them in a deep bowl. Cover them with honey and let stand for 10 to 12 hours. Strain out the onion and take 1 tablespoon of the syrup four or five times a day. Or finely chop an onion, mix with ½ cup of granulated sugar, and let stand overnight. Take

Honey

1 tablespoon of the resulting syrup every 4 to 5 hours.

■ **Dry skin.** Honey has been used since ancient Egyptian times as a beauty aid. Applied as a mask, it moisturizes skin and leaves your face soft and dewy. Just smooth it on your face, leave it on for 20 minutes or so, and rinse with warm water.

■ **Colds.** Try a hot toddy as a cold rescue. Before hundreds of cold remedies became available at the supermarket, certain home remedies were probably a lot more fun to take—and if you took enough, they absolutely worked, because pretty soon you just couldn't feel your cold anymore. There are many variations on the hot toddy, which apparently originated in Scotland. Start with juice, honey, or tea and add the liquor of your choice.

■ **Queasiness.** In traditional Indian medicine, common spices are used to quiet a roiling stomach. Try eating ½ cup of plain yogurt to which you've added 2 pinches of cardamom and ½ teaspoon of honey, suggests Vasant Lad, M.A.Sc.

Just What the Doctor Ordered!

Put Moisture Where It Counts

Good, old-fashioned honey can gently moisturize vaginal tissues. While you may need to use it daily at first, over time, you should be able to decrease the frequency. For ease of application and extra benefit, add several drops of vitamin E oil to the honey. Avoid raw honey.

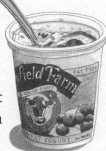

Honey 221

Soothing Sips

SING OUT FOR HONEY

When you've lost your voice due to laryngitis, enjoy a cup of warm tea flavored with lemon and honey. It really works—and it's definitely better than cold or hot water, which can further inflame the vocal cords.

■ **Hangover.** If you really want to bypass a hangover, the experts at the National Headache Foundation suggest that you eat honey on a cracker or piece of toast before or after drinking. Honey contains as much as 40 percent fructose, a sugar known to speed the metabolism of alcohol.

■ **Herpes.** An active herpes eruption can last a heartbreaking week or two, but researchers in the Ukraine found that using a topical ointment containing propolis, a nutrient-rich substance made by honeybees that contains antiviral flavonoids, can cut the duration of lesions to just three days. That's almost half the time it took for lesions to heal with standard medication. Apply three or four times a day.

■ **Eczema.** If your tiny tyke has sensitive skin or maybe a touch of eczema, this soothing bath is a perfect before-bed treat. Fill the bathtub with warm water, adding 1 tablespoon of honey and 2 tablespoons of colloidal oatmeal as the tub fills. Let the youngster soak and play, and when she's had enough, follow with a thorough rinse in clear, warm water.

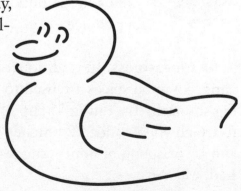

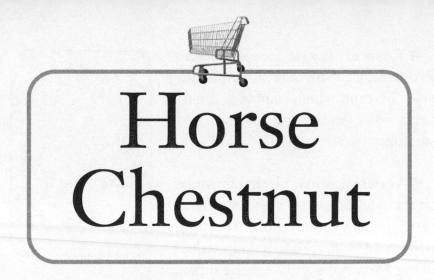

Horse Chestnut

PONY UP FOR HEALTH

Sometimes it seems as though there's not a lot you can do to strengthen your circulatory system and tone sagging or leaky veins. There is one traditional remedy that seems to help, however, and it's made from the lowly horse chestnut. Take a look.

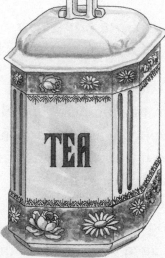

■ **Hemorrhoids.** No one likes to admit they have hemorrhoids, but most people get them from time to time. The leaves, bark, and seeds of the horse chestnut tree contain aescin, a compound that helps block enzymes that weaken veins, even when applied externally. "Dabbing horse chestnut tea onto hemorrhoids can be soothing as well as strengthening," says Jerry Gore, M.D. First, make some horse chestnut tea according to the package directions, then soak a small, soft cloth in the cooled liquid and apply it after each bowel movement.

223

■ **Rosacea.** If your face is reddened by rosacea, try using a cream containing horse chestnut, which improves the tone of vein walls. Applying it twice a day may minimize the redness.

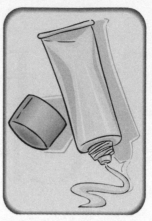

■ **Varicose veins.** Herbal formulas that include the classic vessel strengtheners butcher's broom, horse chestnut, yarrow, and stoneroot may help reduce leaking from veins and decrease inflammation inside them. That's important when you have varicose veins. The catch is, if you're prone to varicose veins, you may need to stay on these herbals forever to be sure they don't return. Women who are pregnant or breastfeeding shouldn't take formulas containing horse chestnut.

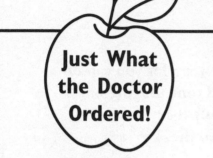

Just What the Doctor Ordered!

Take the Pain Out of Sprains

You can keep a sprain from turning black and blue by applying a gel that contains horse chestnut extract. A substance in the herb called aescin helps keep blood from seeping out of damaged blood vessels, thus minimizing discoloration.

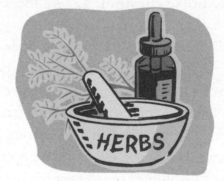

Horseradish

SWEAT AND SOOTHE

If the only time you eat horseradish is when you whip up a roast beef sandwich, it's definitely time to put more spice in your life. This tongue-burning condiment is one hot healer! Here's why.

■ **Stuffy nose I.** Wasabi, the powerful Japanese horseradish that can almost blow the lid off a manhole, will empty your sinuses when you're congested. Eat ¼ teaspoon of wasabi or regular horseradish three times daily or make your own by grating 1 teaspoon of fresh root into a cup of hot water and steeping for 5 minutes. Strain and drink three cups a day.

■ **Stuffy nose II.** Why buy over-the-counter decongestants when you have nature's own nose-

MAGIC MIXES

OUT, DARNED SPOTS!
You can bleach age spots with a combination of 1 teaspoon each of grated horseradish, lemon juice, and vinegar and three drops of rosemary oil. It has a strong odor, but it will make spots fade swiftly.

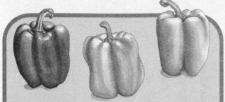

Fabulous Food Fix

A Hot Tip for Aching Ears

When congestion is backing up into your ears, try this potent (some would say desperate) treatment. Spread ½ teaspoon of horseradish or mustard on three or four slices of raw garlic. Then eat them, washing the concoction down with a cup of peppermint tea.

clearing medicine in your refrigerator? The chemicals in horseradish stimulate the nerve endings in your nose and make it flow like a faucet when you're stuffed up due to a cold or the flu. Plus, horseradish has antiviral properties. "I suggest patients take a teaspoon of freshly grated root or a half-teaspoon of horseradish extract three times a day," says Michael DiPalma, N.D.

■ **Bronchitis.** To get mucus flowing and break up chest congestion, try this broncho-buster cracker spread suggested by James A. Duke, Ph.D. Mix small amounts of garlic, ginger, mustard, turmeric, chopped chile peppers, and horseradish into a

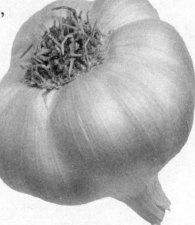

paste. Spread very small amounts on crackers and nibble gingerly, one tiny bite at a time. The ingredients will make everything run, promises Dr. Duke—your eyes, your nose, and even the thick mucus clogging your bronchial tubes.

■ **Cancer.** Horseradish is packed with isothiocyanates, chemical compounds that seem to deactivate other chemicals before they can trigger cancer. Scientists think that isothiocyanates may be especially helpful in staving off cancers of the mouth, pharynx, lung, stomach, colon, and rectum.

Horseradish

■ **Food poisoning.** There's some evidence that the chemicals in horseradish help fight *Listeria*, *E. coli*, and other harmful bacteria that cause food poisoning. There's no telling when these bacteria may end up in your food, especially sandwiches, so why not top your sandwich fillings with some horseradish? It'll taste great, and you can rest a little easier.

■ **Heart disease.** Vitamin C is an essential nutrient for preventing heart disease, mainly because it helps stop harmful molecules (free radicals) from damaging the linings of arteries and encouraging the accumulation of cholesterol deposits. Just 2 tablespoons of fresh or prepared horseradish provides 12 percent of the vitamin C you need daily.

■ **Poor appetite.** You need good nutrition when you're recovering from a respiratory infection, but it's hard to eat when you're so congested that you can't taste a thing. Garlic, onions, chile peppers, and horseradish are packed with potent flavors that break through to your taste buds when nothing else will. That means you can eat and enjoy the healthy foods that will get you back on your feet again, fast.

Horseradish 227

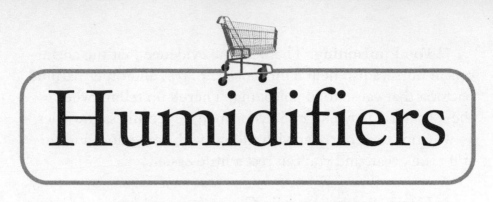

Humidifiers

THE MAGIC OF MOISTURE

Your body is composed mainly of water, but you sure wouldn't know it during the cold months, when the combination of cold air and indoor heat sucks just about every drop of moisture from your skin and mucous membranes. The solution, of course, is to head for the health and beauty aids aisle and pick up a humidifier. Here's how it can help.

■ **Dry eyes.** Use a humidifier if your eyes are bone-dry due to allergies, but be sure to keep it clean so you don't add allergens such as mold spores to the air.

■ **Itchy skin.** You can combat winter itch by keeping a healthier moisture balance in the air. Experiment with the settings on your humidifier to see which one is right for you.

■ **Laryngitis.** If you have an extreme case of laryngitis, try resting in a warm room with high humidity for a day or two, letting your worn-out throat soak up some moisture while you sleep.

■ **Postnasal drip.** Dry indoor air can thicken mucus and make postnasal drip even worse. The best approach is simply to plug in a humidifier, which will help thin mucus.

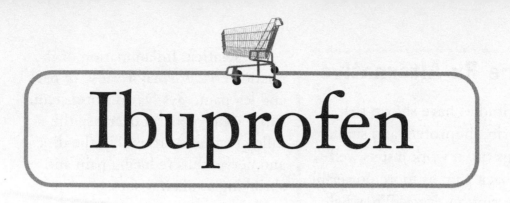

Ibuprofen

THE LITTLE PILL WITH A BIG PUNCH

Aspirin had a lock on the pain-relief market for a long time, but these days, ibuprofen is often the pain reliever of choice. It's just as effective as aspirin at reducing pain and inflammation, and it's less likely to cause side effects. Best of all, it brings relief for hundreds of conditions. Although kids who are allergic to aspirin shouldn't take it, for the rest of us, it's an amazing drug. Here's a sample of what it can do.

■ **Painful intercourse.** For some women, the uterine contractions from an orgasm can cause pain that puts a damper on the pleasure of sex. According to doctors at the Florida Hospital Family Practice, you can prevent this by taking ibuprofen prior to intercourse.

ON THE SHELF
- ✓ Advil
- ✓ Motrin
- ✓ Proflex
- ✓ Nurofen

■ **Menstrual pain.** Ibuprofen blocks the production of pain-producing prostaglandins, natural chemicals that cause menstrual cramps by increasing uterine contractions, says Mary Ellen Mortensen, M.D.

229

The Rx Alternative

Studies have shown that aspirin, ibuprofen, and similar drugs often work just as well for back pain as more powerful prescription drugs. They help in two ways: They're analgesics, which means they work directly on the pain, and they have anti-inflammatory effects that reduce painful swelling.

■ **Sciatica.** Inflammation of the sciatic nerve is a major cause of back and leg pain, says David Borenstein, M.D. Ibuprofen can decrease the inflammation surrounding the disk and nerve, thus reducing pain and shrinking swollen tissues.

■ **Shingles.** Over-the-counter remedies can help control the pain of shingles. Take ibuprofen (or aspirin) according to your doctor's instructions.

■ **Lupus.** Whether your lupus is active or inactive, the idea is to stop flare-ups of this autoimmune disease and keep symptoms bearable. To that end, you may need to take drugs to reduce inflammation, including corticosteroids and nonsteroidal anti-inflammatory drugs such as ibuprofen. Check with your doctor for the right dose and formulation.

■ **Burns.** You'll probably need some ibuprofen or another pain reliever when you have a burn. These drugs won't help the burn heal, but they're very effective at reducing pain while nature takes its course. Just follow the package directions.

■ **Arthritis.** What's the best pill to reach for when you need relief from arthritis? There's no clear answer. Most doctors advise patients to start with ibuprofen, although some people do better with aspirin or naproxen. You'll just have to try different painkillers until you find the one that works best for you. If you're going beyond the guidelines on the label, or you have any chronic health problems besides arthritis, consult your doctor first.

■ **Earache.** Ibuprofen quickly eases ear pain and helps control the fever that often accompanies infections. Unless you're sensitive to it, take it every 4 hours or as directed on the label.

Hangover Helper

Sometimes, all a hangover headache needs is an over-the-counter analgesic. As long as you're not sensitive to it, take 600 milligrams of ibuprofen two or three times daily.

■ **Migraines.** It's generally fine to take ibuprofen at the first sign of a migraine. Over-the-counter treatments are surprisingly effective as long as you take them before the migraine really gets under way. If the pain doesn't retreat fairly quickly, you should see your doctor, especially if you've had a recent head injury, the pain occurs on both sides of your head, or it's accompanied by difficulty speaking or mental confusion.

■ **Shoulder pain.** Take ibuprofen right away if you suspect your shoulder pain is caused by a rotator cuff tear. It's a good choice because it inhibits the activity of inflammatory substances called prostaglandins.

■ **Anal fissure.** Don't ignore common pain relievers such as ibuprofen if you have an anal fissure. They work!

■ **Bursitis.** Most cases of bursitis will heal by themselves in 7 to 10 days, according to doctors at the Mayo Clinic. In the meantime, take ibuprofen to reduce inflammation and pain.

■ **Groin pain.** Ibuprofen is surprisingly effective at easing groin pain, says Martin Resnick, M.D.

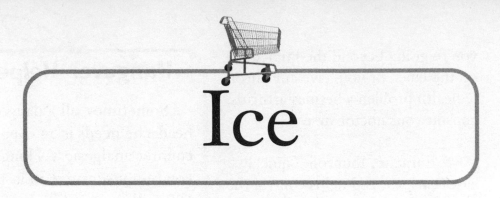

Ice

CHILL OUT!

It's hard to believe that a little frozen water can make such a difference in your health. Even in this age of high-tech medicine, doctors recommend simple ice almost as often as aspirin for easing minor aches and pains—and more. Here's why.

Hemorrhoid Helper

Sit on a bag of ice when you have hemorrhoids. A large plastic bag filled with crushed ice and covered with a towel may not be practical as a long-term seat, but it can numb the pain and swelling for a while and help you feel more comfortable.

■ **Joint injuries.** The best first aid for acute pain from an injured joint is ice. Put some ice cubes in a washcloth or small towel and apply to the sore joint for about 20 minutes. Remove the ice pack, wrap the joint in an elastic bandage to prevent swelling, and elevate your injured limb above the level of your heart. Repeat the treatment every few hours. If you don't feel relief within two days, start to alternate hot compresses or a heating pad with the ice. Use 3 minutes of heat, then 1 minute of cold,

232

alternating for 15 or 20 minutes once or twice a day and always ending with cold.

■ **Itching.** Apply cold packs or ice cubes wrapped in a towel when itching gets the best of you. Cold slows blood circulation, thus reducing swelling and inflammation.

■ **Muscle pain.** A cold pack can ease sore muscles, and the effects of cold last longer than those of heat because it takes longer for your body to warm up than to cool off. To make an ice pack that molds to your contours, fill a zip-close plastic bag with one part rubbing alcohol to four parts water. Put that bag into a second bag so it doesn't leak and put the pack in the freezer. When you ache, pull it out and apply it for 15 to 20 minutes.

■ **Pinkeye.** Ice-cold compresses can soothe your eyes when you have pinkeye. Simply place a damp washcloth that's been chilled in the freezer or just a cool, wet paper towel over your closed eyes for about 10 minutes. Remove it for 30 to 60 minutes, then reapply as often as you feel the need.

■ **Back pain.** Ice is a great analgesic for back pain. It's preferable to aspirin or

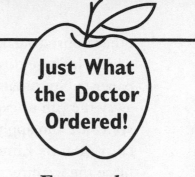

Just What the Doctor Ordered!

Freeze the Mouth Flames

If you've burned your mouth with scorching hot cheese when taking a bite of pizza, you can get quick relief by applying ice to the area. It will strip away residual heat, numb the pain, and narrow tiny blood vessels, which will inhibit inflammation or bleeding under the surface. The best way to use ice is to simply suck on an ice cube for a while. You can also swish ice water around in your mouth for about 20 seconds several times a day.

other nonsteroidal anti-inflammatory drugs such as ibuprofen, which, in large doses, can cause stomach upset. Simply fill a paper or Styrofoam cup with water and freeze it, then peel away the rim to expose the ice surface. Holding the cup, lie on your side and apply the ice directly to the painful area in a circular motion. Limit the massage to about 5 minutes, and don't place the ice directly on the bony portion of your spine.

■ **Hangover.** Put your head on the rocks when you have a hangover. Put some crushed ice in a plastic bag (or grab a bag of frozen peas) and hold it against your head to help shrink the swollen blood vessels that are causing the throbbing. Some experts also recommend placing your feet in a tub of warm water at the same time. Although the remedy's medicinal benefits are hazy, it's bound to feel wonderful.

■ **Poison ivy.** If you've been bushwhacked by poison ivy and live in the eastern United States, look for another plant—jewelweed—to treat it. (The tall, slender plant has oval, slightly toothed leaves and small hanging flowers.) Simply break a stem and rub the juice onto the affected area. Jewelweed can help keep the irritating urushiol oil in poison ivy from binding to your skin and spreading, says Beth Burch, N.D. A few drops of extract will work, too. To keep a reserve handy, mix a few drops of the extract with water and freeze the solution as ice cubes to use on any itchy spots that may crop up.

> ## Pain-Free Piercing
>
> Many ear-piercing services use a topical anesthetic to numb the ears during the procedure. You can get the same effect afterward by rubbing an ice cube on and near the piercing sites.

■ **Arthritis.** When an arthritic joint is inflamed—it may be painful, swollen, or even feel hot—put some ice on the fire. "Ice is very good for inflammation and swelling," says James Herndon, M.D. He recommends putting an ice pack on the sore joint for about 20 minutes at a time. Repeat the treatment once every hour for as long as it seems to help.

■ **Tendinitis and bursitis.** If tendinitis or bursitis is making a joint feel hot and swollen, the first thing you should do is get some ice on it. Applying cold constricts blood vessels and reduces the flow of fluid and inflammatory chemicals to the area. Apply a cold pack or ice cubes wrapped in a washcloth or small towel to the area for about 20 minutes, repeating every hour or two until the pain goes away.

■ **Cancer pain.** You wouldn't think that simple home remedies such as heat and ice would be helpful for cancer pain, but they're surprisingly effective. Each person responds differently to heat and cold, so you'll just have to try both to see which is most effective. For cold treatments, apply an ice pack or ice cubes wrapped in a washcloth or small towel to the painful area. Hold it in place for 20 minutes, then let your skin warm up for 20 minutes. Repeating the treatment once an hour or so will numb nerve endings and help you feel better.

■ **Lyme disease.** When you have Lyme disease, your symptoms may come and go, so you can be fine one day and feel totally awful the next. When you're achy or tired, you may

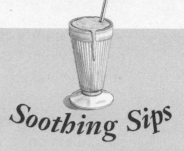

Soothing Sips

HAVE A COLD ONE

Drinking piping-hot liquids swells the uvula—the soft structure that hangs at the back of your throat—and increases your discomfort when you have a sore throat. To help curb a sore throat's swelling and pain, it's better to drink cool or even icy drinks. Just crush some ice in a blender, add your favorite juice, and sip it throughout the day.

want to apply a cold pack or ice cubes wrapped in a small towel to a sore joint or muscle. Hold it in place for about 20 minutes at a time and repeat throughout the day.

■ **Postsurgical pain.** After surgery, you'll probably take painkillers prescribed by your doctor, and that's a good thing. Using a cold pack will probably provide even more relief, according to Cristopher Bosted, N.D. "It generally helps to ice the surgical area during the first 24 to 72 hours," he says.

■ **Shiners.** Nothing is better for a black eye than applying ice right away. Cold causes blood vessels to constrict, or narrow, which reduces internal bleeding, swelling, and those unsightly color changes, says Priscilla Natanson, N.D. It also numbs the area and helps ease the throbbing. Make an ice pack by wrapping some ice cubes in a washcloth or small towel, then gently hold it against the area for 15 to 20 minutes every few hours during the 24 hours following the injury, Dr. Natanson advises.

■ **Toothache.** It may seem strange to think that placing a cold pack (or a washcloth wrapped around some ice cubes) on the outside of your mouth would have much effect on a toothache, but it does seem to help. Hold it

Heat and Cold to Go

If you're constipated, you can get things moving from the outside by alternating hot and cold packs on your lower abdomen. First, heat a damp cloth in the microwave, remove it with tongs, and wrap it in a towel, then place the towel over your lower body. After 3 minutes, replace it with an ice pack wrapped in a towel. Leave the cold pack on for 30 seconds, then repeat the sequence three times. "Your blood vessels will expand and contract, initiating a natural pumping action that will spur elimination," explains Christine Boorean, N.D.

against the tender area for 15 to 20 minutes every few hours until you can see your dentist.

■ **Facial pain.** It doesn't work for everyone, but sucking on an ice pop or ice cube often takes the edge off trigeminal neuralgia, a kind of nerve pain that affects the area around your mouth. As soon as you feel the pain coming on, get something cold in your mouth. Another option is to apply a cold pack to your face, but be gentle, because too much pressure can make the pain worse.

Freeze Out Herpes

When you first feel the burning that signals a herpes outbreak on the horizon, get out the ice tray. Wrap some cubes in a small towel and apply it to the area for 10 minutes at a time several times a day. Not only will the burning subside, says Tori Hudson, N.D., you may even keep lesions from appearing.

■ **Labor pain.** Back pain is very common during labor. Some women apply hot water bottles or heating pads to soothe their lower backs, but ice is often better because it acts as a local anesthetic.

■ **Neck pain.** Applying a cold pack or ice cubes wrapped in a washcloth or small towel is a great way to numb neck pain. At the same time, it will reduce any inflammation, which makes the soreness worse. Another good method is to hold a bag of frozen peas or corn against your neck. In some ways, this is actually the best approach because the bag will conform to the shape of your neck. Either way, apply cold for only 15 or 20 minutes at a time.

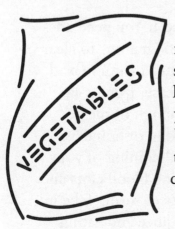

Ice **237**

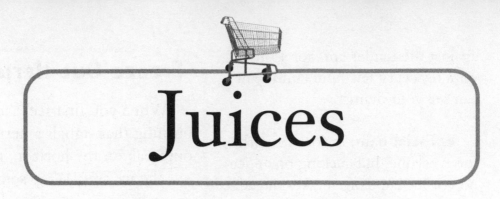

Juices

SWIG A GLASS OF HEALTH

In the 1970s, just about everyone had a juicer on the counter, but within a few years, most of those juicers had disappeared into a cupboard, tucked out of sight behind the Salad Shooters. The juicing craze didn't last very long, but there are some good reasons to put that machine back in action. Here's a sample.

■ **Allergies.** Tomato juice is among the healthiest beverages you can drink, and it does double duty if you have allergies—and you spike it with horseradish. Just grate some into a glass of tomato juice and drink it down; it will perk up your senses and clear the passages from your nose right up into your sinuses.

Sour Flake Fighter

Rinsing your hair with lemon juice after shampooing leaves it squeaky clean and helps remove dandruff flakes.

■ **Heart disease I.** You need adequate amounts of B vitamins to clear excess homocysteine, an amino acid linked to heart disease, from your blood. Without enough of these nutrients, the buildup of homocysteine can damage the lining of your arteries, encouraging blood clots and cholesterol deposits to form. Take in plenty of Bs by swigging down lots of orange juice and eating

238

more beans, whole grains, and fruits and veggies.

■ **Heart disease II.** Light to moderate consumption of wine reduces your risk of developing heart disease or of dying from it. Red wine wins out over white because it contains a number of plant chemicals that help inhibit blood clotting and have other protective properties. Want an alcohol-free alternative? Drink red or purple grape juice. It contains many of the same plant chemicals found in wine.

■ **High cholesterol.** If you live in a desert area with access to pomegranate trees, pick a fruit, squeeze, and sip the juice. An Israeli study suggested that the juice of the pomegranate helps block the process that causes cholesterol to stick to artery walls. These fruits appear now and then in supermarkets, and you may be able to find bottled juice in some stores.

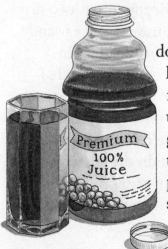

■ **Colds.** There are good reasons that doctors advise cold sufferers to drink gallons of citrus juice. The vitamin C in fruit juices may act like interferon, a natural body chemical that stops virus growth. It's most effective if you use it at the first sign of a sniffle. Most health professionals agree that vitamin C has a slight antihistamine effect, so drinking more citrus juice may also help reduce nasal symptoms.

Fabulous Food Fix

O.J. Boosts Iron

Millions of American women don't have all the energy they should due to iron-deficiency anemia. An easy solution is to enjoy citrus fruit juices with your meals—they'll help you absorb more iron from foods.

Juices

■ **Constipation.** To make a dandy drink that will relieve constipation, puree some dandelion leaves in a blender with water and pour the juice into a glass. Drink up to three glasses of this tonic. Just be sure your leaves come from a lawn that hasn't been blasted with chemicals. People who take diuretics or potassium supplements should avoid dandelion.

■ **Sore throat.** Onion juice mixed with honey or sugar is a traditional sore throat remedy. It's thought that onion stimulates saliva to clear the throat and perhaps reduces inflammation. To make the syrup, cut an onion into rings, place in a deep bowl, and cover with honey. Let stand for 10 to 12 hours, then strain out the onion and take 1 tablespoon of the syrup four or five times a day. You can also mix finely chopped onion with ½ cup of granulated sugar and let it stand overnight. Take 1 tablespoon of the syrup every 4 to 5 hours. Caution: Never give raw honey to children under age 1.

Natural Bone Builder

Chicory is a plant that helps Native Americans heal bones damaged by osteoporosis. Elders who drink lots of juice from cooked or raw chicory say their bone fractures due to osteoporosis heal faster.

■ **Earache.** To ease the pain of ear infections, crush a couple of mullein leaves in a sieve and collect the juice. With a dropper, put two drops of the juice in the painful ear and seal it with a cotton ball. This method also works with bottled mullein flower oil (made by steeping the flowers in olive oil), which you can keep in the refrigerator. The only thing you do differently is warm the dropper by rubbing it in your hands first so your ear isn't shocked by the cold! The oil helps kill the bacteria that caused the ear infection.

■ **Bloating I.** Potassium and magnesium counterbalance sodium and help reduce excess fluid in your body—good news when you're feeling bloated. To get plenty of potassium, enjoy orange, grape, or vegetable juices. You can get lots of magnesium by eating whole grains and nuts.

■ **Bloating II.** Asparagus juice is an effective diuretic that can help reduce premenstrual fluid retention. When you steam asparagus, save the water, let it cool, and gulp it down.

■ **Alzheimer's.** According to a study, not getting enough of the B vitamin folate could cause your brain to atrophy. Folate, as well as vitamins B_6 and B_{12}, may keep your gray matter intact by keeping levels of homocysteine, a by-product of natural body functions, in check. Since excess homocysteine is associated with Alzheimer's disease, it pays to pad your diet with folate-rich orange juice, along with plenty of vegetables.

■ **Poor digestion.** Living in our toxic world can overburden your liver and compromise its ability to metabolize fats and cholesterol. Perk it up a bit by squeezing a lemon into your daily water ration. The lemon juice helps prod your digestive system, including your liver, encouraging it to go to work.

Just What the Doctor Ordered!

Do the Vanishing Act

Lemon juice is a mild bleaching aid that works as well on age spots as it does on fabric stains. Mix equal parts of lemon juice and water, apply some to each spot, and leave it on for 5 minutes before rinsing. Repeat three times a week, and the brown spots may fade to taupe. Use more lemon juice and less water as your skin gets used to the preparation. Your goal is to be able to apply the juice "straight up."

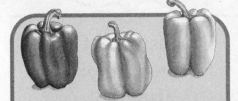

Fabulous Food Fix

Sweeter Feet

Applying radish or turnip juice to your feet can help reduce odors because the juices are natural deodorants.

■ **Age spots.** Mushroom juice contains kojic acid, a lightening agent derived from Japanese mushrooms that has been found to block the overproduction of melanin. "It's just as effective as hydroquinone for fading age spots without overlightening or irritating skin," says Jeanette Jacknin, M.D.

■ **Weak nails.** Carrot juice contains loads of calcium and phosphorus and is great for strengthening nails. Try replacing your O.J. with the other orange-colored juice several times a week.

■ **Burns.** As long as you don't have kidney or stomach problems, you can take 1,000 milligrams of vitamin C daily from juice or in supplement form to reduce cell damage caused by burns.

■ **Chemo side effects.** Chemotherapy patients often experience a lot of stomach upset. Fruit and vegetable juices are easy to get down, and they provide high concentrations of antioxidants and chlorophyll, both of which may help neutralize toxins from chemotherapy or radiation.

■ **Tooth stains.** Fresh strawberry juice is said to whiten teeth over time. Paint the juice on your teeth and leave it on for 5 minutes, then rinse with warm water to which you've added a pinch of baking soda.

■ **Canker sores.** Rinse your mouth with 1 to 3 tablespoons of aloe juice three times a day to dull the pain and reduce bacteria in your mouth. Be sure to get aloe juice, not gel.

■ **Hemorrhoids.** Is blood from hemorrhoids staining the toilet water red? Simply mix a few ounces of cranberry juice with an equal amount of pomegranate juice and drink it between meals. Both are hemostatics, which help stop bleeding.

■ **Heartburn.** To reduce heartburn and soothe indigestion and gassiness, drink a cup of papaya juice to which you've added 1 teaspoon of organic sugar and two pinches of cardamom. Both aid digestion and reduce gas and cramping.

■ **UTIs.** Cranberry juice contains bacteria-fighting compounds called proanthocyanidins, condensed tannins that have been shown to keep the bacteria that cause urinary tract infections (UTIs) from attaching to the urinary tract, even in people with antibiotic-resistant strains. At the first sign of burning, start drinking 2 cups of unsweetened cranberry juice every hour.

■ **Gallbladder problems.** Because the gallbladder is intimately involved in digestion, it makes sense that food therapies can help it work a little better. A traditional way to boost its function is to drink vegetable-juice cocktail that includes celery, parsley, beets, carrots, radishes, and lemon. Rowan Hamilton, Dip.Phyt., recommends combining any or all of the ingredients to suit your taste and drinking about two cups a day.

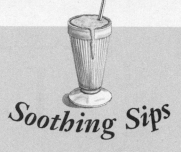

Soothing Sips

GET UP AND GO WITH PRUNES

Ounce for ounce, prunes are packed with more fiber than almost any other fruit or vegetable—including dried beans. What's more, they contain dihydroxyphenyl isatin, a natural laxative. Down a glass of juice before bed to encourage a morning bowel movement.

Juices 243

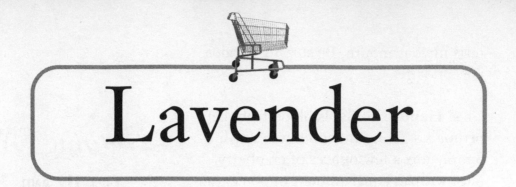

Lavender

SWEET SMELL, STRONG MEDICINE

Lavender is one of the best-smelling garden herbs, and one of the most powerful. It's traditionally been used to ease depression and lift the spirit, but scientists have recently found that it's just as effective for the body as it is for the mind. Take a look.

■ **Sunburn.** Lavender is an antiseptic, cooling herb that can relieve the sting of sunburn and protect against secondary infections. Fill an 8-ounce spray bottle with cold water and add 6 drops of lavender oil. Shake well, then spray on the burned areas.

Relax and De-Stress

A few drops of lavender oil added to your body lotion can be a source of anxiety-preventing aromatherapy all day long. For a more dramatic effect, add a drop of lavender oil to a dab of your favorite salve and rub it into your temples or solar plexus as a reminder to relax and breathe deeply.

■ **Aches and pains.** For general pain, try a soothing soak. First, put ⅓ cup each of chamomile, lavender, and lemon balm into a muslin bag and put it in the tub while you run the water. Then pour in 2 cups of Epsom salts and swirl the water to dissolve the salts. Soak in the tub for 10 to 15 minutes or until you break a healthy sweat.

244

■ **Joint pain.** To relieve sore joints, add a few drops of arnica oil to a warming wintergreen, lavender, or rosemary salve. All three can help increase circulation to the area. Use three or four drops of oil for each ½ teaspoon of salve and apply to sore joints three or four times a day. Arnica is for external use only; do not use on broken skin.

■ **Thinning hair.** Barbers have long known that massaging the scalp with lavender oil simulates circulation, feeding both oxygen and nutrients to hair follicles and perhaps stimulating hair growth. Add six drops of lavender oil to ½ cup of warm almond, soy, or sesame oil (all of which easily penetrate the skin) and massage the mixture into your scalp for 20 minutes, then wash it out with shampoo to which you've added three drops of bay oil.

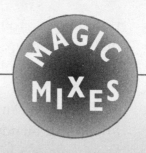

MAGIC MIXES

FABULOUS FOOT TONIC
Tired feet? Pamper them at the end of the day with a relaxing soak in a basin of warm water to which you've added some Epsom salts and a few drops of lavender, chamomile, or peppermint oil. The oils reduce inflammation as well as muscle spasms.

■ **Burns.** Ever since French perfume chemist René-Maurice Gattefossé healed his burned hand by plunging it into a vat of lavender oil, this scented herb has been used to guard against infection and prevent burn scars. Apply several drops of oil directly to your burn throughout the day.

■ **Earache.** Rubbing oil behind your ear (where your lymph glands are located) or placing an oil-saturated cotton ball inside your ear may soothe an earache and help stimulate the lymph glands to remove infectious agents. You can make your own oil by mixing several drops of lavender oil with a few tablespoons of olive oil.

■ **Corns.** Any oil softens the skin, but herb-infused oil blends stimulate circulation and help keep your feet healthy and ache-free, says Pamela Taylor, N.D. She recommends a blend of the following oils: Add two drops each of peppermint oil and carrot seed oil to an ounce of calendula oil, then mix in five drops each of lavender oil and geranium oil. Store the mixture in a small bottle and massage it into your feet once a day—more often when your corns are aching.

■ **Ingrown toenail.** To treat an ingrown nail, put a quart of water in a saucepan, then add 1 cup of dried calendula flowers, 1 tablespoon of dried thyme, and ½ cup of dried lavender flowers. Simmer the mixture for 5 minutes, let it cool to room temperature, and pour it into a basin. Soak your foot for about 5 minutes to fight infection and reduce painful swelling.

■ **Boils.** Tea tree and lavender are two of the most powerful herbal oils for killing bacteria and helping boils heal more quickly. Add a few drops of either to a cup of warm water, then moisten a washcloth and hold it on the boil for about 10 minutes several times a day.

Just What the Doctor Ordered!

Steam Away Acne

You can prevent blemishes with an antiseptic herbal steam. Just place 1 tablespoon of lavender flowers in a pot of hot water. Bend over the pot so the steam bathes your face (but don't get close enough to burn yourself). Let the lavender vapors steam your face for 15 minutes, then rinse with cool water and pat dry.

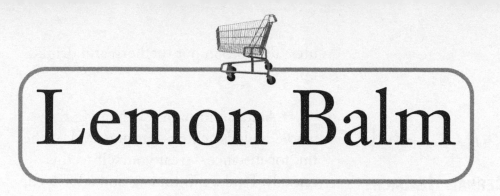

Lemon Balm

A SWEET-SMELLING HEALER

A lemon-scented member of the mint family, lemon balm (melissa) has been a favorite of herbalists for centuries. It smells (and tastes) a heck of a lot better than modern medicines, and in some cases it's just as effective. Here's why.

■ **Colds.** Immune-stimulating and astringent herbs can help ease the discomforts of a cold. Combine equal parts of yarrow, lemon balm, licorice root, ginger, eyebright, and rose hips, then add 1 heaping teaspoon of the mixture to a cup of hot water. Steep for 10 minutes, strain, and drink two or three cups per day. Don't use licorice root if you have high blood pressure or kidney disease.

■ **Hangover.** Ease your poor self to the kitchen when you have a hangover. Lemon balm tea is delicious and will help ease your headache and lift your sagging spirits. Put 2 teaspoons of dried leaves in 1 cup of boiling water and steep for 10 min-

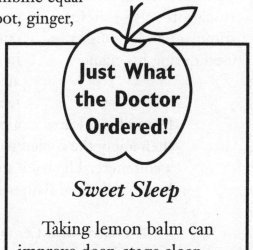

Just What the Doctor Ordered!

Sweet Sleep

Taking lemon balm can improve deep-stage sleep. Follow the label directions.

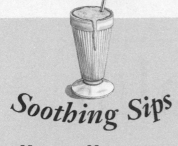

Soothing Sips

HERBAL HEADACHE HEALER

When a headache is starting up, prepare a tea of feverfew, lemon balm, and ginger with 1 teaspoon of dried herb per cup of hot water. Steep for 10 minutes, then strain. Drink up to three cups daily. Feverfew may cause mouth irritation in sensitive individuals. It's also a uterine stimulant and shouldn't be used during pregnancy.

utes, then strain out the herb and drink up.

■ **Aches and pains.** When your whole body is aching—from a cold or the flu, for instance—treat yourself to this remedy. Find a muslin bag and add ⅓ cup each of chamomile, lavender, and lemon balm. Start to run the water in the tub, then toss in the bag. Add 2 cups of Epsom salts and swirl the water to dissolve them. Get into the tub and soak for 10 to 15 minutes, or until you start to sweat.

■ **Cold sores.** Studies show that lemon balm helps cold sores heal quickly with less crusting. "Lemon balm contains at least four antiviral compounds," explains Jeanette Jacknin, M.D., "so it's considered by some to be a first-choice herbal treatment." The key is to apply it at the first inkling of an outbreak. Make a tea by steeping 2 to 4 teaspoons of dried lemon balm leaves in a cup of hot water for 10 minutes or so, then apply the cooled solution directly to the sore. Or look for a commercial lip balm that contains lemon balm and slather it on.

■ **Heartburn.** Lemon balm is a time-honored relaxant that can help soothe jangled nerves—and that's good for your insides. Heartburn can pop up at any time, but it's a lot more common

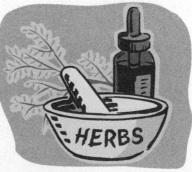

Lemon Balm

when your stress levels are reaching the combustion zone. When you defuse stress, you almost automatically reduce the risk of heartburn, so try this stress-easing tea. Steep 2 to 3 teaspoons of dried lemon balm leaves in a cup of hot water for 10 minutes, then strain and sip one to three times a day.

■ **Herpes.** To help cut the healing time for genital herpes, find an ointment that contains lemon balm and apply it two to four times a day. The herb contains a variety of antiviral chemical compounds that can help knock out the infection and promote faster healing.

■ **Shingles.** Just as lemon balm exudes a heavenly scent in your garden, you can use it to get heavenly relief from the itching of shingles— and perhaps even heal more quickly. Simply wrap some moist leaves in a damp cloth and apply it to your blisters. You can also drink lemon balm tea, made by steeping 1 to 2 teaspoons of dried leaves in a cup of hot water for 10 to 15 minutes. Strain out the herb and sip three cups of tea a day.

■ **Intestinal spasms.** This sweet-smelling herb can help relax muscles and calm a roiling digestive tract. Add 6 to 12 drops of lemon balm extract to a glass of water and drink it three times a day.

MAGIC MIXES

RUB AND RELAX
An abdominal massage can help release nervous tension and emotional stress, both of which are often held in the belly. Just add four to six drops of lemon balm or chamomile oil to 1 tablespoon of massage oil. Using gentle pressure, smooth the oil over your abdomen in wide circles. Then, beginning at your belly button, massage in small clockwise circles with your fingertips and gradually expand to bigger circles.

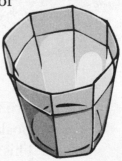

Lemon Balm

Lemons

PUCKER POWER

A squeeze of lemon gives zip to just about any recipe, and nothing beats a tall glass of lemonade on a hot summer day. But there's more to lemons than mouth-puckering tartness. As it turns out, there's a lot of healing power beneath that brash yellow skin. Here's what we mean.

■ **Cranky gut.** If your digestive system isn't working as well as it should—maybe you get heartburn a little too often, or you feel bloated and heavy after eating—sip a little lemon water. It jump-starts the digestive process and helps it work more efficiently. Simply add a squeeze of lemon juice to ½ cup of warm water and drink it before each meal.

■ **Coughs.** Here's a traditional (and delicious) remedy for nagging coughs: Heat a little red wine, add lemon, cinnamon, and sugar, and sip it before bed.

■ **Sore throat.** Here's an inexpensive remedy for a sore throat: Soak half a lemon in saltwater, then suck on it for a while. This treatment moistens your throat and relieves soreness (but it's not recommended for people with high blood pressure).

■ **Dull hair.** A lemon rinse makes your hair squeaky clean and shiny, and it helps remove dandruff flakes. Dilute 2 ounces of juice in a quart of water and rub it in well after shampooing.

■ **Dull nails.** Clean up dingy, tired-looking nails with a lemon scrub. Cut a lemon in half and dig your fingers into the juicy flesh. Just be sure that your fingers don't have cuts or scrapes on them, or you'll be in for a stinging surprise!

■ **Queasiness.** If you're feeling nauseated, try this traditional remedy from India. Simply grab a lemon, scratch into the peel, and inhale the fresh citrus aroma.

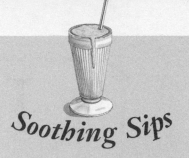

Soothing Sips

PICK UP THE IRON

Ever wonder about the Southern habit of spicing up greens with vinegar? Acidic condiments, such as vinegar and lemon juice, help liberate the iron in greens so it's more easily absorbed by your body—and that can help reverse iron-deficiency anemia.

■ **Age spots.** Age spots may be a natural skin change, but that doesn't mean you have to put up with them. Try cutting a lemon in half and rubbing the exposed fruit along the backs of your hands several times a day. The spots will gradually start to fade.

■ **Dragon breath.** Lemons are a great remedy for bad breath because they boost the flow of saliva and help flush away odor-causing germs. Squeeze the juice of half a lemon into ½ cup of water, then swish and spit.

■ **Laryngitis.** When you have laryngitis, enjoy a few cups of tepid tea with lemon and honey. It's very soothing for your larynx.

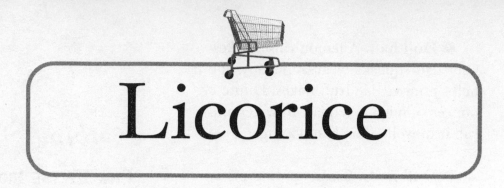

Licorice

ROOT FOR YOUR HEALTH

Forget the licorice candy that you eat at the movies. Real licorice—a root used in herbal medicine for thousands of years—is 50 times sweeter than sugar. People with high blood pressure or kidney disease should steer clear of it, but for the rest of us, the benefits are sweet indeed. Check 'em out.

■ **Infections.** If you're getting medical treatment for an infection, you can help strengthen your immune system. Combine equal parts of echinacea, goldenseal, and licorice root and steep 1 heaping teaspoon in 1 cup of hot water for 15 minutes. Strain and drink two or three cups daily.

■ **Dragon breath.** Forget the plastic bristles: You can make your own cleansing herbal toothbrush. Peel a length of licorice root and chomp on it. Fray the ends for an instant mouth freshener.

Just What the Doctor Ordered!

Cream the Cankers

Licorice gel contains a chemical compound that helps ease canker sores by thickening the mucous lining of the mouth. "When my patients use licorice gel, their canker sore pain disappears in 30 seconds," says Jennifer Reid, N.D.

■ **Bronchitis.** For quick relief from bronchitis, make a soothing tea by soaking 2 heaping tablespoons of marshmallow root in 1 quart of cold water overnight. Strain, then bring 1 cup of the tea to a boil. Add ½ teaspoon each of licorice root and thyme, cover, and steep for 15 minutes. Drink three or four cups per day.

■ **Heartburn.** Chewable tablets of deglycyrrhizinated licorice (DGL), which have had the blood pressure–raising component of licorice root removed, can help soothe heartburn. Chew two to four tablets before meals or follow the package directions.

■ **Sore throat.** Here's a blast of natural relief for a sore throat: First, buy yourself a new plant mister. Then make a triple-strength tea by adding 3 teaspoons each of dried slippery elm, echinacea, and licorice to 3 cups of water. Bring it to a full boil, then reduce the heat and let it simmer for 10 to 15 minutes. Strain out the herbs and pour the brew into your new spray bottle. Open your mouth, stick out your tongue, and spray the back of your throat as needed during the day. Ahh, relief!

■ **Eczema.** The glycyrrhizin in licorice works like a topical steroid to reduce the inflammation of eczema. Simmer 2 table-

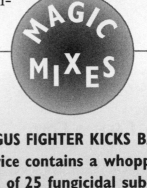

FUNGUS FIGHTER KICKS BACK
Licorice contains a whopping total of 25 fungicidal substances, just what you need when you have athlete's foot or any other fungal foot infection. Too bad munching on licorice whips won't do the trick. What you need to do is add 6 teaspoons of powdered licorice to a cup of boiling water and simmer for 20 minutes. Strain out any residue, let the tea cool, and dab it on your inflamed toes three times a day.

Soothing Sips

CALM A COLD

When you have a cold, the steam from hot licorice tea will speed the flow of mucus from your nose, and ingesting the herb will stimulate production of interferon, which helps the body defend against viral invaders, brings mucus up from the lungs, and soothes a scratchy throat.

spoons of ground, dried licorice root in 2 cups of water for 15 minutes, then strain the solution, let it cool, and apply it to your eczema. You can also buy glycyrrhetinic acid cream and apply it to itchy areas three or four times a day.

■ **Low libido.** Want to perk up your sex drive? Take a whiff of Good and Plenty licorice candy. According to studies at the Smell and Taste Treatment and Research Foundation, when women sniffed it, their vaginal lubrication—and libido—increased.

■ **Herpes.** To help cut the healing time for genital herpes outbreaks, dab on an ointment that contains glycyrrhetinic acid, one of the active chemicals in licorice, several times a day.

■ **Arthritis.** Licorice root is a friend indeed when your arthritis flares up, because it can counteract the inflammation. Brew a cup of tea by steeping 1 teaspoon of dried licorice in 8 ounces of water. Sip it twice a day for up to three weeks.

■ **Flu.** Drinking just about any herbal tea feels good when you have the flu, but licorice tea is especially good because of its antiviral properties. Drink a cup or two a day until you feel better. To make the tea, add a teaspoon of licorice to a cup of hot water, steep for 10 minutes, and strain.

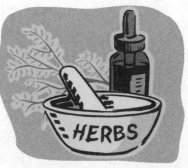

Licorice

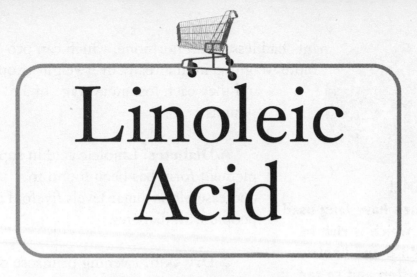

Linoleic Acid

A FRIENDLY FAT

These days, there's almost a collective, horrified gasp if you even mention the word *fat*. It's true that some fats, especially saturated and trans fats, are bona fide health wreckers. Other fats, however, including linoleic acid, are actually good for you—and may, in some cases, reverse some potentially serious health problems. See what you think.

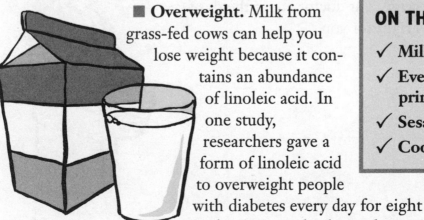

■ **Overweight.** Milk from grass-fed cows can help you lose weight because it contains an abundance of linoleic acid. In one study, researchers gave a form of linoleic acid to overweight people with diabetes every day for eight weeks. As a result, the study partici-

ON THE SHELF

✓ Milk
✓ Evening primrose oil
✓ Sesame seeds
✓ Cooking oils

255

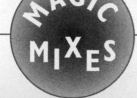

pants had less leptin hormone, which can promote weight gain in already overweight people, and they each lost an average of 3.5 pounds.

OPEN, SESAME!
Indian women have long used sesame oil, which is rich in both vitamin E and linoleic acid, to moisten and soften dry, cracked hands and feet. Pour 1/2 cup of sesame seeds and 1/4 cup of warm water into a blender and process for 3 minutes. Strain the lotion, apply it to your skin, and leave it on for as long as possible. Rinse with warm water, then cool water, and blot dry.

■ **Diabetes.** Linoleic acid in supplement form has been found to decrease blood sugar levels fivefold in people with diabetes.

■ **Dry skin.** Evening primrose oil contains two forms of linoleic acid, both of which may alleviate dry skin. Take 1,000 milligrams (about a tablespoon) of oil three times a day, or get gel caps and follow the dosage instructions on the label.

■ **Cancer.** There's a chance that linoleic acid may inhibit tumors in the breasts, ovaries, lungs, and colon.

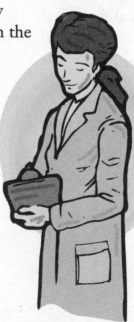

Talk with your doctor about the dose that's right for you.

Linoleic Acid

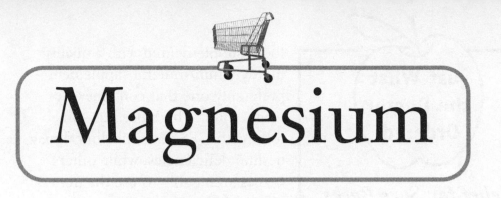

Magnesium

ONE MIGHTY MINERAL

The solution to many of our most serious health threats doesn't come from a high-tech laboratory; it's magnesium, one of nature's most common minerals. It's found in abundance in dozens of your favorite foods—and the list of its potential benefits just keeps on growing. If you feel that your diet doesn't provide enough and you're considering supplements, check with your doctor first.

■ **Heart disease.** Studies show that the magnesium in walnuts, almonds, and pecans can protect your heart. As a bonus, these same nuts can also lower cholesterol, according to a report in the *Journal of the American Dietetic Association*. In fact, people who eat nuts regularly have a much lower risk of heart disease and heart attack than those who don't eat them.

■ **CFS.** If you have chronic fatigue syndrome (CFS), you will benefit by eating mostly natural plant

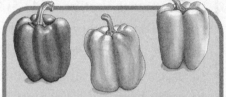

Fabulous Food Fix

The Muscle Mineral

Spinach (as well as other leafy greens, dried beans, lentils, and avocados) is loaded with magnesium, which is important for stoking energy and relieving muscle pain. In fact, people who get frequent muscle cramps may have a magnesium deficiency.

257

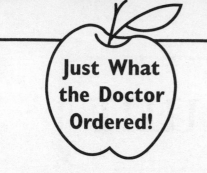

Just What the Doctor Ordered!

Relief for Sore Backs

Supplements that contain both calcium and magnesium can encourage your tense back muscles to loosen and relax. Look for combination supplements that provide 500 to 1,000 milligrams of calcium and 200 to 400 milligrams of magnesium. Capsules tend to work better than tablets because they're easier for the body to break down.

foods supplemented with a quality multivitamin/mineral supplement—preferably one that contains extra magnesium. That's because some folks with CFS have subclinical magnesium deficiencies, while others' bodies aren't able to use the mineral efficiently.

■ **Bloating.** Potassium and magnesium counterbalance sodium and help reduce fluid in your body when you're feeling a little bloated. To get plenty of potassium, enjoy grapes, orange juice, vegetable juices, and—of course—bananas. Most of us get enough magnesium in the food we eat, but if you suspect you don't, add some wheat germ, whole grains, and nuts to your diet.

■ **Magnesium deficiency.** According to the *Journal of the American Dietetic Association*, chocolate cravings may be a result of magnesium deficiency. When your body's under stress, it uses more magnesium, and that can make you feel down. Since having a little chocolate may stabilize both your mood and your magnesium levels, you can think of it as a good reason to indulge (as if you needed one!).

■ **Brittle nails.** Calcium and magnesium are essential to nail health. Make your own herbal mineral potion by mixing together equal parts of

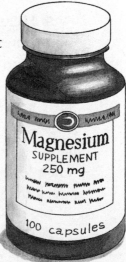

Magnesium

nettle, horsetail, and oats. Steep 1 heaping teaspoon in 1 cup of hot water for 10 minutes, strain, and drink one or two cups daily. If you use fresh nettle, be sure to wear gloves to avoid the stinging hairs.

■ **Brain fog.** For mental alertness, we all need minerals such as magnesium, potassium, and boron because they help brain cells communicate more efficiently. Millet, dark leafy greens (such as collards, kale, and broccoli), and figs are full of them. Include these foods in your diet every day.

■ **Osteoporosis.** There's magic in magnesium when you're trying to protect your bones. Along with calcium, you need this mineral to prevent osteoporosis, the bone-thinning disease that affects millions of women after menopause. Good sources of magnesium are potatoes, seeds, nuts, legumes, whole grains, and dark green vegetables, and supplements are an option if you don't think you're getting enough in your diet.

■ **Stiff blood vessels.** Kale, mustard greens, and turnip greens are all loaded with magnesium, a mineral that relaxes

Defend Your Airways

If you have asthma, think of magnesium, a mineral found in dark leafy greens, whole grains, nuts, and fish, as "a sedative for your bronchial tubes," suggests Anna Szpindor, M.D. According to studies, a diet deficient in magnesium may contribute to more frequent and severe flare-ups. If you go the supplement route, take 400 milligrams each of magnesium gluconate and calcium citrate (which can guard against the bone thinning that may result from long-term use of corticosteroids, often used to treat asthma) twice a day, suggests Dr. Szpindor.

Magnesium 259

the body's smooth muscles, including those that encircle blood vessels. "Magnesium is critical for keeping blood vessels toned so they're less likely to seize up with exertion," says Robert Bonakdar, M.D. Since magnesium can cause loose stools in some people, Dr. Bonakdar suggests starting with 200 milligrams daily between meals and then slowly building up to 400 milligrams twice a day if your bowels can tolerate it.

■ **Constipation.** There's a reason one of the best-known laxatives is called milk of magnesia: A magnesium deficiency can cause constipation. Make it a point to eat magnesium-rich greens regularly, and if you're frequently constipated, you may want to add supplements.

■ **Dizziness.** Calcium and magnesium act as antispasmodics to ease open narrowed blood vessels that may cause dizziness by reducing blood flow to the inner ear, says Michael D. Seidman, M.D. You can probably take a "cal-mag" supplement, with a goal of getting 400 milligrams of magnesium and 1,000 milligrams of calcium a day.

■ **Injuries.** Although many foods are high in magnesium, you need extra-large amounts after an injury because the mineral relaxes muscles and promotes healing. You might consider taking a magnesium supplement until your injury heals.

■ **Angina.** Magnesium has a variety of critical functions, and one of them is keeping the heart healthy and strong. When you have angina, make an extra effort to get plenty of magnesium. It's probably fine to take supplements.

Magnesium

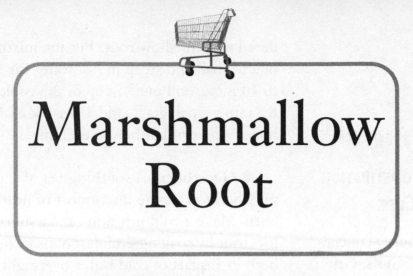

Marshmallow Root

SLIPPERY AND SMOOTH

If your only experience with marshmallow is setting one on fire at the end of a stick, you're in for a surprise. This herbal remedy isn't part of a graham-cracker-and-chocolate treat. It's a natural soother and moisturizer that you really shouldn't do without. Here's why.

■ **Dry hair.** Marshmallow is a great natural moisturizer for dry hair. Put 2 teaspoons of dried marshmallow root into 1 cup of boiling water and steep for about 15 minutes. Strain out the herb and let the solution cool in the refrigerator before using it to rinse your hair.

■ **Gas.** To relieve gas, crush 1 tablespoon of dried bee balm leaves with 1 teaspoon of pow-

Splinter Be Gone!

Marshmallow ointment can coax a stubborn splinter to the surface of your skin. Dab some on the site, cover with a bandage, and leave it alone for a few hours. When you remove the bandage, the splinter will have inched close enough to the surface for you to easily pluck it out with a pair of sterilized tweezers.

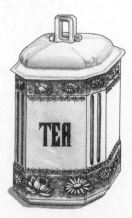

Soothing Sips

SLICK CONSTIPATION CURE

This slippery concoction softens stools. Grind equal parts of marshmallow root, flaxseed, and slippery elm in a coffee grinder. Stir 1 rounded teaspoon into an 8-ounce glass of water and drink immediately. Repeat once or twice daily, following each dose with another full glass of plain water. For added benefit, mix in unfiltered apple juice for bowel-soothing pectin.

dered marshmallow root. Put the mixture in a tea ball and steep in hot water for 5 to 10 minutes. Pour ½ cup of the cooled tea into a small glass, add 1 teaspoon of honey, and drink it before each meal.

■ **Heartburn.** A soothing tea of slippery herbs eases the discomfort of heartburn. Make a cold infusion of marshmallow root by soaking 2 tablespoons of the herb in 1 quart of cold water overnight. Strain, then drink throughout the day.

■ **Sore throat.** To ease a raspy, irritated throat, make a marshmallow tea base by soaking 2 tablespoons of marshmallow root in 1 quart of cold water overnight. Strain, then bring 1 cup of the tea to a boil. Add ½ teaspoon each of licorice root and thyme, cover, and steep for 15 minutes. Drink three or four cups a day. One caveat: People with high blood pressure or kidney disease should avoid licorice root.

■ **Cranky gut.** Marshmallow tea soothes inflamed tissues and helps heal the lining of the gut. Make a cold infusion by soaking 2 tablespoons of marshmallow root in 1 quart of cold water overnight. Strain and drink throughout the day.

■ **Queasiness.** Marshmallow tea is a traditional tummy soother. Simply steep 1 to 2 tablespoons in a cup of hot water for 10 minutes, then strain and drink.

Marshmallow Root

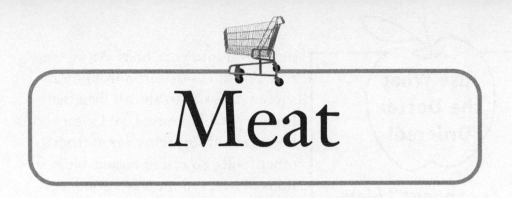

Meat

AN OCCASIONAL TREAT

Millions of Americans have cut back on meat in order to lower cholesterol and keep their weight under control, but you don't necessarily have to give up meat altogether. Lean beef as well as chicken, pork, and other meats are loaded with essential nutrients that you need for—well, just about everything. Take a look.

■ **Alzheimer's.** Meats and poultry are rich in B vitamins, which your brain needs to function properly. In particular, vitamins B_6 and B_{12} and folate may keep your gray matter going by keeping homocysteine levels in check. Since excess homocysteine, a by-product of metabolism, is associated with Alzheimer's disease, pad your diet with meats and poultry for B_6 and B_{12} and enjoy orange juice, broccoli and other cruciferous veggies, avocados, and legumes for a daily serving of folate.

■ **Anemia.** If you have iron-deficiency anemia, you may find it difficult just to work up the energy to get through each day. It's possible that blood loss is causing your symptoms, so you'll want to see your doctor, but you may simply need to get

263

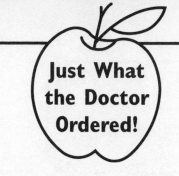

Just What the Doctor Ordered!

Zinc about This

Lean meats are rich in zinc, a mineral that may minimize age-related tinnitus and hearing loss. The recommended intake is 15 milligrams a day, which you can easily get simply by including lean meats in your diet. Alternate them with fish, which is also a good source of zinc.

more iron into your body. Most research shows that iron from meat sources is easier to absorb than that from vegetable sources, and meat boosts the absorption of iron from other foods, so eating reasonable portions of lean red meat is a good way to boost your iron stores.

■ **Angina.** Red meat provides carnitine, an amino acid that may help strengthen the heart muscle. That's important if you have angina, in which blood flow to the heart is restricted by narrowed arteries. Only super-lean cuts will help, however. Less-than-lean cuts are loaded with saturated fat—the stuff that your body turns into cholesterol and glues to your coronary arteries. Try one or two servings a week (a serving is a piece of meat the size of your fist that weighs 3 or 4 ounces).

■ **Weakened immunity.** You need plenty of protein to keep your immune system healthy. This is always important, but especially when you have an infection of some kind. To make sure you're getting enough, divide your weight by 2.2 to get your weight in kilograms, then eat 1 gram of protein daily for each kilogram of body weight. Lean meat is a good source of protein, as are beans and fish.

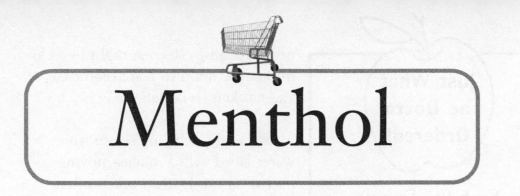

Menthol

HEAD-CLEARING GOODNESS

If you think that the penetrating smell of menthol is just for stuffy noses, you're not up to date on some of the latest news. That head-clearing pungency is just what the doctor ordered for all sorts of problems—including, of course, congestion. Here's what else it can do.

■ **IBS.** Peppermint is a natural menthol and antispasmodic herb. Doctors sometimes recommend it for patients with irritable bowel syndrome (IBS), which can cause painful intestinal cramps as well as sudden, gotta-go bouts of diarrhea. Try a cup of calming peppermint tea to relax the muscles of your digestive tract and relieve the spasms that trigger diarrhea. Just stir 1 teaspoon of mint leaves (fresh or dried) into 1 cup of hot water and steep for 10 minutes. Strain out the leaves and enjoy. Drink as many as three cups a day after meals.

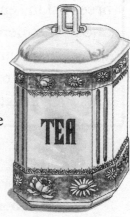

■ **Lung infections.** To protect your lungs during a cold or the flu, use a chest rub containing menthol or eucalyptus. Better yet, make your own rub with 1 teaspoon of olive oil and three or four drops of thyme oil. The warming vapors keep your respiratory passages open and moist even as they fight infection with their antiseptic action. Plus, they make it a lot

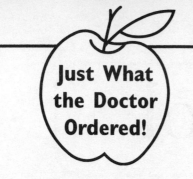

Just What the Doctor Ordered!

Stop the Sweats

If you're getting hot flashes, look for an over-the-counter menopause cream that relieves flushing with cooling ingredients such as menthol. When your body temperature begins to rise, just rub on the cream for a breezy skin sensation. Or try one of the menthol cooling sprays that come in palm-size canisters and tote it in your purse for instant heat relief.

easier to get to sleep at night by helping mucus drain so you breathe easier and awaken less often.

■ **Colds.** Inhaling steam from water laced with a mucus-moving herbal oil can help shrink swollen throat and nasal tissues, which will make you feel a lot better when you have a cold or sinusitis. Your partner will appreciate it, too, because this remedy can stop noisy snoring. Boil a pot of water to which you've added a few drops of peppermint (its menthol will give you the sensation of free-flowing air). Put the pot on a table or counter and lean over it (but not so close that you burn your skin). Drape a towel over your head and shoulders to capture the steam, then inhale deeply through your mouth and nose.

■ **Bug bites.** "I tell patients never to go camping or walking in the woods without a bottle of peppermint oil to carry along," says Sharol Tilgner, N.D. When you apply it to a bite, the cooling menthol will distract you from pain and encourage blood flow to the area to flush out the venom and disperse the inflammatory chemicals that have rushed to the site. The swelling and itch should fade pretty fast, Dr. Tilgner says. In a pinch, mint toothpaste will work, too.

■ **Foot aches.** Don't forget the menthol when your feet are sore or swollen. "Anything that has menthol or camphor in it will stimulate the flow of blood to the feet and wash away the inflammation that causes soreness," says Pamela Taylor, N.D.

■ **Sinus headache.** Here's a fast way to stop the pain of sinus headaches: Add a few drops of menthol or eucalyptus oil to hot water (just about as hot as you can stand it). Soak a small towel, wring it out, and drape it over your eyes, nose, or wherever else you hurt. The heat breaks up congestion and provides nearly instant relief.

■ **Cranky gut.** Since peppermint is bursting with natural menthol, it can quell stomach spasms, help digestion, and even kill bacteria. Sip a cup of peppermint tea after meals.

■ **Bugs.** Smooth mentholated rub onto your arms, legs, and neck to repel mosquitoes, ticks, and other bad biting bugs.

■ **Nail fungus.** Are you battling nasty toenail fungus? Massage mentholated rub into the skin around the nail twice a day until the fungus is gone. If you're prone to nail fungi, use the rub daily to prevent outbreaks.

A Must for Bad Backs

There are plenty of topical ointments that can help ease the muscle aches that accompany disk pain. Look for products that contain camphor or menthol, which produce a cooling sensation and decrease pain and inflammation. The sooner you knock out inflammation, the sooner you'll find yourself moving normally again.

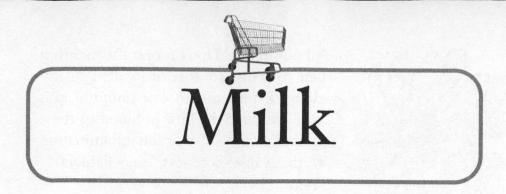

Milk

IT DOES DO A BODY GOOD

Milk has been called the perfect food, although that's certainly a bit of exaggeration by the dairy industry. It is true, though, that milk is packed with goodness that can benefit your body inside as well as out. Take a look.

■ **Poison ivy.** To ease the discomfort of poison ivy, dip a soft cloth in milk and gently wash the affected skin. Keep repeating the treatment throughout the day until the rash is healed. This remedy also works for irritation caused by handling hot peppers.

Save That Tooth!

If you've had a tooth knocked out, keep it moist by putting it in a glass of milk. Proteins in the milk will help keep the tooth alive until you can get to a dentist.

■ **Rough hands.** Do your hands feel like sandpaper? You can soothe them by rubbing a little warm milk into your skin each night.

■ **Eye irritation.** Are your eyes swollen, tired, or irritated (maybe from too many hours in front of the computer)? Soak two cotton pads in ice-cold cream or whole milk, then lie down in a comfortable place, put one pad over each eye, and relax for 10 minutes or so. Rinse with warm water, then cool water. The fat content of the liquid will soothe and moisturize the delicate skin around your eyes.

■ **Blackheads.** For a quick and easy facial cleanser, mix 2 tablespoons of whole milk with 2 tablespoons of warm (not hot) honey. Rinse your face with water and massage the cleanser in for a couple of minutes, then rinse it off and pat your face dry. This mixture doesn't keep well, so make it as you need it.

■ **Fatigue.** Folate is a key player in red blood cell production. If these cell levels drop, you'll feel draggy and fatigued—not just for an hour or two but possibly for weeks or months at a time. You can easily add more folate to your diet by having a few daily glasses of milk. If you're thinking of getting pregnant, plan ahead to focus on folate, since your need will double during pregnancy.

■ **Aging skin.** For ages, women have enjoyed lolling in milk baths—more specifically, in buttermilk baths, because of buttermilk's high lactic acid content, which is good for the skin. A tubful would probably mean you'd need your own cow, but many

MAGIC MIXES

MILKY NERVE MENDER
When you're tired and irritated, try this simple soother. In a blender, mix 2 cups of nonfat dry milk, 1 cup of cornstarch, and (if you like) your favorite scented oil. Add ½ cup of the mixture to your bathwater, sink into the tub, and relax. Store the remaining mixture in an airtight container at room temperature.

women simply bathe their face or hands in buttermilk once or twice a day to keep the skin soft and smooth.

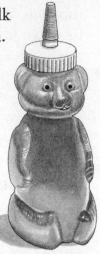

■ **Colds.** Before hundreds of commercial cold remedies became available, there were some home remedies that were probably a lot more fun. If you took enough, you got to the point where having a cold just wasn't a problem anymore. One traditional remedy is simply to drink warm milk and honey with a little booze mixed in.

■ **Weak bones I.** You need plenty of calcium to prevent osteoporosis, a serious, bone-thinning disease that affects millions of women after menopause and is a leading cause of hip and spinal fractures. The daily adult requirement is 1,200 milligrams (1,500 milligrams for post-menopausal women). Some of the best dairy sources are 8 ounces of milk (300 milligrams), 1 ounce of Cheddar cheese (200 to 300 milligrams), and 1 cup of yogurt (275 to 325 milligrams). Milk is generally fortified with vitamin D, which you need to help your body absorb calcium.

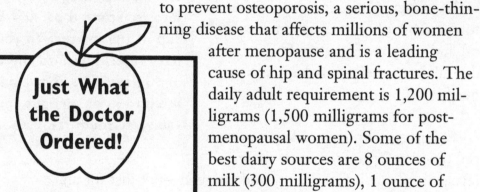

Just What the Doctor Ordered!

Bessie for Burns

Dabbing whole milk on sunburn for 15 minutes every 2 to 4 hours can be ultra-soothing. It's the fat content that does the trick, but don't try it until the heat has gone out of the burn, or you'll feel as if you've jumped into a fire.

■ **Weak bones II.** Vitamin D, which helps your body build strong bones, is stored in body fat and manufactured naturally in your body when you're exposed to sunlight. We often rely on the vitamin D supply we build up during the summer months, but in winter, some housebound folks may need a daily supplement. Drink at least one glass of vitamin D–fortified milk every day.

■ **Dry skin.** A milk and honey massage is one way to start your day off on the right foot, especially when your skin is as parched as desert air. Mix equal parts of honey and milk and, starting at your feet, massage the lotion into your thirsty skin. It's probably best to try this in the shower, where you can simply rinse off when you're done. Also, applying it when you're damp will lock all of that extra moisture into your skin, where you need it most.

■ **High blood pressure.** Potassium prevents thickening of the artery walls and works with sodium, an electrolyte, to regulate your body's fluid levels. That's important because too much fluid in your arteries can raise your blood pressure. Studies have shown that people who get enough potassium can sometimes get their blood pressure back to normal levels. Milk, along with bananas, apples, string beans, peas, and beans, will help you do it.

■ **Thinning hair.** While vitamins and minerals don't do a thing to jump-start hair growth in men, studies show they may prove helpful for some women. It's especially important to beef up the protein content of your diet by having plenty of milk and other protein-rich foods, such as poultry and fish, suggests Jeanette Jacknin, M.D.

■ **Insomnia.** Oats have long been used to soothe the nerves and treat insomnia, and milk further invites drowsiness, since

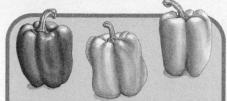

Fabulous Food Fix

Swish and Feel Better

Swishing milk around in your mouth will coat a canker sore and protect it from acids and other irritating substances, says David A. Sirois, D.M.D., Ph.D.

it's loaded with tryptophan. This amino acid is necessary for production of the brain chemical serotonin, which controls sleep patterns and helps you relax and unwind, so have a bowl of warm oatmeal before bed.

■ **Hangover I.** Fatty foods aren't good for your cholesterol levels, but they can protect your head when you're drinking. Alcohol enters your system more slowly when you have food in your stomach, and fatty foods are particularly good at delaying the absorption of alcohol. To help prevent morning-after misery, have some milk or indulge in some cheesy snacks.

■ **Hangover II.** Protein helps your brain cells regenerate when you have a hangover. A nice, cool glass of fat-free milk is the perfect way to get started.

■ **Tennis elbow.** When you're recovering from tennis elbow, you need a lot of protein, the nutrient that your body uses to repair muscle damage. The usual rule is to get 0.8 gram of protein for each kilogram of body weight. Here's an easy way to figure out how much you need: Divide your body weight by 2.2 (there are 2.2 pounds per kilogram), then multiply that number by 0.8 to get your daily target for protein. Thus, if you weigh 150 pounds, you'll need 54 grams of protein. That's roughly the amount you'd get in a cup of tuna salad, a cup of long-grain white rice, and a cup of milk.

■ **Pepper in the eye.** If you inadvertently get a few grains of pepper in your eye, flush it out with a few drops of milk.

Milk

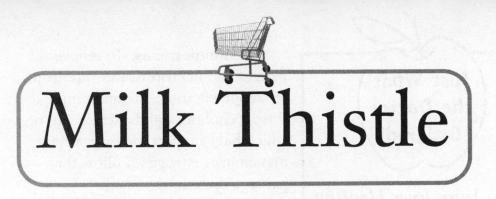

Milk Thistle

AN HERBAL POWERHOUSE

Herbalists traditionally used milk thistle to protect the liver and help with digestive problems. Studies have confirmed that it really works for liver health—and more besides. Here's the lowdown.

■ **Rosacea.** Silymarin, a component of milk thistle, can help reduce the inflammation of rosacea, says Gail L. Nield, M.D. It's especially effective when combined with vitamin E. If you use it when your face is merely pink, it could prevent it from progressing to the red stage. Follow the package directions.

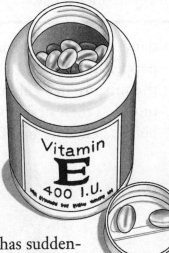

■ **Hormone imbalance.** If your hair has suddenly become either very oily or very dry, take 20 milligrams of milk thistle daily. It will help your liver rebalance your hormones.

■ **Lazy liver.** Using milk thistle occasionally tones the liver. Put 1 teaspoon of the dried herb into 1 cup of hot water, steep for 15 minutes, and strain. Drink one cup between meals.

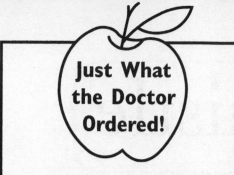

Just What the Doctor Ordered!

Keep Your Eyes Healthy

Milk thistle is a powerful antioxidant herb that may help protect vision and eye tissues. To use it, grind 1 teaspoon of milk thistle seeds and add them to your cereal or a smoothie once a day.

■ **Endometriosis.** To relieve the pain of endometriosis, use "lipotropic" supplements that contain milk thistle, choline, and dandelion, all of which help support the liver, which metabolizes estrogen. Follow the package directions.

■ **Hangover.** Bitters may help your liver metabolize alcohol and prevent morning-after miseries. Make some by mixing equal parts of

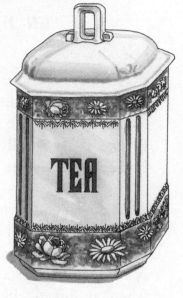

dandelion root, gentian, milk thistle, and peppermint. Steep 1 heaping teaspoon of the mixture in 1 cup of hot water for 20 minutes, then strain. Sip the tea slowly before bed and again first thing in the morning. People who take diuretics or potassium supplements shouldn't use dandelion.

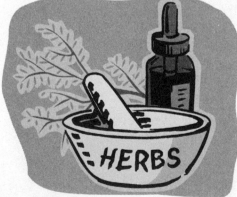

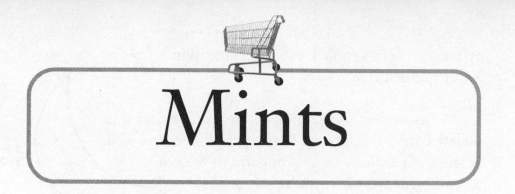

Mints

MEDICINES WITH A REFRESHING BLAST

Forget for a moment the mouth tingle that you get when you suck on peppermint candy or chew a piece of spearmint gum. Real mints, the kind that grow in your garden, are an entirely different story. They stimulate digestion, encourage circulation, and even knock out some of our most common infections. Take a look—but remember to be cautious when using essential oils internally.

■ **Queasiness.** The volatile oils in peppermint can help counteract nausea. Simply uncap a vial of peppermint essential oil and inhale for a few seconds. If you're feeling up to a bath, add four to six drops to your tub. Just remember to breathe deeply while you're soaking.

■ **Hives.** You may find some temporary relief from hot, itchy hives by dabbing them with cool mint tea. Stir 1 teaspoon of dried or fresh leaves into 1 cup of boiling water and simmer for 10 minutes, then strain out the herbs.

A Tangy Tummy Tamer

Placing a single drop of peppermint oil on your tongue may help calm stomach upset that often accompanies a hangover—and it tastes a whole lot better than that pink stuff or other over-the-counter remedies.

275

After the tea has cooled, rub it on your skin as a healing lotion.

■ **Insomnia.** You've probably heard of valerian, a sedative herb that no one likes to drink because, well, it smells like stinky socks. Peppermint tea is a tasty alternative when you're struggling with insomnia because it helps promote restful sleep.

MAGIC MIXES

OILY CORN FOILER

Any oil softens the skin, but herbal oil blends encourage blood flow and help keep your feet healthy, says Pamela Taylor, N.D. She recommends the following mixture. To an ounce of calendula oil, add two drops each of peppermint oil and carrot seed oil, then mix in five drops each of lavender oil and geranium oil. Store the blend in a small bottle and rub it into your feet once a day—more often when your corns are bothersome.

■ **Leg pain.** If you occasionally get leg cramps during exercise, there's a good chance that blood isn't flowing into your legs as efficiently as it should. To stimulate circulation, exercise your blood vessels with cold herbal wraps of yarrow and peppermint. Make a strong infusion by steeping 2 tablespoons of each herb in 2 cups of hot water, covered, for 15 minutes, then strain and chill. Meanwhile, prepare several lengths of gauze, muslin, or cheesecloth. When the infusion is thoroughly chilled, saturate the cloths, wrap them around your lower legs, and relax with your legs elevated for 20 minutes. Do this daily for several weeks.

■ **IBS.** If your digestive system isn't working the way it should, take capsules of peppermint oil three times a day between meals. This mint is especially helpful if you have irritable bowel syndrome (IBS)

Mints

because it's a powerful antispasmodic and pain reliever. If capsules aren't available, try using peppermint leaves to make tea. Steep 1 heaping teaspoon in a cup of hot water, covered, for 10 to 15 minutes. Strain and drink three cups daily between meals.

■ **Bug bites.** Don't go into the great outdoors without a bottle of peppermint oil. In fact, you may want to keep peppermint handy somewhere in your yard or other outdoor areas during the warm months. When you apply it to an insect bite, the menthol in mint provides a cooling sensation that distracts you from pain, and it encourages blood flow to the area to flush out the venom and disperse the inflammatory chemicals that have rushed to the site. Swelling and itching should subside pretty quickly.

■ **Stuffy nose.** You can make your own nasal balm to ease congestion. Place ¼ cup of petroleum jelly in a small saucepan and warm it until it melts. Remove it from the heat and stir in 10 drops each of peppermint essential oil, eucalyptus essential oil, and thyme essential oil. When the balm reaches room temperature, pour it into a clean jar for storage. Apply a small amount to your nostrils one to three times daily. The petroleum jelly prevents the essential oils from being

Mint Some Headache Relief

Studies show that if you rub peppermint oil—a proven anesthetic—on your forehead, you may be able to relieve the pain and reduce the sensitivity associated with tension headaches. What's more, if you use the oil daily, you may even be able to sidestep future headaches. Simply mix peppermint oil with an equal amount of rubbing alcohol and apply no more than a couple of drops to your forehead and temples. Wait 15 minutes, then massage the area for 3 minutes. Repeat three times a day.

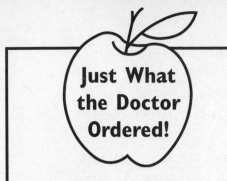

Just What the Doctor Ordered!

Hand It to Mint

This simple routine will help soften rough, dry hands. Mix 1 teaspoon of castor oil and 1 drop of lemon or peppermint oil. Massage it into your skin before bed, then sleep with cotton gloves on.

absorbed into the skin, so you can inhale the volatile oils for a prolonged period.

■ **Gas.** Ever wonder why restaurant waiters leave peppermints along with the check? It isn't, as you might suspect, a bribe for a fat tip but rather a nod to peppermint's ability to boost the flow of digestive juices and reduce gassiness and cramps. Too bad restaurants don't dispense them before meals! One study showed that nearly 80 percent of people who took peppermint capsules or tablets three or four times daily before meals had less flatulence. Look for enteric-coated peppermint capsules, which are less likely to cause heartburn and are just as effective for gas.

■ **Constipation.** To ease constipation, lie on your back and place a drop or two of peppermint oil on your abdomen. Press your palms firmly into your stomach and massage for 5 to 10 minutes in a clockwise motion to mimic the direction that food moves when passing through the digestive system. This approach is a lot safer than over-the-counter laxatives, and it feels better, too!

■ **Rashes.** A good Rx for any itchy rash is to mix gel from an aloe leaf with a drop of peppermint oil, then smear it on the affected area.

■ **Snoring.** Do you do some intense log sawing at night? To stop the racket, try inhaling steam from water laced with mucus-moving peppermint oil. First, add a few drops of oil to a pot of boiling water. Put the pot on a table or counter and lean over it (but at a safe distance so you don't burn your face). Drape a towel over your head and shoulders to capture the steam, then inhale deeply through your mouth and nose. The menthol in peppermint will give you the sensation of free-flowing air and shrink swollen throat and nasal passages.

■ **Yeast infections.** Peppermint oil is a powerful fungus fighter. If you get frequent yeast infections, pick up some capsules and take them according to the label directions. Be sure the oil is meant for internal use, and don't put it anywhere but in your mouth.

■ **Foot aches.** Peppermint is good for achy feet. Fill a basin with warm water, spike it with Epsom salts and a few drops of peppermint oil, then sit and soak your tired tootsies. The mixture helps reduce inflammation as well as muscle spasms.

■ **Canker sores.** An herbal tea made with peppermint is a great way to calm cantankerous cankers. Put several tea bags in a saucepan, cover them with water, and simmer, covered, for about 30 minutes. Let the tea cool to room temperature, swish it around in your mouth for 30 to 60 seconds, and swallow it, suggests John Hibbs, N.D. Repeat the treatment several times a day until the sore is completely gone.

Minty Breath Freshener

Bad breath is often caused by deposits of plaque on the teeth and at the gum line. Look for breath-freshening products that contain zinc gluconate and peppermint oil, one of nature's best neutralizers, along with coenzyme Q_{10}, a substance that tightens gum tissue so plaque can't become trapped there.

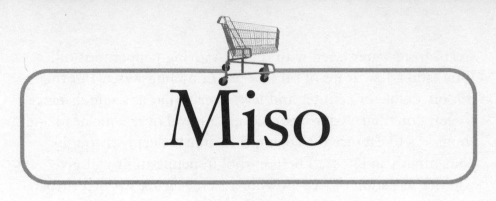

Miso

SOY GOOD

This rich, salty condiment made from soybean paste is a flavoring ingredient often used as a base for delicious Asian soups—and each spoonful provides a good-health bonus as well. Here's a sampling.

■ **Anemia.** Fermented soy foods such as miso aid your body's absorption of iron from foods and can help prevent iron-deficiency anemia.

■ **Chemo side effects.** If you're undergoing chemotherapy and keeping solid foods down is a problem, sip miso soup. Soups can help replenish the electrolytes (minerals necessary for normal heart rhythm, muscle contraction, and a whole host of other regular body functions) you lose when you vomit.

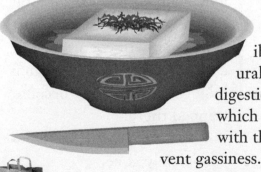

■ **Gas.** Miso is a great source of fructo-oligosaccharides, indigestible dietary sugars that feed the natural "friendly" bacteria that facilitate digestion. If you're taking antibiotics, which wipe out these good bacteria along with the bad, eating miso could help prevent gassiness.

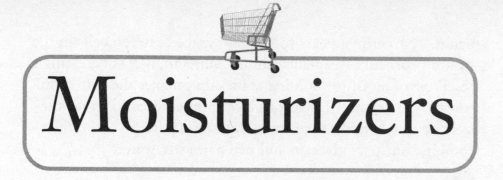

Moisturizers

PACK IN THE WATER

Your skin protects your body from every conceivable environmental assault, from bacteria and viruses to the sun's burning rays. But it can't do its job when it's as dry and crinkly as an old paper bag. Moisturizers can make a real difference in how your skin holds up over time—and, of course, they can make you feel (and look!) a whole lot better. Here's how.

■ **Dry skin.** For years, dermatologists have lauded petroleum jelly as the thickest emollient and therefore the best treatment for very dry skin. The problem, of course, is that its thick, greasy texture isn't the most pleasant thing to have on your skin. There is an alternative, though. There's evidence that moisturizers with large amounts of glycerin (which has a less greasy feel) may work just as well, if not

---

Homemade Tanning Oil

In a blender, mix the juice of a lemon with ¼ cup each of strong black tea and salt-free mayonnaise. Pour the mixture into a container with a lid, squeeze the contents of five vitamin E capsules (400 IU each) into it, and stir. Cover the container and keep it in the refrigerator, then slather on the lotion before you head out to bask in the sun. Just don't stay out too long—there's no sunscreen in this!

better. "Glycerin appears to increase space between cells in the stratum corneum," explains Leslie Baumann, M.D., "creating a reservoir of moisture-holding ability that makes the skin more resistant to drying." Look for glycerin in commercial moisturizers or simply make your own. Buy some pure glycerin, then combine one part glycerin and two parts rosewater.

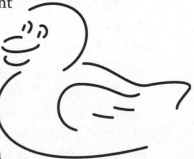

■ **Calluses.** Foot calluses aren't much to look at, and they can rub against the sides of shoes and create painful friction. If you have calluses, apply moisturizers that contain vitamin E oil, cocoa butter, or lanolin. They make calluses softer and less painful.

■ **Vaginal dryness.** It's common to lose vaginal moisture and lubrication over time, a process that accelerates in the years preceding menopause. Even more effective than lubricants are over-the-counter nonhormonal moisturizing gels, such as Replens. They hydrate the cells of the vaginal lining and allow them to build up a continually moist protective layer. In most cases, these products significantly increase moisture, acidity, and elasticity after a few months of use. Each application lasts up to three days; follow the package directions.

■ **Eczema.** Moisturizers can help prevent flareups of eczema, but among the different types, the American Academy of Dermatology says that ointments are best, creams are less helpful, and lotions, because they are made of mostly water, are least helpful. Whichever you choose, use it within 3 minutes of bathing to lock in the moisture from the bath.

Moisturizers

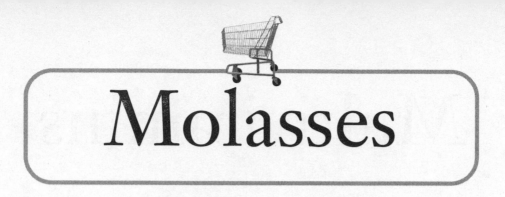

Molasses

A SWEETIE OF A HEALER

You can't have delicious gingerbread or pecan pie without the savory sweetness of molasses. This thick, syrupy liquid is better for you than plain sugar, and it actually has some impressive health benefits. Check 'em out.

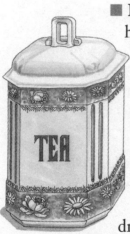

■ **Pregnancy aches.** In the latter half of pregnancy, women often experience aching and cramping in their legs. You can prevent the pain by eating foods rich in calcium and magnesium, including molasses. Make a tea by stirring 1 teaspoon of blackstrap molasses into 1 cup of hot water, then drink a cup every day.

■ **Weak nails.** Want to make your fingernails and toenails harder and stronger? Eat 1 tablespoon of molasses daily. It's rich in sulfur—one of the keys to maintaining healthy nails.

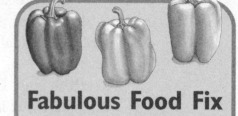

Fabulous Food Fix

Do Some Ironing

Blackstrap molasses is a great source of iron. In the old days, folks often slathered it on whole grain bread for breakfast. If you enjoy the taste, try eating about 2 tablespoons of molasses daily; you'll get about 10 milligrams of iron—nearly 40 percent of the daily requirement— and just 85 calories.

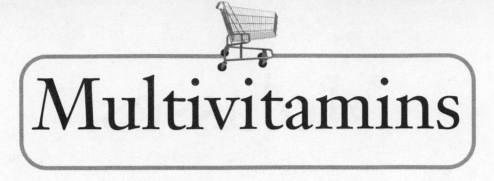

Multivitamins

HEALTH INSURANCE IN A PILL

Doctors have known for a long time that taking a multivitamin is the easiest way to prevent deficiency diseases caused by low levels of vital nutrients. Now, there's also good evidence that taking a daily multi can ward off dozens of other health threats besides. Here's how.

■ **Restless legs.** If you have restless legs syndrome, in which your legs go a little haywire and jerk, twitch, or tingle at night—you have to make sure your nerves get the nutrients they need to function properly. Take a high-potency multivitamin/mineral supplement that contains zinc and folic acid, suggests Andrew Weil, M.D. He also recommends taking a calcium/magnesium supplement at bedtime to help calm nerves and muscles. Ask your doctor about the dose that's right for you.

Safer Surgery

When you have surgery, taking vitamin and mineral supplements will ensure that your body's repair systems are working at peak efficiency. A daily multivitamin can help, so start taking it ahead of time.

■ **Clogged pores.** Vitamins A, C, and E are collectively referred to as antioxidants because they protect the body from oxygen-related free radicals that damage skin cells and promote inflammation, which can lead to blocked pores. Be sure your daily multivitamin/mineral tablet provides all three nutrients to fight free radicals before they do their dirty work.

■ **CFS.** A well-balanced diet is essential if you have chronic fatigue syndrome (CFS), but let's face it, it's hard to eat a proper diet when you're tired and dragging all the time. One way to boost your intake of key nutrients is to take a daily multi. It will give your body a good foundation to fight symptoms and repair any damage that may have occurred.

Just What the Doctor Ordered!

A Hormonal Helper

If you're gaining weight and feel sluggish, depressed, and cold, and a blood test indicates low levels of thyroid hormone, follow your doctor's orders, which may include taking a high-potency multivitamin that contains 800 IU of vitamin D (necessary for thyroid hormone production).

■ **Dull hair.** For healthy hair, some doctors suggest a high-potency multivitamin/mineral supplement that contains the B-complex vitamins, 1,000 milligrams of vitamin C, 400 IU of vitamin E, 15 milligrams of zinc, and 1.5 milligrams of copper. Check with your doctor about taking these supplements and ask about taking iron, especially if you have hair loss following crash dieting or physical trauma.

■ **Itchy scalp.** The B vitamins, particularly biotin, are essential to a healthy scalp, so make sure your multivitamin contains biotin, or take a B-complex supplement that contains 300 micrograms of biotin.

■ **Weak nails.** If your nails bend or break easily, you may have a deficiency of zinc, iron, essential fatty acids, or silica and other trace minerals. Try popping a multivitamin/mineral supplement and see if your nails improve. Look for a formula that contains 1,200 milligrams of calcium and about 15 milligrams of zinc, both of which contribute to nail strength.

■ **Sore throat.** Load up on vitamins A and C when you have a sore throat. Both strengthen immunity and increase the activity of specialized cells that fight infection. Take a multivitamin that contains both, plus (if you don't have stomach or kidney problems) 500 milligrams of vitamin C twice a day.

■ **Cuts and scrapes.** Skin injuries can take forever to heal, and ouch—they hurt! If you're not taking a daily multivitamin already, this is a good time to start. The extra nutrients will ensure that your body has all the raw materials it needs to repair your cut or scrape.

■ **Bruises.** When you have a bruise, your body's need for nutrients increases dramatically, particularly for zinc, vitamin A, and selenium. You'll get plenty of these and other healing vitamins and minerals by taking a

Where's the Boron?

Raisins, pears, apples, and other fruits, as well as nuts and beans, all contain the trace element boron, which can relieve pain and joint stiffness and actually appears to protect against arthritis. If you don't eat fruit on a regular basis or don't live in a particularly arid area, where concentrations of boron in the soil and water are highest, consider taking a daily multivitamin supplement that provides 1 to 3 milligrams of boron.

multivitamin every day until the bruise is gone.

■ **Bursitis and tendinitis.** That multivitamin you take every day with breakfast is especially important when you're coping with bursitis or tendinitis. There are a lot of nutrients that are important for connective tissue health, and a multivitamin provides them all.

■ **Canker sores.** Folic acid and vitamin A, along with the mineral zinc, are especially important if you have canker sores, since your body uses these nutrients to strengthen and maintain healthy membranes. You'll get plenty of protective nutrients just by eating a healthy diet, but taking a daily multivitamin is also a good idea.

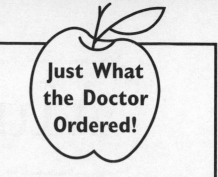

Just What the Doctor Ordered!

Supplement for Stones

It hasn't been proven, but there's some evidence that people who don't get enough vitamin B_6 in their diets are more likely to get kidney stones. If you've had kidney stones in the past, an easy preventive strategy is to take a daily multivitamin that contains the full Daily Value for B_6. Check the label of your multivitamin to make sure it says "100 percent."

■ **Gum disease.**

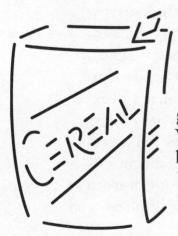

The B vitamin folic acid helps repair and replenish gum cells that have been damaged by gingivitis. The best way to get enough (the recommended amount is 400 micrograms a day) is to take a daily multivitamin. You can also get a good supply of this vitamin by eating plenty of plant foods, along with breakfast cereals fortified with it.

Mushrooms

MAKE ROOM FOR 'SHROOMS

Those tasteless button mushrooms sold in most supermarkets have about as much healing power as an office envelope. If you broaden your culinary horizons and load up on other mushroom varieties, however, you'll get an abundance of powerful chemical compounds—and, of course, some great tastes. Here's what they can do for you.

Pack In the Nutrients

You've probably noticed that when you cook mushrooms, they nearly vanish. That's because they're like little sacs full of water that leak when heated—and that's okay. It makes for tasty broth, and it concentrates nutrients so you get more per forkful.

■ **Heart attack and stroke.** Chinese tree ear mushrooms may help prevent circulatory diseases. One study showed that a single tablespoon of soaked mushroom taken three or four times a week may be as effective as daily aspirin for preventing strokes and heart attacks. What's more, the mushroom won't irritate your stomach as aspirin may. So load your plate—and try to eat them several times a week.

288

■ **Anemia.** Since folate is a key player in red blood cell production, it's essential for preventing anemia. You can easily add more to your diet by eating plenty of mushrooms, along with citrus fruits, dark green vegetables, liver, eggs, milk, wheat germ, and brewer's yeast. Because this B vitamin is destroyed by heat and light, eat your fruits and veggies fresh and cook them as little as possible. Also, if you're considering having a baby, start to get more folate now; your need will double when you're pregnant.

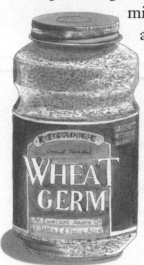

■ **Age spots.** Mushroom juice contains kojic acid, a lightening agent derived from Japanese mushrooms that has been found to block the overproduction of the skin pigment melanin. "It's just as effective as hydroquinone for fading age spots without overlightening or irritating skin," says Jeanette Jacknin, M.D. While juice from your portobello burger probably won't do the trick, any over-the-counter skin lotion that contains kojic acid will. Simply apply it twice daily, and your age spots may fade significantly in less than two months.

■ **UTIs.** Most supermarkets offer several tasty varieties of gourmet mushrooms. If you have a urinary tract infection (UTI), you should definitely eat them daily because they boost the ability of your immune system to combat infections. "Different mushrooms stimulate different aspects of the immune system, so it's good to combine them and get a broad spectrum of effects," says Crystal Abernathy, N.D. Look for shiitakes, reishis, and maitakes.

■ **Cancer.** Maitake, reishi, and coreolis mushrooms contain components that stimulate the immune system and may play a role in preventing cancer. So eat 'em and stay healthy!

■ **High cholesterol.** Eat shiitake mushrooms if you're watching your cholesterol. They have a slight but definite ability to lower very low density lipoprotein (VLDL) cholesterol, a particularly dangerous type. Also, both shiitake and maitake mushrooms appear to lower blood pressure.

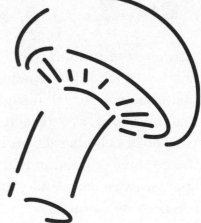

Fabulous Food Fix

Win the Cold War with Interferon

Smoky-tasting shiitake mushrooms amp up production of interferon, a protein that girds the body to defend against viral invaders, while reishi mushrooms may help ease respiratory tract inflammation. When you have a cold, either add these 'shrooms to your therapeutic chicken soup or look for them combined in extract form and follow the label directions, advises John Hahn, N.D., D.P.M.

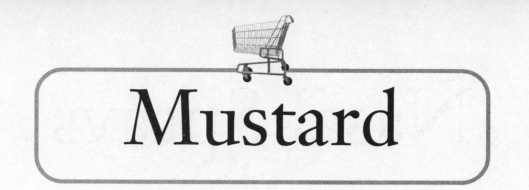

Mustard

A HOT YELLOW HEALER

If you think of mustard as mainly a way to zip up the taste of ballpark 'dogs, you're in for a surprise. It turns out that this brash yellow condiment has all sorts of healing powers, so open that jar and get started!

■ **Coughs.** Those little packets of hot mustard that accompany Chinese takeout can come in handy when you have a cough because they liquefy mucus and stop your barking.

■ **Stuffy nose.** When your nose and head are clogged to the max, spread ½ teaspoon of mustard or horseradish on three or four thin slices of ginger or garlic. By the time you're done eating, your congestion will be gone!

■ **Chest congestion.** An old-fashioned mustard poultice can ease a tight chest. Just add a few drops of water to a little dry mustard to create a thin paste, then apply it to your chest. Cover it with a layer of flannel and a heating pad set on low. Lift a corner of the cloth every 5 minutes to check for redness, and don't use the poultice for longer than a total of 15 minutes.

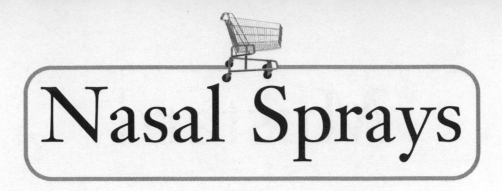

Nasal Sprays

SWIFT SNIFFER SOOTHERS

When your head's so congested it feels as if it's stuffed with cotton balls, reach for a nasal spray. Unlike pills, decongestant and anti-inflammatory sprays go to work almost instantly. And because the medicine goes right where it's needed, the sprays are among the safest remedies you can use. Check out these top picks from doctors.

Spray Away Sinusitis

For quick relief from sinusitis, use a saline nasal spray several times a day to remove mucus that could harbor bacteria. If you can find one that contains eucalyptus, so much the better. Eucalyptus kills bacteria, and it helps clear congestion that gives you that stuffed-up feeling.

■ **Colds.** Research indicates that zinc spray may cut the duration of colds by about two days. Spritz an over-the-counter zinc nasal spray into each nostril four times a day within 48 hours of the first inkling of a cold.

■ **Allergies.** Doctors often recommend starting to use an anti-inflammatory nasal spray a few weeks before the allergy season starts. These sprays are designed to short-circuit allergic reactions by blocking your body's release of histamine, a body chemical that causes congestion. You'll have less discomfort if you can block histamine before your allergies get a running start.

■ **Postnasal drip.** To wash away annoying postnasal drip, use a nasal douche or a Water Pik with a nasal nozzle. Make a solution of 1 teaspoon of baking soda or salt to 1 pint of warm water and irrigate your nose two to four times a day. If this treatment seems too elaborate, try using a simple saline nasal spray often to keep your nasal membranes moist, suggests the American Association of Otolaryngologists. This will minimize irritation that can kick mucus production into high gear.

■ **Dragon breath.** Using a saline nasal spray regularly helps thin out mucus from postnasal drip and keeps it from collecting on the back of your tongue. Bacteria use this protein-rich gunk to make smelly sulfur molecules and leave a sour taste in your mouth. The quicker you get rid of it, the less likely you are to experience room-clearing bad breath. You can buy a spray or make your own solution by dissolving ½ teaspoon of table salt in a glass of warm water. Put it in a bulb syringe and spritz your nostrils.

Just What the Doctor Ordered!

Fly the Ear-Friendly Skies

To avoid in-flight earaches, take an over-the-counter decongestant as soon as your flight is announced. Then, an hour before descent, use a decongestant nasal spray to help clear things up. It's also a good idea to drink plenty of water during the flight because dehydration from dry air in the aircraft cabin causes mucus to thicken.

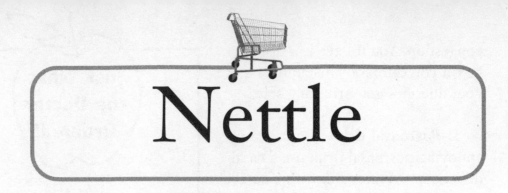

Nettle

SOOTHING SPINES

You wouldn't think that an herb that's loaded with sharp little spines could do so much good, but nettle, spines and all, deserves a place in every herbal medicine chest. Here's how to "get the point." If you use fresh nettle, be sure to wear gloves to protect your hands.

■ **Allergies.** Spring greens and flowers often make the best potions for allergy relief. Look in your backyard for nettle, eyebright, cleavers, and elderflowers. Pick them fresh, mix equal parts of each, and steep ¼ cup in 1 quart of water overnight. Strain the solution and drink it throughout the day.

■ **Dandruff.** Steaming your scalp with nutritive herbs is a deep cleansing treatment that fights dandruff. Mix together equal parts of fresh or dried rosemary, nettle, and peppermint leaves. Add 2 tablespoons of dried herb (½ cup fresh) to 2 cups of hot water and steep, covered, for 10 minutes. Strain the infusion, cool slightly, and apply it carefully to your scalp. Cover your hair with a shower cap and wrap your head in a hot, wet towel. Sit and chill out for 30 minutes, then rinse with an herbal rinse.

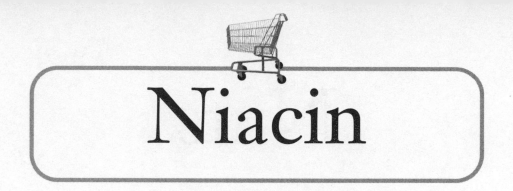

Niacin

A VITAL VITAMIN

Niacin, one of the B vitamins, is an essential nutrient—you can't live without it. In recent years, however, scientists have also found that niacin acts almost like a drug and can be used to prevent and treat several conditions. Here's a sample of what this powerful B can do.

■ **Raynaud's disease.** If you have Raynaud's, a condition that can cause your hands and feet to feel cold and change color due to impaired blood flow, your doctor may advise you to take a form of niacin called inositol hexaniacinate to improve circulation.

■ **Ear noise.** If tinnitus makes you hear ringing or other sounds in your ears, taking a B-complex supplement may minimize your symptoms, possibly by improving nerve function in your ears.

■ **Low energy and poor digestion.** A multivitamin supplement that contains niacin can boost your energy and even improve digestion. People who don't get enough of this key B vitamin may even feel mentally disoriented or have diarrhea.

295

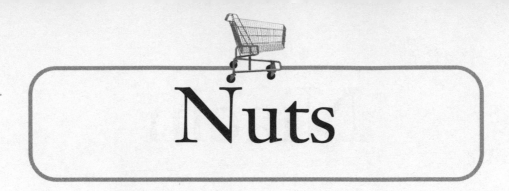

Nuts

NOTHING NUTTY ABOUT 'EM

A lot of people avoid nuts because these crunchy snacks are among the most concentrated sources of fat in the plant world, with up to 25 grams in $^1/_3$ cup. Don't let this hold you back, though, because the fats in nuts are better for you than those in meat, and there's good evidence that nuts are among the most powerful foods you can eat. So get crackin' and have a handful a day!

■ **Sunburn.** The next time you have a sunburn, load up on nuts. They contain antioxidants, beneficial chemical compounds that block some of the harmful effects of sun damage and can even reduce your risk of skin cancer.

Put Out the Brain Flames

Regularly eating nuts and other foods high in omega-3 fatty acids can reduce brain inflammation and help you maintain better focus and memory.

■ **High cholesterol.** Make an effort to eat a handful of nuts daily if your cholesterol reading is on the high side. Studies have shown that both walnuts and almonds can lower cholesterol, and a report in the *Journal of the American Dietetic Association* revealed that pecans can, too. The theory is that the monounsaturated fat in nuts can protect against heart disease. In fact, walnuts can lower cholesterol even more effectively than olive oil, according to a study reported in the *Annals of Internal Medicine*. These nuts lowered the risk of coronary heart disease by 11 percent, according to lead researcher Emilio Ros, M.D.

■ **Macular degeneration.** Nuts are loaded with vitamin E, a nutrient that appears to reduce the risk of macular degeneration, the leading cause of blindness in older people. Eating nuts regularly will help keep your vision sharp year after year.

■ **Weak bones.** To keep your bones healthy and strong, you need magnesium. The best food sources are potatoes, seeds, nuts, legumes, whole grains, and dark green vegetables.

Fabulous Food Fix

A Nutty Moisturizer

Dry skin, especially in the winter, can be the result of too little fat—the right kind of fat, that is. The skin is the place where water and oil meet, and both are essential to good skin health. Make sure your diet includes one or more servings a day of the omega-3 fats found in almonds, walnuts, and pecans.

■ **Leg swelling.** If your legs or feet swell, you may need to balance electrolytes such as potassium and magnesium, which counterbalance sodium and help reduce excess fluid in your body. For potassium, have grapes, orange juice, vegetable juices, and bananas. If you suspect you're not getting enough magnesium, add some wheat germ, whole grains, and nuts to your diet.

■ **Dandruff.** One of the B-complex vitamins, biotin, is essential for healthy hair and can help discourage dandruff.

All you need to do to get enough is eat a handful of nuts a day, says Jeanette Jacknin, M.D.

■ **Joint pain.** Here's a tasty remedy for sore joints. Nuts and beans, along with raisins, pears, apples, and other fruits, all contain the trace element boron, which can relieve pain and joint stiffness and actually appears to protect against arthritis.

■ **Asthma.** Nuts can help you breathe easier if you have asthma because the magnesium they contain acts like a sedative for the bronchial tubes.

■ **Gum disease.** The vitamin E in nuts fights cell damage caused by renegade oxygen molecules called free radicals. The more nuts you eat, the less your risk of having serious gum disease.

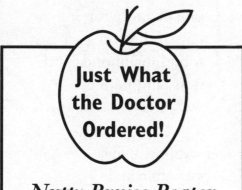

Just What the Doctor Ordered!

Nutty Bruise Beater

When you have a bruise, eat a handful of Brazil nuts. They're loaded with skin-repairing selenium.

■ **Depression.** Tryptophan, an amino acid in foods such as turkey and nuts, is ultimately converted into serotonin, a mood-regulating neurotransmitter, in the body. In one study, when women who were depressed feasted on tryptophan-rich foods such as nuts, their depression eased without the help of medication.

■ **Psoriasis.** To soften scaly areas of skin on your hands and feet caused by psoriasis, lace your bathwater with Epsom salts and soak for a while. After patting the itchy areas dry, rub them gently with some warm peanut oil and top the oil with a paste made with baking soda and castor oil. Finally, put on white cotton gloves or socks and get into bed. If you do this for a few nights, your scales should soon disappear.

■ **Ear noise.** Low levels of magnesium may constrict inner ear arteries and lead to tinnitus, that annoying ringing or other "ghost" noise in the ears. You may find that the sounds diminish when you start eating more nuts, which are rich in magnesium.

■ **Heart disease.** Many of us don't get nearly enough selenium, a trace mineral that appears to play a role in keeping arteries clear. Nuts are loaded with it, and unlike selenium supplements, which can be dangerous, they're perfectly safe!

■ **Frostbite.** If you're hibernating to heal frostbite, plan on eating like a squirrel. That means nuts—lots of them. They're a great source of vitamin E, the nutrient that's essential for repairing damaged skin. Sunflower seeds and almonds have the most, so eat 1/4 cup a day until your skin's completely healed.

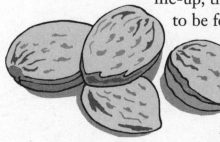

■ **PMS.** Many women crave sugar and chocolate when they're premenstrual. While a sweet treat may be a quick pick-me-up, the sudden rise in blood sugar is bound to be followed by a crash that will make you miserable. If you do indulge your sweet tooth, include some protein (chocolate with nuts, for example) to reduce the sugar's negative effects.

> ## Eat Hearty
>
> Peanuts are packed with a miracle elixir called coenzyme Q_{10}. It appears to bring oxygen to the heart and, if you have heart problems, may even help curb the damage caused by lack of oxygen.

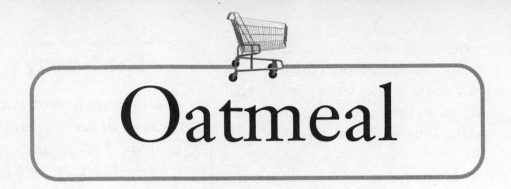

Oatmeal

IT'S JUST GOOD HORSE SENSE

A few hundred years ago, most people had never tasted oatmeal because oats were given almost exclusively to horses. In some parts of the world, though, this nutritious grain made the journey from the stable to the kitchen table—and our health today is better for it. Here's what doctors say about this beneficial cereal.

■ **High cholesterol.** Oatmeal is a great source of soluble fiber, the kind you want more of when you're trying to lower cholesterol. Just 1 cup a day can reduce your cholesterol levels pretty quickly.

■ **Constipation.** Oatmeal is just the thing when you're dealing with constipation. It contains a gummy type of fiber called mucilage that soaks up water, which makes stools larger and softer. Starting the day with a bowl of oatmeal will make stools easier to pass, with less straining.

■ **Yeast infections.** A quick way to ease the discomfort of a yeast infection is to soak in warm water. Just fill the bathtub, add a handful of colloidal oatmeal (the kind intended for soaking, so it won't gunk up the drain), and relax for a while.

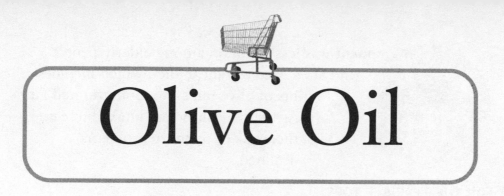

Olive Oil

ONE FABULOUS FAT

About 50 years ago, scientists first noticed that people in Greece and other Mediterranean countries had heart disease rates that were a fraction of those for people in the United States. Was it the wine they drank? The produce they ate? All that exercise going up and down hills? The answer to each of these questions was yes—but there was something else. Olive oil, it turns out, can almost literally turn back the clock on disability and disease. Take a look for yourself.

■ **Colds.** Using poultices when you have a cold is a good way to make yourself rest. Make a chest rub by adding three or four drops of herbal oil (try eucalyptus, lavender, or thyme) to 1 tablespoon of olive oil. Apply it liberally to your chest, cover with a clean cloth, and settle into a comfy chair with a cozy afghan and a good book.

■ **Mental decline.** A daily splash or two of olive oil will help keep your mind healthier. An Italian study of diet and cognitive decline found that cognitive impair-

The Cutting Edge

If you're fresh out of shaving cream, slather on some olive oil before picking up the razor. (Ladies, this will make shaved legs sleek and smooth.)

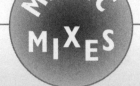

ment was less common among elderly people who ate a Mediterranean diet, which includes lots of olive oil, a monounsaturated fat. As their "healthy fat" intake increased, their risk of memory problems declined.

HELP FOR THE TERRIBLE TOES
Native American healers suggest using a mixture of equal portions of garlic oil and olive oil as a remedy for foot fungus. Since over-the-counter remedies for athlete's foot don't always work very well, this traditional approach is certainly worth a try. Of course, there's no telling what it does for foot odor! You may not want to try it unless you live alone.

■ **Stress.** When you're stressed out, try a peppermint–olive oil foot rub to restore your vitality. Add three or four drops of peppermint oil to 1 tablespoon of olive oil, then massage it into your clean feet and give in to the sensation!

■ **Heart attack.** The risk of heart attack among people who live in the Mediterranean region is half that of Americans, although they actually eat a bit more fat than we do. The reason may be that the fats in their diets are usually unsaturated types,

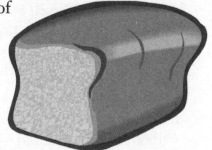

such as olive oil. People who eat a lot of olive oil tend to have lower levels of harmful LDL cholesterol while maintaining higher levels of beneficial HDL. In addition to olive oil, your heart-protective diet should include whole grain breads, cereals, and pasta.

■ **Stuffy nose.** To open your nasal passages, apply oil to your sinuses once or twice daily. First, soak a washcloth in hot water and apply it to your face to increase circulation to the area. Keep the cloth in place for 5 minutes, resoaking it in hot

Olive Oil

water to keep it as hot as you can tolerate. Then apply a thin layer of olive oil on the frontal bone above your eyes, below your eyes, on your cheekbones, and on the bony part of your nose. Next, place a couple of drops of eucalyptus oil on your fingers and rub it into the same areas. Finally, place the hot washcloth over your face again and rest for 15 minutes.

■ **Dry lips.** Herbal lip balms rich in olive oil will prevent dry lips.

■ **Earache.** Putting a few drops of olive oil in the ear canal may reduce inflammation and help promote drainage when you have an earache. Just drop the oil into your sore ear, then lie with that ear on a heating pad set on low and covered with a small towel. About 10 to 15 minutes is enough. (Don't try this with kids, though—they may get burned.)

■ **Dry skin.** Looking for the perfect skin moisturizer? Look no further—reach for virgin olive oil for super-soft skin.

■ **Bursitis.** If bursitis in your shoulder is restricting your activities, you can relieve the pain by massaging olive oil into your shoulder or upper arm once a day.

■ **Thinning hair.** Old-timers used to swear by this treatment for hair loss. Once or twice a week, beat a raw egg with about 1 tablespoon of olive oil and massage it into your hair and scalp. Leave it on for a few minutes, then rinse with warm water.

■ **Constipation.** Taking 1 to 3 tablespoons of olive oil acts as a mild laxative and can help get you moving again—without resorting to more powerful drugs.

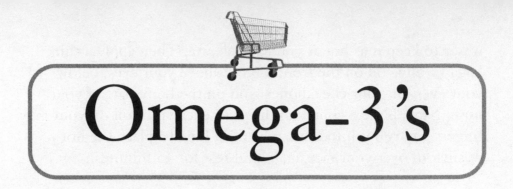

Omega-3's

THE LATEST FISHY FINDINGS

It seems that the more scientists study omega-3 fatty acids, the more health benefits they uncover. To put it simply, the omega-3's—which are found mainly in oily cold-water fish such as salmon and tuna, flaxseed, and a few other foods—affect nearly every part of the body in some remarkable ways. Here's the latest. Just be sure to check with your doctor first if you're taking aspirin or blood-thinning medication.

ON THE SHELF

✓ **Fish**
✓ **Flaxseed**
✓ **Nuts**
✓ **Tofu**

■ **Bruises.** The next time you're banged up and bruised, try some fish oil to reduce inflammation in and under the skin. Take a tablespoon or two daily until the bruise is gone.

■ **Heart disease.** The omega-3's in fish may play a key role in preventing heart disease. Ironically, the fattiest fish with the most omega-3's—salmon, sardines, and herring—are best for you, but all fish have some. According to the *American Journal of Cardiology*, the heart benefits of fish are so impressive that doctors should consider recommending fish oil cap-

sules. Aim for three or four servings of
fatty fish weekly or 1 gram of fish oil a
day. The Japanese, who have the lowest
rate of heart disease in the world, eat fish
nearly every day.

■ **Wrinkles.** Fatty acid deficiency can
leave your skin looking dried out and
wrinkled. Be sure to eat one serving of
omega-3–rich food every day (salmon,
almonds, and sesame seeds are good
sources), or take omega-3 supplements.
Flaxseed oil, black currant oil, borage oil,
and evening primrose oil are all good
choices, too. Take 1 gram once or twice
daily.

■ **Depression and Alzheimer's.**
Brain cells are 60 percent fat, which is
needed to transmit the impulses that
carry thoughts. In a healthy brain,
omega-3 fatty acids predominate. In fact, low levels of omega-
3's have been linked to depression and the risk of Alzheimer's
disease. How do you get these healthy fatty
acids? They're plentiful in oily fish, walnuts,
and flaxseed. To benefit your whole
body, add a handful of nuts, a
serving of fish, or 2 tablespoons
of freshly ground flaxseed to
your diet every day.

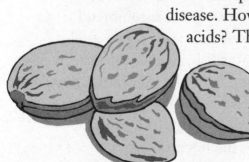

■ **Asthma.** Omega-3's not only inhibit inflammation but
may also repair airway damage. If you eat fish regularly, take 1
to 3 grams of fish oil daily to minimize asthma symptoms. If

Fabulous Food Fix

Purslane Clobbers Cholesterol

The next time you're in
the specialty produce aisle,
check out the purslane.
This leafy green botanical
is a rich source of alpha-
linolenic acid, a plant-
based omega-3 fatty acid
that may help reduce cho-
lesterol in the arteries—
and perhaps prevent leg
cramps while walking. Try
steaming it like spinach.

you don't eat fish often or are sensitive to it, as many people with asthma are, down 3 tablespoons of flaxseed oil a day. Try drizzling it on salads.

■ **Stroke.** If you're concerned about your stroke risk, you may want to take up fishing—or at least get friendly with your local fishmonger. The results of the 14-year Nurses' Health Study, published in the *Journal of the American Medical Association*, revealed that women who ate fish two to four times a week reduced their stroke risk by a whopping 27 percent.

■ **Arthritis.** Researchers at Johns Hopkins Medical Center have developed a bone-and-joint diet that, according to a report from the medical center, can help alleviate the stiff, inflamed joints common to both osteoarthritis and rheumatoid arthritis. The experts recommend eating two or more servings a week of cold-water fish, such as salmon, herring, cod, and blues, because the omega-3 fatty acids in these fish enhance joint health. In a study of 41 people, the doctors observed a 25 percent improvement in swollen joints, morning stiffness, and overall discomfort in the subgroup who took the omega-3 fatty acids.

Fish for Better Sight

An Australian study found that omega-3 fatty acids may help reduce the risk of macular degeneration, a vision-robbing eye problem. To get more fish in your diet, try this chowder recipe: Place two white potatoes, cubed; two large carrots, sliced; one onion, diced; seafood seasoning (Old Bay is good); and at least 1 pound of fish in a pot and add enough water to cover plus 1 inch more. Bring to a boil, then reduce the heat and simmer until the veggies are cooked and the fish is opaque.

■ **Allergies.** The omega-3's in fish inhibit the inflammation that often accompanies allergies. Fish also provide vitamin A, which boosts IgA, an antibody that's released in saliva and attaches to allergens to keep them from invading your system. The recommended dose of fish oil for allergy relief is 1 to 3 grams daily if you eat fish regularly. If you'd rather avoid fish, you can take 3 tablespoons of flaxseed oil, another excellent source of fatty acids, daily.

■ **Chemo side effects.** The omega-3's in flaxseed help reduce the inflammation that results from chemotherapy, so grind some seeds and add a few teaspoons to your morning smoothie or yogurt. As a bonus, flaxseed also promotes intestinal function, which may be impaired by chemo.

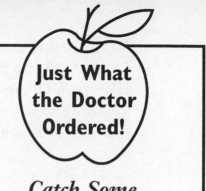

Just What the Doctor Ordered!

Catch Some Heart Health

For people with heart disease, taking at least 1 gram of fish oil a day is a good strategy. The oil improves blood flow, helps lower triglycerides—blood fats that can clog arteries—and helps stabilize insulin resistance, a major factor in heart disease.

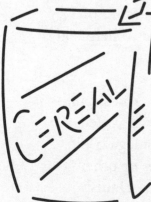

■ **Brittle hair.** If your hair is thin or brittle, you may be deficient in omega-3's. In order to make up the deficit, you'd need to eat fish several times a week. If that's too much fish for you, though, Andrew Weil, M.D., suggests buying whole flaxseed (keep it refrigerated), grinding it, and sprinkling 2 tablespoons a day on cereal or a salad.

■ **High blood pressure.** Omega-3's can help lower blood pressure, but you need about 5 grams a day for the best effect. To reach your quota, Darin Ingels, N.D., suggests asking your doctor about taking fish oil capsules along with 400 IU of vitamin E to offset any fishiness. You could also opt for 1 to 3 tablespoons of flaxseed oil daily.

■ **CFS.** Try to eat fish or flaxseed at least a few times a week if you have chronic fatigue syndrome (CFS). Their omega-3's will help minimize pain.

■ **Eczema.** If your skin is itchy and inflamed from eczema, taking 3 to 6 grams of evening primrose oil may help by correcting a fatty acid imbalance. Other options include taking 3 to 6 grams of flaxseed oil or using a flaxseed compress. Simply grind flaxseed to make a paste, apply it to a piece of gauze, and hold it against your rash.

Cold Fish, Warm Hands

If you have chilly fingers caused by inflammation of the blood vessels that reduces circulation to your extremities, eating lots of cold-water fish, which contain omega-3 essential fatty acids, could increase your tolerance to cold by inhibiting inflammation.

■ **Lupus.** Protein from land-based animals may encourage inflammation in people with lupus, but the beneficial omega-3's in trout, salmon, and other cold-water fish can squelch it. Add more of these fish to your menu to help control flare-ups.

■ **Menstrual pain.** You should definitely eat more fish, flaxseed, and other foods with omega-3's if you have severe cramps or other menstrual discomfort. A Danish study found that women who had severe menstrual pain tended to seldom eat fish.

Omega-3's

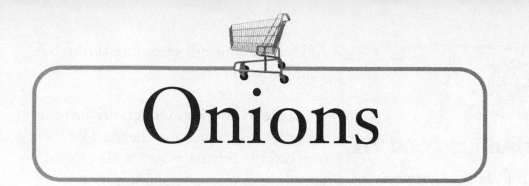

Onions

NOTHING TO CRY ABOUT

Many people don't eat a lot of onions (or their eye-watering cousins, shallots, leeks, and scallions) because of their strong taste and tear-jerking potential. You may want to grab a hanky and start peeling, though, because onions are among the most medically powerful foods you can eat. Take a look at the latest headlines.

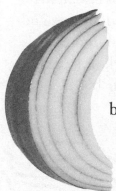

■ **Warts.** You can help eliminate warts by rubbing them with half an onion that's been dipped in salt. Use this treatment twice a day until the warts disappear.

■ **Bronchitis.** Onions are an old-time remedy for bronchial problems. Science has validated this use in recent years after discovering that onions are a rich source of quercetin, an anti-inflammatory compound. Make a pot of onion soup or eat them raw (if you dare)

Onions and Ulcers

Having an ulcer is no reason to hold the onions. In fact, it's all the more reason to add them to salads, sandwiches, soups, and so forth. Onions contain compounds that seem to help eliminate ulcer-causing bacteria, so try to include them in at least one meal a day.

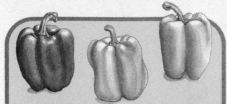

Fabulous Food Fix

Cry Away Congestion

Is your stuffed-up nose keeping you awake? There's no need to get dressed for a trip to the drugstore. Just grab your robe, go to the kitchen, and munch a slice of raw onion. It's a powerful decongestant that's almost guaranteed to unclog your nose.

and feel the warmth spreading through your chest and lungs.

■ **Heart disease.** Onions are just the thing for protecting your heart. The quercetin in onions, which is also found in red wine, tea, and apples, is more powerful than vitamin E at blocking the harmful effects of free radicals, oxygen molecules that damage tissues throughout the body and greatly increase the risk of heart disease. Eating onions daily provides enough quercetin to help prevent free radicals from damaging LDL cholesterol, the process that makes it more likely to gunk up your arteries.

■ **Heart attack and stroke.** Chemical compounds in onions—adenosine and paraffinic polysulfides—keep blood platelets from clumping together to form clots that can trigger a heart attack or stroke. Eating onions more often will help ensure that your blood flows freely where it's needed.

■ **High triglycerides.** One study showed that students fed a high-fat diet actually had a drop in triglycerides—blood fats that increase heart disease risk—when they added big slices of onion to their burgers. So don't cry—just slice and dice!

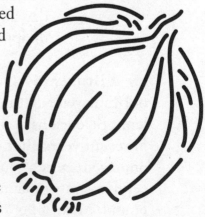

■ **High blood sugar.** In one study, blood sugar levels in diabetic rats that were fed a diet high in onions were controlled as

Onions

well as those of rats given insulin and other diabetes drugs. And they got a bonus: They created less cholesterol than the rats on drugs. It's not certain that people will get the same benefits, but evidence suggests that adding onions to your diet will help keep your blood sugar levels healthier.

■ **Acne.** Have you (or your favorite teenager) broken out in pimples? Reach for this heirloom helper: Mix 1 teaspoon of onion juice with 2 tablespoons of honey and apply it to your face. Leave it on for 10 to 15 minutes, then rinse with warm water followed by cool water.

■ **Faintness.** When you feel faint, hold a cut onion under your nose until the wooziness passes.

■ **Athlete's foot.** Relieve the itch and burn of athlete's foot by massaging onion juice into your tootsies twice a day. Test a small area first to be sure your skin isn't too tender.

■ **Clogged arteries.** Many people don't get nearly enough of the trace mineral selenium, a powerful antioxidant that appears to play a role in keeping arteries clear. Onions, nuts, whole grains, and shellfish contain quite a bit of selenium, so load up and keep your blood flowing.

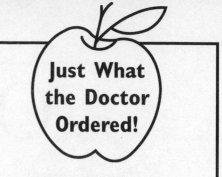

Just What the Doctor Ordered!

Slice and Soothe

You can ease the pain of a minor burn with an onion. First, run cold water over the burned area, then apply a slice of raw onion. The same chemicals that make you cry also block the substances that make you feel pain. And here's a bonus: Onion juice has antibacterial properties that may help prevent infection.

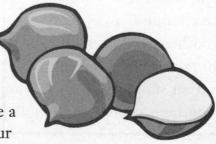

Oranges

THE POWER OF CITRUS

Forget for the moment that oranges are nature's version of fast food, prewrapped and ready to eat at a moment's notice. Forget, too, the deliciously tangy taste. There are more important reasons to enjoy these citrus delights. Here's what the experts have to say.

■ **Gallstones.** One study examined data from 13,000 people and found that women with low levels of vitamin C were more likely to get gallstones than those with higher levels. To get as much as you can, have lots of citrus fruit and juices, which are the best C sources. A whole orange, for example, offers 70 milligrams.

■ **Heart disease.** If you don't get enough B vitamins, the amino acid homocysteine can build up and damage the lining of your arteries, encouraging the formation of

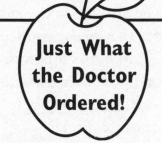

Just What the Doctor Ordered!

Stop the Sagging

To prevent wrinkles, eat plenty of oranges (and stay out of the sun, of course). The vitamin C in oranges and other produce helps maintain collagen, the protein that supports and strengthens skin.

blood clots and cholesterol deposits. Since homocysteine has been linked to heart disease, take in plenty of Bs by downing a glass of orange juice at every opportunity.

■ **Colds.** While vitamin C has yet to be proven to cure a cold, some say it acts similarly to interferon, a natural body chemical that stops the growth of viruses. It's most effective at the first sign of a sniffle, so stock up on oranges—and squeeze yourself one glass of pulpy juice a day.

■ **Allergies.** Most doctors agree that vitamin C has a slight antihistamine effect. The next time your allergies flare up, drink more O.J. or enjoy some juicy oranges. You may find that it helps your nasal symptoms.

■ **Bloating.** If you tend to bloat a bit near your period, be sure to get plenty of potassium, which counterbalances sodium and decreases excess fluid. Oranges are a great source.

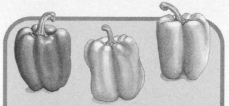

Fabulous Food Fix

Good to the Bone

The Framingham Heart Study found that women whose diets were rich in potassium had denser bones in their spines and hips than women with potassium-poor diets. So load up on bananas and oranges; they're terrific sources of this mineral.

■ **Cancer I.** The pulpy white membrane on orange wedges provides pectin, a kind of fiber that may help reduce the spread of cancer, so don't be too neat when you eat. Get as much of the membrane as you can.

■ **Cancer II.** Oranges are a good source of cryptoxanthin, one of the beta-carotene cousins,

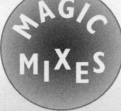

MAGIC MIXES

which may fight cervical cancer. Canned mandarin oranges are loaded with it.

■ **CFS.** Many people with chronic fatigue syndrome (CFS) are deficient in glutathione, a chemical compound that helps your body rid itself of toxins. Since it's questionable how well it works when taken on its own, John Reed, M.D., suggests loading your diet with oranges and other vitamin C–rich foods, which help the body produce glutathione.

■ **Anemia.** If you have iron-deficiency anemia, eat more oranges. Their vitamin C helps your body absorb more iron from other foods.

■ **Weak bones.** Food (rather than supplements) is the best source of calcium because it probably contains other, as-yet-undiscovered bone-building ingredients, so drink plenty of calcium-fortified orange juice. One glass has about as much calcium as a glass of milk.

■ **Sore throat.** Juices are a great way to give your body the extra fluids and natural healing substances it needs to help a sore throat. All fruit juices are beneficial, but orange juice is especially good because it's loaded with vitamin C.

■ **Muscle pain.** Forget the chips, pretzels, and other salty foods when you're coping with muscle pain. Salt makes your body retain water, which can increase painful swelling in your

SOAK AND DE-STRESS
Here's the perfect way to relax: First, cut the leg from a pair of pantyhose and wrap a few chamomile tea bags in it (you can also use a piece of gauze). Next, cut an orange into thin slices. Hang the tea pouch from the bathtub spigot and let warm water flow over it as you fill the tub. Put the orange slices in the water, climb into the tub, and let your troubles float away.

Oranges

muscles. If you need a quick snack, fill up on orange slices, which are naturally low in salt. They also contain a lot of water, which will help sore muscles stay hydrated and heal more quickly.

■ **High cholesterol I.** The white pith just under an orange's skin is packed with pectin, a soluble fiber known for lowering cholesterol—and it's higher in vitamin C than the juice is. If you eat a little of the pith along with your orange, that's a good thing.

■ **High cholesterol II.** Here's something to think about if you're trying to control your cholesterol. In one small Canadian study, women who drank orange juice daily got a big surprise: Their levels of good high-density lipoprotein (HDL) cholesterol rose by 21 percent, a very unusual occurrence. You may get the same benefit by starting your day with a tall glass of juice. Remember that it's HDL cholesterol that removes bad LDL cholesterol from your arteries.

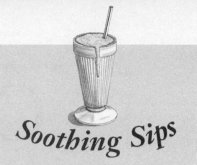

Soothing Sips

CITRUS FIGHTS CANCER

The oil in orange peel is 90 to 95 percent limonene, a natural chemical that's been linked to preventing breast and cervical cancers, at least in test tubes. Limonene ends up in the O.J. you buy because commercial machines squeeze the oranges so hard, so fill your shopping cart with delicious juice!

■ **Gum disease.** The vitamin C that practically drips from oranges toughens gums, reduces swelling, and squelches infection if you have gingivitis. A few daily servings of oranges and other citrus fruits will go a long way toward keeping your gums healthy.

Oranges

Oregano

MORE THAN A PIZZA SPICE

You probably use oregano more than any other kitchen spice, and that's good: Its pungent aroma comes from high-powered chemicals that can do more for your health than a basketful of high-tech drugs. Here are some of the best reasons to spice up your life.

Aromatic Burn Beater

You love oregano on your pizza, and if you have a burn, your skin will love it, too. Oregano oil contains vitamins A and C as well as minerals such as calcium, phosphorus, iron, and magnesium. When rubbed on the skin, it helps heal minor burns, so you'll recover more quickly and have a lower risk of infection.

■ **Gas.** If you get gas from beans and other starchy foods, simply sprinkle on some tasty carminative (gas-reducing) seeds, such as dill, fennel, or caraway. For more gas-fighting oomph, stir in a carminative herb, such as basil, rosemary, oregano, or sage.

■ **Anal itching.** Too much yeast in your system can cause anal itching and burning. To soothe the area, make a strong infusion of oregano by steeping 1 heaping tablespoon of fresh leaves in a cup of hot water, covered, for 15 minutes. Strain, then pour the liquid into a peribottle. Keep the bottle by your toilet, and after each visit to the bathroom, squirt your bottom with the solution.

■ **Sinus headache.** The next time your sinuses start pounding, melt away congestion with an herbal steam. Put a few cups of water in a saucepan and bring it to a boil. Add 2 to 3 teaspoons of aromatic herbs, such as thyme, rosemary, oregano, or basil. It's also good to add a few drops of eucalyptus oil. Then carefully put the pot on a table or counter, drape a towel over your head to trap the steam, and lean over the pot (but not close enough to burn your face). Breathe deeply, inhaling the steam through your nose and exhaling through your mouth. Do this for 10 to 15 minutes two or three times a day.

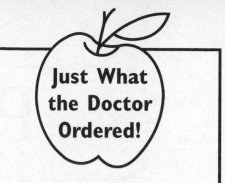

Just What the Doctor Ordered!

Spit and Soothe

For a rash of unknown origin, simply chew a fresh oregano leaf (a strong antiseptic), spit the mash into your hand, and slather it on your rash, suggests Sharol Tilgner, N.D. If you prefer a less primitive method of application, use a few drops of oregano oil.

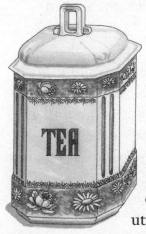

■ **Athlete's foot.** Severe athlete's foot must be treated from the inside out. For starters, try a tea made with equal parts of echinacea, oregano, calendula, and cleavers. Use 1 heaping teaspoon of the mixture per cup of boiling water and steep, covered, for 15 minutes. Strain and drink up to three cups per day. To make an external wash, use ½ cup of herbs per quart of water. Soak your feet for 15 to 20 minutes, then dry well.

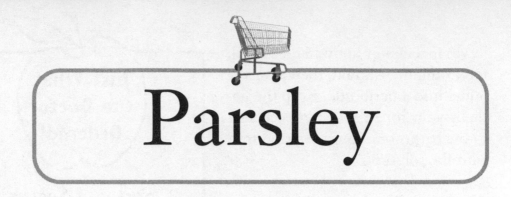

Parsley

MUNCH A BUNCH

Restaurants routinely arrange fresh parsley sprigs on dinner plates, and diners just as routinely shove them aside. Well, cut it out! The next time you go out to eat, be sure to munch that pretty herb. It will freshen your breath and do wonders for your health. Here's how.

■ **Cancer.** The vitamin payload in parsley, especially vitamins A and C, has an important range of health benefits. These two vitamins act as antioxidants, which destroy substances that can damage your cells before they trigger cancer. Why not mince some parsley and garlic and mix it with rice and a dash of olive oil for a quick tabbouleh? Add it to your diet on a regular basis, and you've got an anticancer cocktail!

■ **Weak bones.** Parsley also supplies vitamin K, which may help strengthen your bones. A Harvard study found that women who had the least vitamin K in their diets were about 70 percent more likely to have hip fractures than those who had the most—so dish up more of this vitamin-rich herb!

■ **Heart disease.** Researchers have been studying certain plant compounds in parsley called terpenoids. Preliminary results suggest that these substances can reduce levels of bad low-density lipoprotein (LDL) cholesterol—the stuff that sticks to artery walls and increases the risk of heart disease and other vascular conditions. If you're trying to protect your heart, get into the habit of adding parsley to salads and other dishes.

■ **Anemia.** As many as one-fifth of all vegetarian women are anemic. If you don't eat meat, try your best to prevent iron-deficiency anemia by loading up on salads made with iron-rich kale, beet greens, collard greens, chard, and parsley.

■ **Dragon breath.** Some Native American traditions call for chewing parsley leaves as a breath freshener and digestive aid. You may want to carry a sandwich bag or pouch of parsley leaves so you can munch on them periodically throughout the day.

■ **B.O.** Some body odors are caused by what you eat. The well-known smells of garlic and onions, for example, can come right through your pores, but there's no need to boycott these favorites. Just neutralize their potent aromas by eating parsley and other green leafy vegetables with chlorophyll, a natural deodorant. (That's the origin of the parsley-as-garnish tradition.) If you keep it up, you'll begin to notice the difference in just a few days.

Fabulous Food Fix

Drain Away Bloat

Hot flashes are just one problem associated with menopause. Bloating is another—and parsley is the key to getting rid of all that extra fluid that accumulates and makes you look like Wanda the Whale. To experience the benefits, simply add parsley leaves to your salads or parsley seed to your soups. And, of course, eat your garnish!

Parsley

319

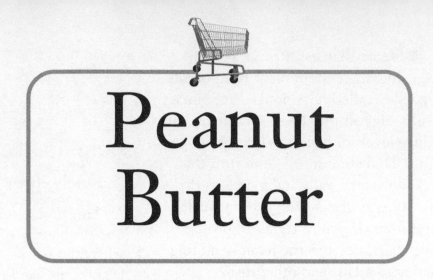

Peanut Butter

SPREAD TO GET AHEAD

You may think that peanut butter serves mainly as a foundation for a big glob of jelly pressed between bread slices, but there's actually a lot of healing power in this thick, creamy spread. Don't believe it? Read on.

The Better Butter

Clinical research shows that eating peanuts and peanut butter can lower bad low-density lipoprotein (LDL) cholesterol and triglycerides without lowering good high-density lipoprotein (HDL) cholesterol. That's a profile that's healthy for your heart.

■ **Brain fog.** "A higher-protein, lower-carbohydrate diet will actually promote concentration," says psychiatrist Daniel Amen, M.D. While carbohydrates cause your energy levels and focus to soar, then quickly crash, protein helps make the neurotransmitter dopamine, which sharpens focus. Keep protein-packed munchies—such as celery stalks filled with peanut butter, string cheese, or protein bars—on hand. You'll be surprised at how just a few high-protein morsels can stimulate your concentration.

■ **Heart disease.** Ounce for ounce, peanuts contain the same amount of monounsaturated fat as tree nuts such as walnuts, pecans, and almonds, which have been shown to protect against heart disease. What's more, peanuts have almost as much protein as beans, so don't dismiss peanut butter as an "empty" snack. Fix yourself a sandwich whenever your stomach's growling.

■ **Injuries.** If you've been injured, you need to get enough protein in your diet to help heal damaged tissue. Typically, a few daily servings of protein-rich foods, such as peanut butter, will give you most of what you need.

■ **Cancer.** Peanuts are packed with sterols, the plant version of cholesterol. Although that sounds as if it could be a problem, it's not. Since plant sterols are absorbed very slowly, they get in the way of the cholesterol from foods and keep it from being absorbed. Sterols have also been shown to inhibit the growth of colon, prostate, and breast cancer cells and to cause cancer cells to die. While Asians and vegetarians (who rarely get those cancers) get about 400 milligrams of phytosterols daily, Americans average only 80 milligrams a day. Adding 2 tablespoons of peanut oil or peanut butter or ¼ cup of roasted peanuts to your daily fare will give you about 50 milligrams of phytosterols.

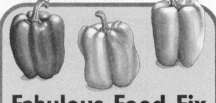

Fabulous Food Fix

Weight a Minute

If you eat a ton of peanut butter, you may gain weight, but if you eat it in moderation, you shouldn't have a problem. In a weight-loss study at Brigham and Women's Hospital, participants who ate peanut butter and other healthy fats lost weight and kept it off more successfully than those on a very low fat diet.

Peppermint

REFRESHINGLY STRONG

All mints have a distinctive, tongue-tingling taste, but peppermint is in a class by itself. Apart from its penetrating flavor and aroma, it triggers changes throughout the body that can keep you healthy. Take a look at the latest findings.

■ **Gas.** Restaurant managers may need to rethink the practice of leaving peppermints for diners at the end of their meals. A study showed that nearly 80 percent of people who took peppermint capsules or tablets three or four times daily before meals had less flatulence. You may want to try enteric-coated peppermint capsules, which are less likely to cause heartburn and are just as effective for gas.

Natural Yeast Control

Peppermint oil capsules, taken by mouth, are powerful fungus fighters that can help control vaginal yeast infections.

■ **Insomnia.** If you're going through a cycle of insomnia—due to stress, changes in the weather, or just bad luck—sip some peppermint tea at bedtime. It will help you drift into dreamland.

■ **Leg pain and swelling.** If you have frequent leg cramps or swelling, you may need to stimulate your circulation. Make a strong infusion of peppermint and yarrow by steeping 2 tablespoons of each herb in 2 cups of hot water, covered, for 15 minutes, then strain and refrigerate. While the solution is chilling, prepare several lengths of gauze, muslin, or cheesecloth. Saturate the cloths in the cold liquid, wrap them around your lower legs, and relax with your legs elevated for 20 minutes. Do this daily for several weeks.

■ **IBS.** Irritable bowel syndrome (IBS) is one of the great mysteries of medicine. No one knows for sure what causes it, and there's no cure. Over-the-

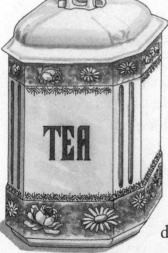

counter and prescription drugs can help a little, but you may get some extra relief with peppermint oil. Taken in capsule form between meals, it's a powerful antispasmodic and pain reliever. If capsules aren't available, try using peppermint leaves to make tea. Steep 1 heaping teaspoon in a cup of hot water, covered, for 10 to 15 minutes, then strain. Drink three cups daily between meals.

■ **Stuffy nose.** To make a decongestant nasal balm, place ¼ cup of petroleum jelly in a small saucepan and warm it until it melts. Remove from the heat and stir in 10 drops each of peppermint oil, eucalyptus oil, and thyme oil. When the balm has

Settle Your Stomach

To cool heartburn, take enteric-coated capsules of peppermint oil three times a day between meals. People with heartburn and other digestive complaints often report quick improvement once they start taking peppermint.

Soothing Sips

CALM THE CANKERS

To relieve the pain of canker sores, make a peppermint mouth rinse. Put several tea bags in a saucepan and add enough water to cover. Cover and simmer for about 30 minutes, then remove the tea bags. When the tea has cooled to room temperature, swish it around in your mouth for 30 to 60 seconds, then swallow it, suggests John Hibbs, N.D. Repeat several times a day until the sores are healed.

reached room temperature, pour it into a clean jar for storage. Apply a small amount to your nostrils one to three times daily. The petroleum jelly prevents the oils from being absorbed into the skin, so you can inhale their aroma for a prolonged period and soothe a sore nose at the same time.

■ **B.O.** Body odor can sometimes be the result of sluggish or poor elimination, but gentle herbs can help clean your body on the inside. Combine equal parts of peppermint, red clover, yarrow, cleavers, and calendula, then steep 1 heaping tablespoon of the mixture in 1 quart of warm water for 15 minutes. Strain and drink throughout the day.

■ **Dandruff.** To deep clean your scalp and reduce dandruff, try an herbal steam treatment. First, mix equal parts of fresh or dried rosemary, nettle, and peppermint leaves. Next, steep 2 tablespoons of the dried mixture (or ½ cup fresh) in 2 cups of hot water, covered, for 10 minutes. Strain the solution, let it cool slightly, and apply it carefully to your scalp. Put on a shower cap, wrap your head in a hot, wet towel, and leave everything on for 30 minutes. Afterward, use an herbal rinse.

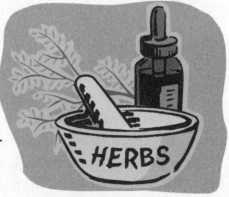

■ **Constipation.** Make an anticonstipation decoction by simmering 1 teaspoon each of burdock root and dandelion root in 2 cups of boiling water for 20 minutes. Remove from the heat and add 1 teaspoon of peppermint, then cover and steep for another 10 minutes. Strain and sip ½ cup first thing in the morning and before each meal. If your constipation is due to stress, add 1 heaping teaspoon of catnip or lemon balm to the mixture. In most cases, you'll be more regular within a day or two. Don't use dandelion if you take diuretics or potassium supplements.

■ **Diarrhea.** Peppermint contains menthol and has antispasmodic properties. To relax the muscles of your digestive tract and calm the spasms that trigger diarrhea, try a cup of peppermint tea. Stir 1 teaspoon of fresh or dried leaves into 1 cup of boiling water and simmer for 10 minutes., then strain and enjoy. You can drink as many as three cups a day after meals.

■ **Bug bites.** When peppermint oil is applied to a bug bite, its cooling menthol lessens pain and stimulates blood flow to the area to flush out the venom and disperse inflammatory chemicals. It also reduces swelling and itching. Try to carry some peppermint oil when you're hiking or camping, but if you forget, mint toothpaste will work, too.

MAGIC MIXES

SCOTCH THE SCRATCHING
Have an itchy rash? Take some gel from an aloe leaf and combine it with a drop of peppermint oil, then smear it on your rash.

■ **Headache.** Studies show that rubbing peppermint oil—a proven anes-

Rub Away Fatigue

Feeling tired and out of sorts these days? Welcome to the club—millions of Americans go through life feeling a little fatigued, as though their zest for life simply left. To refresh your body and restore your vitality, try a peppermint oil foot rub. Add three or four drops of peppermint oil to 1 tablespoon of olive oil, then rub it into your clean feet.

thetic—on your forehead may relieve the pain and reduce the sensitivity associated with tension headaches. Even better, using the oil daily may help prevent future headaches. Just mix equal amounts of peppermint oil and rubbing alcohol, then apply no more than a couple of drops to your forehead and temples. Leave it on for 15 minutes, then massage the area for 3 minutes. Repeat three times a day.

■ **Dragon breath.** To reduce bad breath, look for products that contain zinc gluconate combined with peppermint. Zinc-containing compounds interfere with bacteria's ability to produce sulfur compounds, and peppermint oil is one of nature's best neutralizers.

■ **Queasiness.** To help counteract nausea, simply open a vial of peppermint oil and inhale for a few seconds. If you feel well enough for a bath, add four to six drops of the oil to the bathwater, climb in, and breathe deeply while you're soaking.

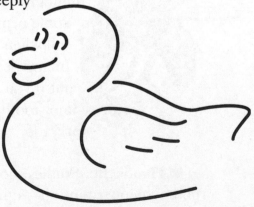

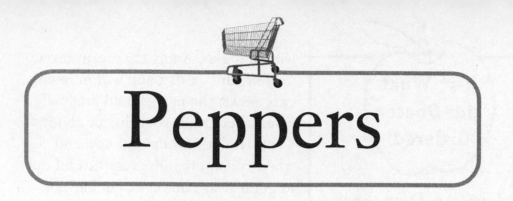

Peppers

COLOR THEM HEALTHY

From green to yellow to red, from crunchy, sweet, and juicy to fiery hot and spicy, the variety offered by peppers is pretty remarkable. Even better, the range of chemicals and nutrients in all types of peppers can do your body good. Here's a look at the latest findings on their exciting benefits.

■ **Toothache.** You can relieve a toothache by rubbing a drop or two of hot pepper sauce onto the gum at the base of your sore tooth.

■ **Macular degeneration.** Eat more peppers to protect your eyes. They're jam-packed with vitamin C, the nutrient you need most to prevent macular degeneration, one of the leading causes of vision loss.

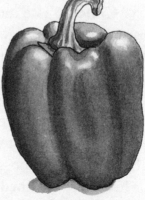

■ **Shingles.** Rubbing hot pepper ointment on your shingles may not sound as though it would put out the fire, but apparently, it does. The American Academy of Dermatology says that creams made with capsaicin, the substance that provides the heat in hot peppers, help some people

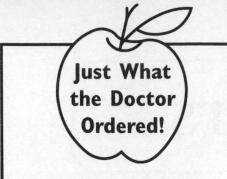
C Fatigue Disappear

If you have chronic fatigue syndrome, John Reed, M.D., suggests that you load up on vitamin C–rich red peppers. Other good food choices include broccoli and oranges and other citrus fruits.

with shingles. Apply the cream three or four times a day, and within one to two weeks, the pain should gradually ease. Check with your doctor about what strength product to buy, and when you apply it, be very careful not to get it near your eyes, genitals, or any area of broken skin.

■ **Joint pain.** Call it chile pepper, call it cayenne, call it capsaicin. Just call it—this cream is really hot stuff! Just smooth it on your aching joints, and you'll begin to feel relief. The heat from the active ingredient brings more blood circulation to your joints, and with it, more healing oxygen. The best creams contain 0.025 to 0.075 percent capsaicin. Use it up to three times a day.

■ **Cancer.** The more nutrients you receive during cancer treatment, the stronger and less prone to infections you'll be. "Relying strictly on supplements can place too much stress on the immune system," says Cynthia Thompson, R.D., Ph.D. She suggests loading your plate with a spectrum of red, yellow, and green foods to get the most cancer-fighting nutrients possible. For instance, on a bed of dark leafy greens (such as spinach or kale), toss some red peppers (for vitamin C), carrots (for beta-carotene), and several cruciferous veggies, such as broccoli or

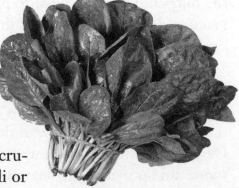

cauliflower (for isothiocyanates, which are potent cancer-fighting compounds).

■ **Gas.** Raw fruits and vegetables are notorious gas promoters in people with irritable bowel syndrome, but you can get your fiber (which will also ease constipation) and nutrients without triggering the gasworks by roasting or grilling fresh peppers and other produce, says Gary Gitnick, M.D.

■ **TMD.** For relief from the pain of temporomandibular disorder (TMD), smear your sore jaw with capsaicin cream. It helps deplete the proliferation of pain-causing prostaglandins. Apply the cream with a cotton swab.

■ **Cranky gut.** Eating spicy foods makes some people with intestinal distress feel worse, but for others, a little culinary heat brings some relief. Hot foods, such as chile peppers and ground red pepper, may make your intestine less cranky. Add a dash of cayenne to spice up your meal or cup of tea. Discontinue use if your symptoms persist or worsen.

■ **Chafing.** Chafed skin can take a long time to heal, but vitamin C can speed things up. You know that orange juice is full of vita-

Hot Help for Hair Loss

Here's a mix that may help you keep a full head of hair. Add one or two drops of red pepper (cayenne) oil to 1 ounce of rosemary oil in a clean, small bottle, then massage your entire scalp with the mixture for at least 20 minutes. Afterward, wash your hair with shampoo to which you've added five drops of rosemary oil per ounce of shampoo. Lather up every day.

Soothing Sips

TORCH A COLD

The next time you feel a cold coming on, add some heat. Three or four times a day, mix 10 to 20 drops of hot pepper sauce or a big pinch of red pepper into a glass of tomato juice, then drink to your health. For a sore throat, substitute water for the tomato juice and gargle several times a day.

min C, but did you know that a cup of chopped red peppers provides almost as much C as a 6-ounce glass of juice? That works out to nearly 300 milligrams. Be sure to include this sweet, crunchy treat on your menu when your skin is on the mend.

■ **Joint injuries.** Vitamin C is critical for repairing injured joints. You could take supplements, but a tastier solution is to add some crunch to your next salad. "Green and red peppers are good sources of vitamin C," says Phoebe Yin, N.D.

■ **Mouse shoulder.** Has too much time at the computer left you with a sore shoulder? Obviously, it's a good idea to move your joint through its entire range of motion just to loosen things up a bit. In addition, you can make your own pain-relieving ointment by adding three or four drops of hot pepper sauce to 2 teaspoons of olive oil. Massage the ointment into your shoulder three or four times a day.

■ **Weak heart.** A sprinkling of red pepper helps keep your heart muscle in good shape, so eat it every chance you get!

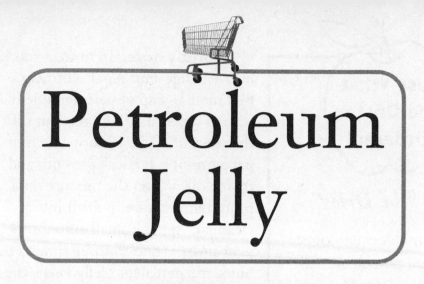

Petroleum Jelly

SMEAR IT ON!

These days, you can spend big bucks on fancy lotions and moisturizers with all sorts of exotic ingredients—or you can use tried-and-true petroleum jelly. You'll get the same or better results at a fraction of the cost. Best of all, it's good for things you've probably never thought of. Check out these tips.

■ **Blisters.** Blisters can develop if your feet are either too sweaty or too dry. If your socks are often soggy, the origin of your blister problem may be that sweaty skin. Try sprinkling a little cornstarch into your socks before you put them on, and dust some between your toes, too. If the skin on your feet is very dry, smooth a thin film of petroleum jelly over them before donning your socks and shoes.

■ **Sore earlobes.** Get pierced earrings into your ears more gently by coating the posts with a little petroleum jelly before you insert them.

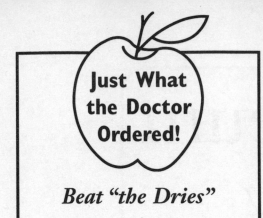

Just What the Doctor Ordered!

Beat "the Dries"

For years, dermatologists have praised petroleum jelly as the thickest emollient and therefore the best treatment for very dry skin.

■ **Stuffy nose.** To make a soothing, decongestant nasal ointment, first melt ¼ cup of petroleum jelly in a small saucepan. Take the pan off the stove and add 10 drops each of peppermint oil, eucalyptus oil, and thyme oil. When the mixture cools to room temperature, pour it into a clean jar. Apply a small amount to your nostrils one to three times a day. Since the petroleum jelly keeps the oils from being absorbed into the skin, it soothes your tender nose while the vapors from the oils help relieve congestion.

■ **Psoriasis.** If you have psoriasis, you already know how hard it is to control skin plaques. There are all sorts of over-the-counter and prescription products, but none of them necessarily work as well as petroleum jelly. Twice a day, bathe the scaly areas, pat them dry, and immediately rub in layer after layer of petroleum jelly or vitamin E oil. Within a week, at least 80 percent of the lesions will disappear, says David Cohen, N.D.

■ **Cold sores.** Petroleum jelly is an easy way to soften the skin surrounding cold sores to prevent cracks or bleeding. Apply a generous layer to the area once or twice a day and keep applying it until the cold sore is gone. If you don't like the smell or consistency of petroleum jelly, vitamin E oil is a good alternative. Open a capsule and spread the oil on the sore and the surrounding area. It's a good moisturizer, and it may speed healing.

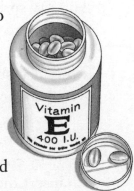

Petroleum Jelly

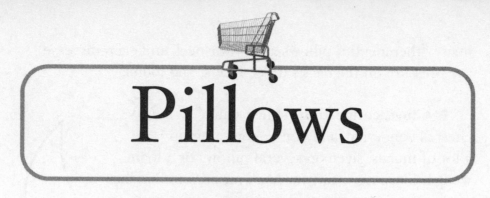

Pillows

KEEP YOUR HEAD UP

You wouldn't think there would be much to say about pillows. Sure, you can sleep on them, pull them over your head, or use them as handy surrogates when you're madder than heck. In fact, though, pillows do all sorts of things besides keep you company at night. Here are a few of their attributes.

■ **Heartburn.** If you have nighttime heartburn, sleeping on a special wedge-shaped pillow raises your upper body and allows gravity to minimize the reflux of stomach contents into the esophagus.

■ **Allergies.** Dust mites are major allergens—and they love to sleep in your bed, so pick up one of the natural citrus laundry detergents and wash your bedding often. If you've ever seen dust mites magnified a million times, you know they're not something you want to sleep with. They live in feather as well as synthetic pillows, but you can wash the synthetics frequently. The citrus will rout the little buggers, and the water will drown them.

■ **Neck pain.** If you have neck pain, using a cervical pillow may relieve it. Choose one with your doctor's advice, since many "therapeutic" pillows arch your neck and even increase the pressure on the neck's disks, facets, and joints.

■ **Chest congestion.** When your chest is congested, and you're coughing up a lot of mucus, sleep on several pillows or a foam wedge. Sleeping with your head raised 6 to 8 inches prevents mucus from pooling in your bronchial passages, thus promoting more peaceful sleep.

■ **Foot and leg pain.** Your dad had the right idea when he came home and propped his feet on the coffee table while he read the paper (or your report card). Raising your feet not only gives them a chance to rest, it also allows gravity to drain away any excess fluid that's contributing to foot or leg discomfort. For this strategy to be really effective, though, you have to raise your feet higher than your head, which usually means lying down and propping your feet on a few pillows.

■ **Varicose veins.** The blood in your legs has to fight gravity to climb all the way back to your heart, which is the reason so many of us get varicose veins. Why not reverse the situation and let gravity work for you? To do it, raise your feet above the level of your heart for a couple of hours each day, or sit with your legs propped up on pillows. About 10 minutes after you elevate your legs, they will feel much better.

Cushion Tension Headaches

Some pillows do an excellent job of supporting your head and neck, while others are so soft that you might as well be sleeping on air. Firm pillows are usually best for preventing tension headaches, but you'll have to experiment to find the type that works best for you.

Pillows

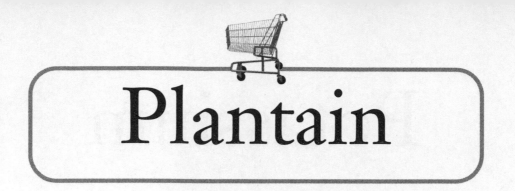

Plantain

NATURE'S BACTINE

The herb plantain is *not* the same as the fruit with the same name! The herb was given its name centuries ago by Roman soldiers who used the plant's broad leaves for their feet—in their language, "plantars." You may not have soldiers' feet, but here's what plantain can do for you.

■ **Asthma.** Teas containing English plantain will help open your bronchial passages when you have asthma or a stubborn case of bronchitis. Steep 1 teaspoon of the herb in a cup of hot water. Let cool and sip three or four times a day.

■ **Burns.** If you have blisters from a burn and they break open, clean the area and apply plantain. It contains the healing agent allantoin and is sometimes called nature's Bactine because it's good for healing all kinds of wounds. Brew a tea, let it cool, and apply it to your burn with a wet cloth soaked in the liquid.

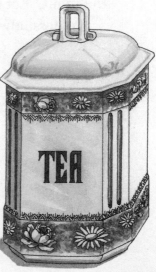

■ **Heartburn.** Plantain tea is an excellent heartburn remedy because it settles your stomach after heavy meals. Sip a cup after eating.

335

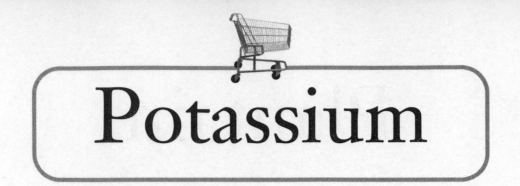

Potassium

BETTER BLOOD PRESSURE—AND MORE

If monkeys eat as many bananas in real life as they do in the movies, you can bet that they don't have to worry about high blood pressure. The reason? Bananas are an incredibly rich source of potassium, a mineral that's been shown to help blood flow through the arteries with less force. What else can this mighty mineral do for you? Check out these tips.

■ **Nighttime restlessness.** Are you up several times during the night? Eat a few dried banana chips during the day. The potassium they supply will help you sleep deeply all night long.

■ **Stroke.** Load up on potassium to protect your brain. According to the FDA, diets rich in potassium and low in sodium may reduce the risk of stroke.

■ **Weak bones.** In the well-known Framingham Heart Study, researchers found that the spines and hip bones of women who ate a lot potassium-rich foods were denser than those of women with potassium-poor diets. Protect your skeleton by eating more bananas and other potassium-rich foods daily.

■ **Vomiting.** If you've been vomiting, keep a few bottles of sports drinks on hand in case you need to restore electrolytes—the sodium, potassium, and other chemicals that keep body fluids in balance.

■ **Bloating.** Taking diuretics, whether herbal or pharmaceutical, to reduce bloating may strip potassium from your body. Instead, you can beat the bloat and retain ample potassium by sipping potassium-rich teas. Parsley is a good choice, as is cleavers, a 19th-century herb once known as bedstraw because it was used to stuff beds.

Prepare for a Brighter Smile

Some tooth-whitening bleaches are okay for sensitive teeth, but if yours are extremely sensitive, you may need to prime them first. One approach is to brush with toothpaste that contains potassium nitrate, such as Sensodyne, for six weeks before your dentist starts treatment.

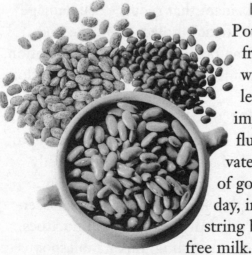

■ **High blood pressure.** Potassium keeps artery walls from thickening and works with sodium to regulate fluid levels in your body. This is important because too much fluid in your arteries can elevate blood pressure. Enjoy lots of good potassium sources every day, including bananas, apples, string beans, peas, beans, and fat-free milk.

Potatoes

SUPER SPUDS!

There's a reason many of us buy potatoes by the sack-ful. You can fry them, bake them, or mash them; you can add them to stews; and you can even puree them to make hearty soups. As for the nutritional payload, well, you could just about live on nothing but potatoes—and get a few extra benefits besides. Check out the latest research.

■ **Macular degeneration.** To protect your eyes, eat more potatoes. They're high in vitamin C, a powerful antioxidant that reduces cell damage from "toxic" molecules in the body and can prevent macular degeneration, one of the leading causes of vision loss.

■ **Constipation.** The next time you're constipated, slurp some potato water. This old-time remedy really seems to loosen things up—even though scientists aren't able to ascertain why. Anytime you boil potatoes, save the cooking water. The next morning, mix 2 tablespoons

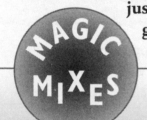

LOSE THE BAGS
To reduce bags and dark circles under your eyes, grate a raw potato and wrap the shavings in two pieces of cheesecloth or pieces cut from pantyhose. Lie down, put one sack over each eye, and relax for 15 minutes. Repeat daily until the circles fade.

of potato water and 2 tablespoons of honey into a mug of hot water and drink it before breakfast.

■ **Weak bones.** Potatoes are loaded with potassium, and studies show that eating potassium-rich foods can help keep your bones strong.

■ **The blues.** The next time you're feeling a little low, leave room on your plate for potatoes. When you eat turkey or other foods high in tryptophan, pairing them with carbohydrates such as potatoes triggers the release of insulin. This allows tryptophan to freely enter your brain and causes an increase in serotonin, a "feel-good" neurotransmitter that helps regulate mood.

Fabulous Food Fix

Drain the Pain

White potatoes contain natural chemicals that seem to help boils drain. Grate a potato and apply it directly to the boil. Leave it on for 10 to 20 minutes, then wash the area well. You can repeat the treatment once or twice a day.

■ **Eczema.** Potato juice reduces inflammation caused by eczema. Just grate a raw potato, dip a gauze pad in the shreds to absorb some of the juice, and gently dab the trouble spots.

■ **Splinters.** You can coax a splinter out of your skin with a raw potato. Tape a slice onto the affected area or, if the sliver is in a finger or toe, hollow out a space that's just the right size and slip the digit into the spud. (Hold it in place with a sock if you need to.) Leave the tater in place overnight, and you'll be able to easily pluck out the splinter out in the morning.

■ **Burns.** Soothe a minor burn by rubbing it gently with the cut surface of a raw potato.

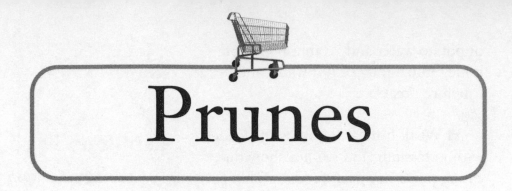

Prunes

MORE THAN A LAXATIVE

To boost the image of prunes, the FDA recently agreed that their name could be changed to dried plums. But as Shakespeare once asked, what's in a name? It's what's inside that counts—and there, prunes are plum beautiful! Here's what experts have to say.

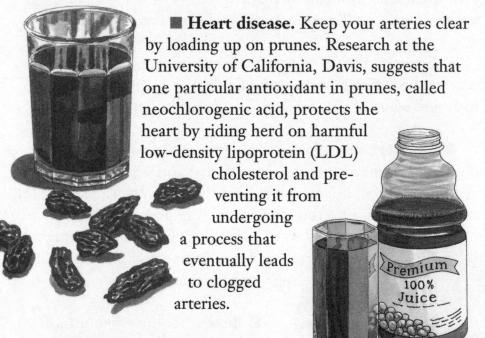

■ **Heart disease.** Keep your arteries clear by loading up on prunes. Research at the University of California, Davis, suggests that one particular antioxidant in prunes, called neochlorogenic acid, protects the heart by riding herd on harmful low-density lipoprotein (LDL) cholesterol and preventing it from undergoing a process that eventually leads to clogged arteries.

■ **Constipation I.** Prunes are packed with more fiber than almost any other fruit or vegetable—including dried beans. What's more, they contain dihydroxyphenyl isatin, a natural laxative. Down a glass of prune juice before bed to encourage a morning bowel movement.

■ **Constipation II.** In hospitals, prunes, bran, and applesauce are frequently mixed together and given to patients to relieve constipation. To make your own cocktail, combine four to six chopped prunes with 1 tablespoon of bran and ½ cup of applesauce. Try it just before bed.

■ **Cancer.** Ounce for ounce, prunes pack more than twice as many antioxidants as raisins do (and raisins are no lightweights!) Antioxidants are valuable compounds because they help fight cancer, so stock up on prunes and enjoy a few daily.

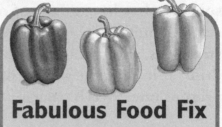

Fabulous Food Fix

The "Anti-Anemia Fruit"

If your energy levels have been on the low side, prunes may help. Along with figs, dates, raisins, and dried peaches and apricots, prunes are brimming with iron, the mineral that you need to prevent (or reverse) iron-deficiency anemia. Eat them every day.

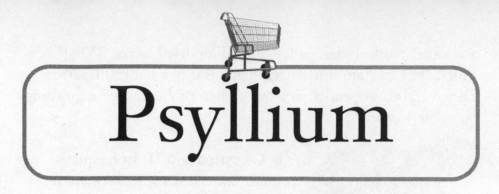

Psyllium

FABULOUS FIBER

Psyllium seeds are loaded with fiber, which makes stools softer and easier to pass. Plus, like other rich fiber sources, they have a host of other health benefits that you really shouldn't ignore. Check out these helpful psyllium strategies, and if you take powdered psyllium, be sure to drink at least eight glasses of water throughout the day to prevent intestinal blockage.

■ **Constipation.** Many doctors recommend powdered psyllium for easing constipation. Take 1 to 2 tablespoons of powder stirred into a glass of water or juice, followed by another full glass of water.

■ **High blood sugar.** Eat more psyllium if your blood sugar tends to be on the high side. Getting 50 grams of fiber daily from psyllium and other foods may lower insulin resistance, one cause of high blood sugar.

■ **Overweight.** Taking a fiber supplement such as psyllium before meals could help reduce the number of calo-

> ### ON THE SHELF
>
> ✓ **Metamucil**
> ✓ **All-Bran Bran Buds**
> ✓ **Kellogg's Guardian**
> ✓ **AIM Herbal Fiberblend**

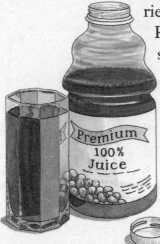

ries absorbed by your body, notes Glen Rothfeld, M.D. Take 1 to 3 tablespoons of psyllium powder dissolved in water or juice three times a day before meals, he suggests.

■ **IBS.** Bulking up the stools with fiber supplements such as psyllium or flaxseed can reduce the severity of colon spasms caused by irritable bowel syndrome (IBS).

■ **Hemorrhoids.** The fastest, most effective way to get the fiber necessary to help shrink hemorrhoids is to mix 2 heaping tablespoons of a commercial psyllium powder, such as Metamucil, into a large glass of water and gulp it down daily.

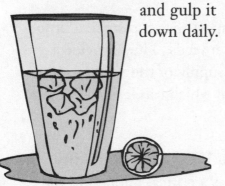

Just What the Doctor Ordered!

No Butts about It

If you've been getting anal fissures but can't seem to get adequate fiber from foods, take advantage of psyllium supplements. They'll prevent those hard, painful stools that frequently cause anal pain.

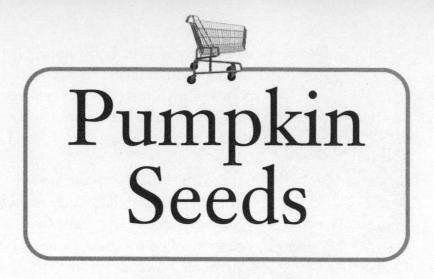

Pumpkin Seeds

NUTRITION WITH CRUNCH

Don't wait for Halloween to scoop these big, slimy seeds from the heart of a jack-o'-lantern. Baked and lightly salted, they're a perfect snack—and you can use them almost like medicine for some common health threats. Here's how.

■ **B.O.** Do you suspect that you smell a little pungent? Eat pumpkin seeds. They provide a good, concentrated supply of the mineral zinc, a deficiency of which can lead to body odor.

■ **Weakened immunity.** Zinc is a critical mineral in the maze of reactions that build immunity against invaders such as viruses and cancer. Just 1 ounce of pumpkin seeds delivers 3 milligrams of this mighty mineral—more than you'll get from 2 ounces of lean beef or 3 ounces of chicken breast.

■ **Fatigue.** Don't go hungry when you're hiking; take along some sunflower and pumpkin seeds. They make crispy, crunchy additions to a power-packed trail mix, and their protein will keep you energized.

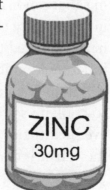

■ **Prostate problems.** Pumpkin seeds are particularly good for men since zinc, one of their major nutrients, is crucial for prostate health. Add them to your salad instead of croutons.

■ **Wounds.** Take advantage of pumpkin seeds when life has literally knocked you around. The minerals in pumpkin seeds, especially zinc, will help your body heal when you have a cut or other injury and especially after you've had surgery.

Fabulous Food Fix

Crunch Away Cramps

Here's a proven remedy for monthly cramps: Eat some pumpkin seeds. They're loaded with fatty acids that lower levels of body chemicals responsible for muscle aches and menstrual cramps.

ZINC
30mg

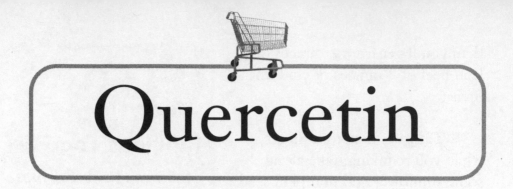

Quercetin

A CHEMICAL YOU CAN COUNT ON

Unless you have an advanced degree in chemistry, it's almost impossible to remember the names of the many beneficial substances in foods without all of them starting to sound alike. One of these chemicals, though, called quercetin, should stick in your mind because it's one of the most amazing "food fixes" ever discovered. Here's what experts have to say.

ON THE SHELF

✓ Onions
✓ Red wine
✓ Grape juice
✓ Apples
✓ Turmeric

■ **Bronchitis I.** Onions have long been a remedy for bronchial problems. After discovering that onions are a rich source of the anti-inflammatory compound quercetin, researchers have validated this use. Anything that decreases inflammation in your respiratory system will help you breathe a little better, so cook up some onion soup or even eat them raw, then enjoy the warmth that spreads through your chest and lungs.

■ **Bronchitis II.** For a healthy, tasty twist, add curry to your recipes, especially if you have allergy-related bronchitis. This Indian spice contains turmeric, a great source of the bioflavonoid-antihistamine quercetin, which can calm reactivity in the airways. Alternatively, you can simply supplement with three 200- to 300-milligram capsules of quercetin a day—one before breakfast, lunch, and dinner—for as long as your symptoms last, suggests Michael DiPalma, N.D.

■ **Heart disease.** Enjoy a little wine with your meals? That's good, because drinking wine in moderation can reduce your risk of developing heart disease or of dying from it. Red wine is more effective than white because it has a number of plant chemicals that help fight oxidation— the process that damages cells and makes cholesterol more likely to stick to artery walls—and reduce the risk of the blood clots that cause most heart attacks. Researchers think that the reason for these effects is quercetin, the pigment in red grape skins. If you'd rather not drink wine, have some red or purple grape juice, which contains many of the same plant chemicals.

■ **Hay fever.** If you have hay fever, start taking quercetin beginning in February. The recommended dose is four 200- to 250-milligram capsules a day between meals.

■ **Sore throat.** The natural pigments (bioflavonoids) that give fruits and vegetables their brilliant hues are loaded with

> ## Just What the Doctor Ordered!
>
> ### *Weep for Stronger Veins*
>
> The stronger your blood vessels, the less likely they are to slacken and lose their ability to push blood uphill— the cause of varicose veins. The quercetin in onion skins helps reduce capillary fragility, so toss an onion—skin and all—into soups and stews so the helpful quercetin leaches into the liquid.

anti-inflammatory agents that can help ease a sore throat. If your poor throat screams every time you eat, it may be easier to take bioflavonoid supplements, and quercetin is one of the best. You'll want to take between 250 and 500 milligrams three times a day.

■ **Allergies.** The quercetin in apples may help inhibit the release of histamine and relieve itching, hives, and other allergy symptoms. If you take quercetin supplements, the suggested dose is 250 to 500 milligrams three 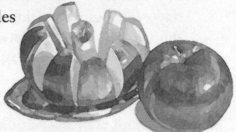 times a day on an empty stomach until symptoms subside. If you take a combination product, follow the directions on the label. Don't take a product that contains bromelain if you take aspirin or prescription blood thinners.

■ **Cataracts.** One study showed that drinking several daily cups of tea (a big quercetin provider) was associated with lower risk of cataracts. Eating onions frequently may help, too, since the amount of quercetin absorbed from onions is double that from tea. Since quercetin survives heat, you can enjoy your onions cooked or raw.

Quercetin Quells Cancer

The quercetin in foods fights cancer, possibly by deactivating carcinogens or causing them to just give up and die. One apple with skin delivers as much quercetin as ½ cup of tea or ⅔ cup of raw onion.

■ **Colds and flu.** The quercetin in onions and other foods is even more powerful than vitamin E for boosting immunity. Be sure to get plenty of quercetin when you've been sick or during cold and flu season, when those nasty viruses are everywhere. It can give your immune system a real boost.

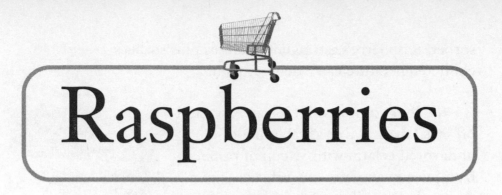

Raspberries

THIS BERRY'S GOT GAME

For thousands of years, herbalists pretty much benched raspberries as minor talent, but scientists today have moved them up to the starting squad because studies show that they do a few things very well indeed. Check these out.

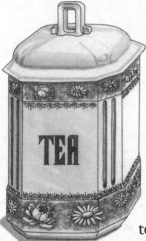

■ **Cramps.** Red raspberry is a uterine tonic that may help relieve cramping and pelvic congestion. If you're sure you're not pregnant, you can steep 1 heaping teaspoon of raspberry leaves in a cup of hot water for 10 minutes, then strain and drink one or two cups daily.

■ **Spotting.** Red raspberry leaf helps to stem heavy bleeding and spotting between periods. As long as there's no possibility that you're pregnant, drink at least two cups of raspberry leaf tea daily.

■ **Sore throat.** The next time you have a sore throat, enjoy a soothing cup of raspberry sorbet. Raspberry's astringent qualities plus sorbet's chilly temperature can ease your pain.

■ **Clogged pores.** Here's an easy, peel-off facial mask. Mix 1½ tablespoons of unflavored gelatin with ½ cup of raspberry fruit juice in a microwave-safe container, then nuke it until the gelatin is completely dissolved. Put the mixture in the refrigerator until it's almost set (about 25 minutes), then spread it on your face, let it dry, and peel it off.

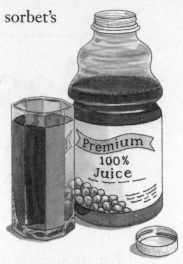

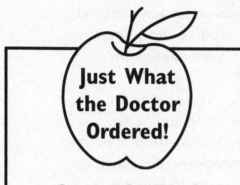

Just What the Doctor Ordered!

Get in the Black

Black raspberries contain 10 to 20 times more plant chemicals called anthocyanins than red raspberries do. Since anthocyanins may help prevent heart disease and cancer, the message couldn't be clearer: Eat more raspberries!

■ **Constipation.** As we get older, our intestinal tracts sometimes start to slow down. The solution? Sprinkle ½ cup or more of raspberries on a bowl of high-fiber cereal every morning. Practiced every day, this little trick can help prevent constipation.

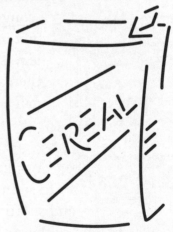

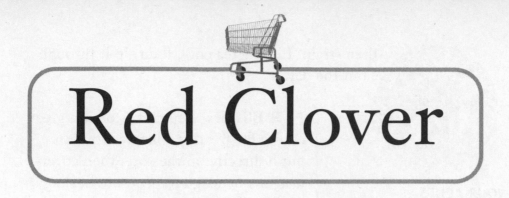

Red Clover

COME OVER, COME OVER!

This pleasantly sweet herb, which grows wild in many fields and along roadsides, has been enjoyed as a tea for thousands of years, and not only for its good taste. Known as a blood purifier, it's used in many tonic and restorative teas and has a history as a woman's herb. It has more than a few important medical benefits that we can take advantage of, although women with breast cancer should avoid it. Here are some of its uses.

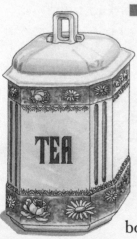

■ **Lyme disease.** Whip up some red clover tea if you're dealing with Lyme disease. The herb has been used traditionally as a blood purifier, for skin health, and for overall constitutional health. Steep $1/2$ cup of fresh red clover flower heads in a quart of boiling water for 10 minutes,

Soothing Sips

COOLING CLOVER

Red clover contains isoflavones, naturally occurring substances that may reduce hot flashes. To make a tea, put 3 teaspoons of dried blossoms in 1 cup of boiling water and steep, covered, for 10 minutes. Strain out the herb and—voilà!—you have a cup of isoflavone tea!

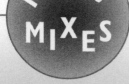

then strain. Let the tea cool, then sip it throughout the day.

■ **Blisters.** Red clover oil is a great choice for treating blisters. You can put it directly on the sore, then cover it with a bandage to promote healing. Repeat the treatment once a day until the blister's gone. Be sure the product you buy is made for topical use. What you don't want is an essential oil, which is too concentrated to apply directly to your skin.

■ **Menopausal discomforts.** Red clover is brimming with phytoestrogens, plant chemicals that have mild estrogenic activity. In fact, it has twice as many phytoestrogens as soy and may be six times more potent. In one study, women who took one tablet of Promensil—the leading red clover supplement—daily for two months had less vaginal dryness. You can make red clover tea by steeping 1 teaspoon in a cup of hot water for 10 to 15 minutes. Strain and drink two cups daily. If you'd like to try Promensil, ask your doctor if it's right for you.

EASE YOUR ACHES
Starting the day with a cup of red clover tea will go a long way toward easing arthritis pain. Add 1 teaspoon of dried red clover blossoms, crushed, and 1 teaspoon of dried alfalfa leaves, crushed, to 1 cup of boiling water. Steep for 5 minutes, strain, and sip. Add a teaspoon of honey if you want to sweeten it up a bit.

■ **Post-illness recovery.** Supporting the body with herbal healing agents when you've been sick can help you recover more quickly. To make a therapeutic tea, mix equal parts of red clover, echinacea, cleavers, prickly ash, and calendula, then add 1 teaspoon to a cup of hot water. Steep for 10 to 15 minutes, strain, and sip.

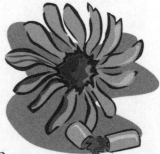

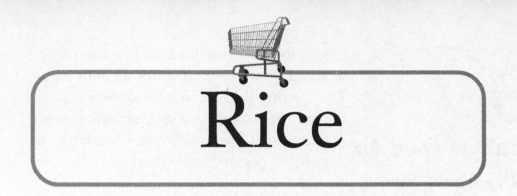

Rice

A GREAT GRAIN FOR HEALTH

Did you know that there are an estimated 40,000 varieties of rice on the world's supermarket shelves? All of them are nutritional powerhouses, but even if you stick to the basic white or brown varieties, you'll get a remarkable array of powerful healing compounds. Here are some of the best reasons to put more rice on your plate.

■ **Gas.** If you often have flatulence, eat more rice and chicken. They're about the only foods that are unlikely to cause gas. In fact, rice is so easy to digest that doctors recommend eating it any time your digestion is upset, such as when you're stressed, you have the flu, or before or after surgery.

■ **Low energy.** All of the B vitamins can help improve energy, along with immune function and mental sharpness, but one of the more important Bs is thiamin pyrophosphate—the activated form of thiamin—which is neces-

Smart Sweets

When your stomach's upset, drinking herbal teas sweetened with regular sugar can actually increase nausea. Next time, when you brew stomach-settling peppermint or ginger tea, use a grain-derived sweetener such as rice syrup. It's easier on your tummy.

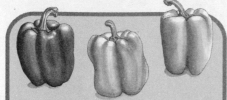

Fabulous Food Fix

Dry Up the Runs

Rice water soothes an irritated intestinal tract and helps replace fluids lost through diarrhea. Boil ½ cup of brown rice in 1 quart of water for 15 to 20 minutes, stirring constantly. Drain and reserve the cooking water, then drink it throughout the day with a little honey added, if you like.

sary for the breakdown and release of energy from carbohydrates. In addition to getting thiamin in a B-complex supplement, eat more of it by choosing rice bran cereal for breakfast and snacking on peanuts, pecans, and walnuts.

■ **Heart disease.** If heart disease runs in your family, make an effort to eat more brown rice. A study at Columbia University showed that women who ate three daily servings of whole grains, such as brown rice, had a 27 percent lower risk of developing heart disease than those who ate only refined grains, such as white rice. This is partly because brown rice is loaded with fiber and because it may have chemical compounds that can knock down your cholesterol numbers.

■ **Diabetes.** A study of more than 65,000 nurses revealed that those who ate large amounts of refined grains had twice the risk of developing diabetes compared with those who consumed mostly unrefined carbohydrates. All rice is good for you, but the brown, unprocessed form is what you want more of to keep your diabetes risk as low as it will go.

■ **IBS.** Two-thirds of people who have irritable bowel syndrome (IBS) are allergic or intolerant to at least one food, and almost half find relief by keeping a food diary, identifying their triggers, and eliminating the offenders. In many cases, switching from foods made with wheat to oat bread and rice cereals can make a huge difference.

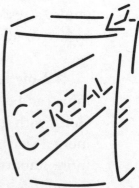

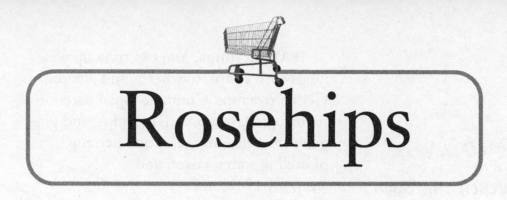

Rosehips

C WHAT YOU GET

Americans have always loved roses, and they appreciate the health-giving properties of vitamin C, so why not combine the two with rosehips? Read on to find out what this combo can do for you.

■ **Colds.** Immune-stimulating herbs can help ease the discomforts of a cold. For a healing tea, combine equal parts of rosehips, yarrow, lemon balm, licorice root, ginger root, and eyebright. Use 1 heaping teaspoon of the herb mixture per 1 cup of hot water, steep for 10 to 15 minutes, and strain. Drink two or three cups per day. Leave out the licorice if you have high blood pressure or kidney disease.

■ **Hemorrhoids.** Rosehips, along with yarrow, horse chestnut, and butcher's broom, can help strengthen your blood vessels and may relieve hemorrhoids. Mix equal parts of each herb, then measure 1 heaping teaspoon into a cup of hot water and steep for 10 minutes. Strain and drink two or three cups a day.

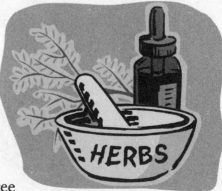

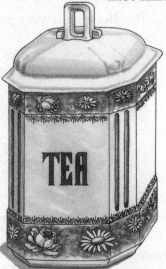

Soothing Sips

QUENCH THE BURN

Heartburn can sometimes be caused by food sensitivities. To help decrease reactions, drink a cup of rosehip tea before meals. Steep 1 heaping teaspoon of rosehips in 1 cup of hot water for 15 minutes, strain, and enjoy.

■ **Weak lungs.** You can tone up your lungs with restorative herbs and vitamin C–rich rosehips. Combine equal parts of thyme, ginkgo, aniseed, rosehips, and ginger. Add 1 heaping teaspoon per cup of boiling water, cover, and steep for 15 minutes. Drink two or three cups per day. People who are taking aspirin or blood-thinning medications should avoid ginkgo.

■ **Shingles.** Hot tea made with rosehips is just the thing when you have shingles because it's high in vitamin C. To make the tea, steep 1 teaspoon of rosehips in 1 cup of hot water, then strain, cool, and sip. Drink several cups daily at the first hint of a shingles outbreak.

Rosehips

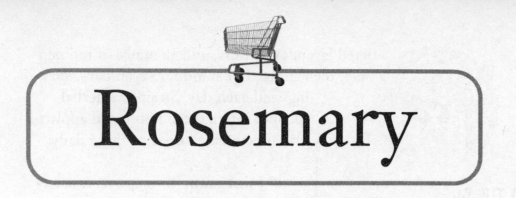

Rosemary

PUNGENT AND POWERFUL

Rosemary is among the strongest-smelling kitchen spices, and, as you may suspect from that penetrating aroma, it's loaded with powerful oils that you can count on for good health. Here are a few good reasons to, well, spice up your life!

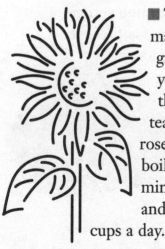

■ **The blues.** Flowers and plants do more than make the world a more beautiful place: Their fragrance, color, and chemical makeup can also lift your mood. To beat the blues, steep 1 teaspoon of dried rosemary in 1 cup of boiling water for 10 minutes, then strain and drink two or three cups a day.

■ **Poor circulation.** A warming herbal liniment may help increase circulation to paralyzed muscles. To a 1-quart bottle of rubbing alcohol, add 2 ounces of powdered rosemary leaves, 1 ounce of pow-

Piney Odor Eater

Pine-scented rosemary is a natural antibacterial herb that can help quash body odor, especially when combined with sage. Mix 1 tablespoon of each herb with 1 cup of baking soda and sprinkle on any odor-causing body part.

357

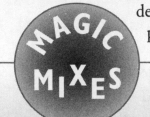

MAGIC MIXES

dered lavender flowers, and ½ ounce of red pepper, then shake. Let stand for seven days, shaking well each day. Strain the herbal alcohol into a clean bottle and apply to the affected area once or twice daily.

BEAT THE BUGS
To cut your risk of infection, wash wounds with rosemary extract. This aromatic herb is a mild antiseptic that appears to penetrate the skin and may allow the wound to dry out better than antibiotic creams and ointments, which can smother the skin and may seal in germs.

■ **Joint pain.** To help increase circulation and soothe aching joints, apply an ointment made by adding a few drops of arnica oil to a warming rosemary salve. For every ½ teaspoon of salve, add three or four drops of arnica. Smooth it on your sore joints three or four times a day. Arnica is for external use only; do not use on broken skin.

■ **Sprains.** The next time you get a sprain, you can help yourself recover with a cooling herbal pack. First, fill a bowl with ice-cold water and sprinkle several drops of rosemary oil into the water. Next, soak a clean washcloth in the bowl, wring it out well, and lay it over the sprained area. Finally, cover the cloth with an ice pack and leave it on for no longer than 20 minutes.

■ **Dandruff.** If you're ever embarrassed by dandruff flakes, try steaming your scalp with nutritive herbs. Mix together equal parts of fresh or dried rosemary, nettle, and peppermint. Add 2 tablespoons of the dried mixture (or ½ cup of fresh) to 2 cups of hot water, cover, and steep for 10 minutes. (If you use fresh nettle, wear gloves while preparing the herbs to avoid being stung by the nettle's sharp spines.) Strain the infusion, cool

Rosemary

slightly, and apply it carefully to your scalp. Cover your hair with a shower cap and wrap your head in a hot, wet towel. Relax for 30 minutes, then use an herbal rinse.

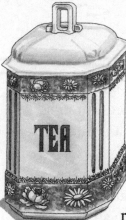

■ **Brain fog.** This lovely tea may not turn you into a wizard, but it will certainly give your brain a healthy workout. Combine two parts ginkgo with one part each rosemary, yarrow, and hawthorn. Use 1 heaping teaspoon of the mixture per cup of hot water and steep, covered, for 15 minutes. Drink one or two cups a day. People who are taking blood-thinning medications or aspirin should avoid ginkgo.

Spice Away Yeast

Many common kitchen spices, including oregano, thyme, and rosemary, have fungus-fighting properties. Use them liberally when preparing meals for as long as you're fighting off a yeast infection. The same herbs can also tackle athlete's foot fungus from the inside out.

■ **Thinning hair.** Gentle scalp massage can enhance circulation and may encourage hair growth. Mix four to six drops of rosemary oil in 1 tablespoon of olive oil and gently rub it into your scalp. For a deeper effect, put on a shower cap, then wrap a hot, wet towel around your head. Either way, leave it on for 30 minutes, then shampoo.

■ **Age spots.** To fade age spots, combine 1 teaspoon of grated horseradish, 1 teaspoon of lemon juice, 1 teaspoon of vinegar, and three drops of rosemary oil, then apply the mixture to your spots. It has a strong odor, but it will make spots fade swiftly.

■ **Bronchitis.** For quick relief from bronchitis, fill your bathtub with hot water and add two drops each of eucalyptus, thyme, and rosemary oil, plus about a cup of Epsom salts. Climb in and relax as the steam increases the flow of mucus to clear your head, the molecules from the oils help dilate your small airways to ease your breathing, and the magnesium from the Epsom salts is absorbed through your skin to further relax your bronchial passages.

■ **Dry skin.** A facial steam can deep-six dryness—especially if you use herbal oil that encourages oil production in your skin, says herbalist Kathi Keville. Simply bring 3 cups of water to a boil, then remove the pot from the stove. Add one drop each of rosemary, geranium, rose, fennel, and peppermint herbal oil. Drape a towel over your head and tuck the ends around the pot so the steam is captured inside a "mini-sauna." Be careful not to get close enough for the steam to burn your face. Limit your steam sessions to about 5 minutes once a week.

■ **Gas.** If beans and other starchy foods make you gassy, simply stir in some rosemary.

Just What the Doctor Ordered!

Coffee, Tea, or Rosemary?

When your energy flags, don't go for a cup of joe—reach for rosemary instead. It induces brain waves normally produced when a person is alert and concentrating, explains Alan Hirsch, M.D. Simply place a rosemary plant on your desk and rub its leaves to help you focus.

■ **Muscle strains.** To soothe the pain of a strain, take a warm shower and use shower gel mixed with a few drops of muscle-soothing rosemary oil. Massage the oil into the meat of your sore muscle, stroking upward toward your heart.

■ **Varicose veins.** When blood vessels lose some of their ability to push blood uphill from the legs back to the heart, some blood remains in the veins, causing the swelling and discoloration that characterize varicose veins. Placing hot, then cold compresses soaked in a solution of circulation-boosting herbs on your problem veins provides a soothing pumping action that facilitates blood flow, says Jeanette Jacknin, M.D. To give it a try, soak a cloth in a mixture of 10 drops each of rosemary, cypress, geranium, ginger, juniper, and lavender oils added to 1 quart of hot water. Hold the compress on your leg for 15 minutes. Soak another cloth in a batch of solution made with the same oils and cold water and apply it for 15 minutes. Finally, massage your leg gently with one or more of the oils, stroking upward toward your heart.

■ **Sinus headache.** If your sinuses are pounding, try an herbal steam to break up congestion. In a saucepan, bring a few cups of water to a boil, then add 2 to 3 teaspoons of rosemary and a few drops of eucalyptus oil. Remove the pan from the stove and put

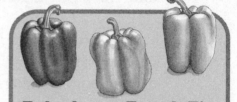

Fabulous Food Fix

Season Your Skin

Studies have shown that consuming an extract of rosemary can help prevent damaging changes to skin—from too much sun, for example, or simply the natural changes that occur as you get older—by protecting the fat in skin cells.

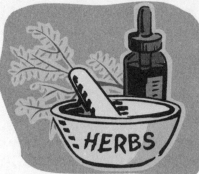

it on a table or counter. Drape a towel over your head to trap the steam, carefully lean over the pot, and breathe deeply for 10 to 15 minutes, inhaling though your nose and exhaling through your mouth. Repeat two or three times a day.

■ **Blisters.** If you're worried about infection from a blister, rosemary and thyme can help because they're powerful bacteria fighters. Add a tablespoon of each herb to a cup of hot water and steep for about 10 minutes. Let the liquid cool to room temperature, pour some on a cloth, and hold it against your blister for about 20 minutes. You can repeat the treatment once or twice a day until the blister is gone.

■ **Cancer.** Adding plenty of rosemary to recipes may reduce your cancer risk. Rosemary is packed with carnosol, a phenolic compound that fights cancer by interrupting inflammation so those evil cells can't get a toehold and grow. Carnosol also appears to boost your liver's production of several cancer-fighting substances, including glutathione-S-transferase.

■ **Heart disease.** When you flavor foods with rosemary instead of lots of butter or sour cream, you protect your heart from saturated fat and your waistline from excess pounds.

■ **Stress.** Rosemary is being explored for its ability to relax you when its aroma is inhaled, so always breathe deeply when cooking with rosemary.

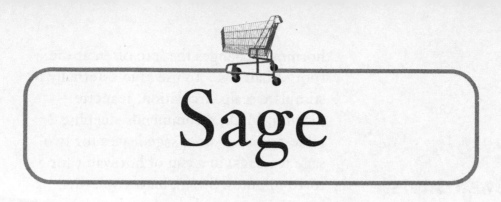

Sage

SUPER SAGE ADVICE

Centuries ago, sage was known as *toute bonne*, French for "all's well." That may be a bit of an exaggeration, but sage does contain aromatic oils that are extremely powerful healers. Here's what experts have to say about this wonderful herb. Women who are pregnant or breastfeeding shouldn't use sage internally.

■ **Runny nose.** The pungent oval leaves of the sage plant aren't just for enhancing turkey stuffing—they can also nip a runny nose in the bud. At the first sign of a drip, steep 1 teaspoon of dried sage leaves in ½ cup of hot water for 10 minutes or so, strain, and sip slowly.

Nix the Night Sweats

At the first hint of night sweats, drink some sage tea, suggests nurse-midwife Carol Leonard. To make the tea, steep 1 tablespoon of dried sage in a cup of hot water for 10 minutes, then strain.

■ **Thinning hair.** It may be especially, well, sage to use sage to encourage hair growth. Taken internally, this pungent culinary herb helps the body adapt to the

Soothing Sips

SWEAT STOPPER

In one study, researchers found that people who perspire heavily can reduce sweating by 50 percent by drinking tea made from dried sage, which seems to help suppress perspiration-prompting nerve fibers. The effects don't kick in for a couple of hours, but they do last for several days. To try the tea, simmer 4 tablespoons (about 20 leaves) of dried sage in a quart of water for 10 to 15 minutes, then strain and sip a cup or two a day.

hormonal changes that are often at the root of hair loss. To use sage externally to stimulate scalp circulation, Jeanette Jacknin, M.D., recommends steeping 2 tablespoons of dried sage leaves (or two sage tea bags) in a cup of hot water for 5 to 10 minutes. Strain, let it cool, then pour it over your hair after shampooing. Leave it on for 5 minutes, then rinse. Repeat daily. You can also add a few drops of sage extract to your favorite shampoo.

■ **Athlete's foot.** Soaking your toes in tinctures of fungicidal plants is a soothing way to knock out athlete's foot with zero side effects, says Daniel DeLapp, N.D. He suggests mixing several drops of tincture of black walnut hulls, thyme, pau d'arco, spilanthes, goldenseal, and oregano in a quart of warm water, then soaking your feet twice daily. Dry your feet thoroughly, then sprinkle with sage powder, a mild antiperspirant, before donning clean cotton socks.

■ **Sore throat.** To relieve sore throat pain, stimulate your immune system to do what it does best. Combine equal parts of sage, echinacea, agrimony, and cleavers, then steep 1 heaping teaspoon of the mixture in 1 cup of hot water for 10 minutes. Strain, then sip the hot tea slowly three or four times a day to give your immunity a boost.

■ **Smelly feet.** If foot odor is a problem, look for sage, tea tree, or green clay, which are all odor neutralizers. Sprinkle some in your shoes, and you'll say sayonara to odor.

■ **Chest congestion.** Warm steam soothes the lining of the bronchial tubes and loosens secretions. To relieve chest tightness, fill a bowl with very hot water and add a few drops of sage oil. Put a towel over your head, lean over the bowl (be careful not to get too close), and inhale deeply through your nose.

■ **Gum disease.** Sage, myrrh, and calendula can protect tissues against gum infection, which is the leading cause of tooth loss—and it can even damage your heart if bacteria slip into the bloodstream. Add five drops of a tincture of each herb to a small amount of warm water, then swish it around your mouth for several minutes two or three times a day.

■ **Dull hair.** Herbal rinses help make hair shiny and relieve scalp irritation. If you have dark hair, traditional herbs to use include rosemary and sage; chamomile and calendula are suggested for

Herbal Deodorant

The tangy-smelling sage you use to season poultry stuffing contains compounds that can fight odor-causing bacteria, and piney rosemary is another natural antibacterial herb. Mix 1 tablespoon of each ground herb with 1 cup of baking soda and dust some under your arms.

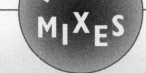

blondes, and cloves are recommended for auburn or red hair. Make a strong tea by adding 4 tablespoons of herb to 1 quart of boiling water and steeping for 15 minutes. Add ¼ cup of apple cider vinegar to the solution to restore the scalp's proper pH, then use as a final rinse after shampooing.

SAGE FOR STINGS
You can make a great poultice to treat stings and swelling using sage and vinegar. Just run a rolling pin over a handful of freshly picked sage leaves to bruise them. Put the leaves in a pan, cover them with apple cider vinegar, and simmer on low until they soften. Remove the leaves, carefully wrap them in a washcloth, and apply it for instant relief.

■ **Laryngitis.** Gargling with red sage tea can soothe the inflamed mucous membranes of your larynx when you have laryngitis. Pour 1 cup of warm water over 1 teaspoon of red sage and steep for 10 minutes. Strain, then gargle.

■ **Stress.** Make your own flower water to spritz on your skin during the day for a fragrant lift. Made from essential oils that mitigate stress, flower water can

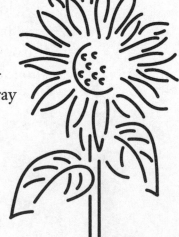

be used whenever the need arises. Mix 10 drops each of lavender, clary sage, and Roman chamomile oil with 5 milliliters of isopropyl alcohol, then add that to 100 milliliters of distilled water. Store in a glass spray bottle and use liberally.

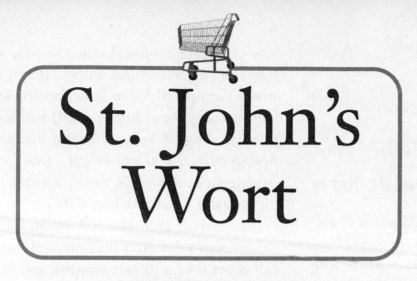

St. John's Wort

A SAINTLY HEALER

Entire books have been written about St. John's wort, an herbal medicine that's been used for more than 2,000 years. Scientists have found that it's among the most effective treatments for minor depression. It's also a powerful germ killer that can be applied topically, and it helps all sorts of injuries heal more quickly. Here's a sample of the many uses for this high-powered herb.

■ **Bursitis.** St. John's wort oil is an excellent pain reliever for bursitis. The next time a wrist, shoulder, or elbow is so stiff you can hardly move it, apply the oil directly to the affected area. For an extra boost, add four to six drops of arnica oil and two or three drops of wintergreen oil.

■ **Depression.** A slew of studies since the 1970s have shown that St. John's wort can ease mild (but not severe) depression, perhaps by inhibiting the reabsorp-

Soothing Sips

DRINK AND BE HAPPY

Native American healers use a "basic herbal cheer" mixture made with St. John's wort flowers, passionflower, and devil's-club bark. To try it, combine equal amounts of each herb in a glass jar, mix well, and close the jar tightly. Then, when you're feeling low, put 1 tablespoon of the herb mixture in a mug and add boiling water, Cover, steep for 10 minutes, and strain. Drink two cups a day.

tion of a brain chemical called serotonin. Researchers have found, in fact, that it works just as well for mild depression as high-powered (and high-priced) antidepressant drugs. Check with your doctor first to be sure you've just got a low-grade case of the blues, then pick up a high-quality brand such as Kira or Nature's Made and take 300 milligrams three times a day. You may not feel its full effect for up to two months, and in some people, it can cause stomach upset, allergic reactions, and heightened sensitivity to the sun. Do not take St. John's wort with other medications.

■ **Irritated nerves.** For inflamed and irritated nerves, add several drops of St. John's wort oil to a few drops of arnica and apply frequently. Arnica is for external use only; do not use it on broken skin.

■ **Burns.** As long as the skin isn't broken, you can apply St. John's wort oil to minor burns two or three times a day to promote healing and ease pain. If you use it immediately after a burn and keep applying it for a few days, there's a good chance that the burn will heal without even causing a blister.

■ **Earlobe pain.** For a sore earlobe—due to a recent piercing, for example—apply tincture of St. John's wort. It's great for healing damaged skin because it quickly kills surface bacteria. Since tinctures are alcohol based, you may feel a little stinging

St. John's Wort

when you use this remedy, but it doesn't last long, and the tincture will help keep the area problem-free.

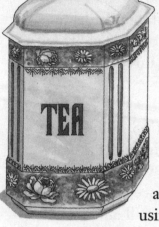

■ **Aches and pains.** To concoct a pain-relieving tea, combine two parts echinacea with one part each of St. John's wort, skullcap, lemon balm, and oatstraw. Add 1 heaping teaspoon of the mixture to a cup of hot water, cover, and steep for 10 minutes. Strain and drink three or four cups a day. If you're taking any medications, consult your doctor before using this tea.

■ **Spinal pain.** As osteoporosis progresses, the bones in your spine can begin pinching the nerves that run between them. St. John's wort oil is specifically indicated for nerve pain. Massage a small amount of oil into any painful areas two or three times daily.

■ **Sciatica.** To help relieve sciatica pain, combine equal parts of St. John's wort oil, arnica oil, and castor oil and gently massage the mixture onto the nerve track, beginning at the buttocks and going down the back of the affected leg. If you have a painful disk problem, use the oil on that area as well.

■ **Neuroma.** Numbness, tingling, and burning on top of the foot during exercise may signal the development of a Morton's neuroma—a

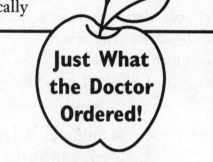

Just What the Doctor Ordered!

Rub and Relax

Many women find it helpful to use massage oils externally to help muscles relax prior to intercourse. St. John's wort oil is a wonderful choice for this purpose.

little tumor along the nerve extending over the ball of the foot that makes wearing lace-up shoes particularly uncomfortable. Use alternating hot and cold footbaths to reduce the inflammation, and apply St. John's wort oil two or three times a day.

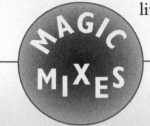

SPIKE THE PAIN

St. John's wort helps fight bacteria and eases the pain of splinters. First, wash the area well with soap and water. If you can, remove the splinter, then apply St. John's wort oil to the area once or twice a day. If you can't get the sliver out, there's a good chance that it will work itself out—and in the meantime, using the oil will greatly reduce the risk of infection.

■ **Cold sores.** Both St. John's wort oil and lavender oil inhibit the activity of herpes simplex, the virus that causes cold sores. Once or twice a day, use a cotton swab to dab a small amount of oil on the sore.

■ **Hand injuries.** If you've bashed your finger or thumb, applying St. John's wort tincture can help. Since the tincture is made with alcohol, it will kill any germs that happen to be lurking inside the wound.

■ **Shingles.** To reduce residual nerve pain after a shingles outbreak, add 30 drops each of extracts of St. John's wort (a wound healer), astragalus (an immune booster), Jamaican dogwood (a nerve sedative), and, unless you have high blood pressure, licorice (an antiviral) to a glass of water, then drink three glasses a day for up to 20 days. You can also apply St. John's wort oil directly to the painful areas two or three times a day to calm the inflamed nerves.

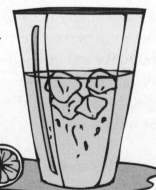

St. John's Wort

■ **Foot pain.** Creams that include the herbs arnica, comfrey, or St. John's wort work well to increase circulation and reduce the inflammation that may be making your feet hurt, according to Pamela Taylor, N.D. You can buy a cream with one or more of these ingredients or add 6 to 12 drops of one of these herbal oils to an ounce of grapeseed, olive, or almond oil to make a soothing liniment.

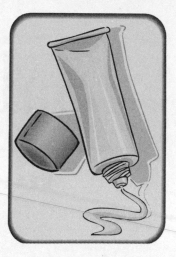

■ **Stubbed toe.** Herbal oils made from arnica and St. John's wort can make a real difference when you've stubbed your toe. They help relieve pain, promote healing, and reduce the risk of infection. Combine 6 to 12 drops of either oil with a few tablespoons of olive or almond oil, then apply the mixture to the sore area a couple of times a day.

■ **Blisters.** St. John's wort is great for killing germs and easing pain when you have a blister. Moisten a square of gauze with an alcohol-based tincture of the herb, then apply it to the blister after you've washed it.

■ **Muscle pain.** To add an herbal soother to your rubdown, try St. John's wort, a traditional treatment for both nerve pain and muscle soreness. Buy some St. John's wort oil and add 6 to 12 drops to an ounce of olive or almond oil, then rub it on.

Soothe the Scrape

If you want to be absolutely, positively sure that abrasions don't get infected, paint on a little St. John's wort tincture. This herb kills just about all of the bacteria it encounters.

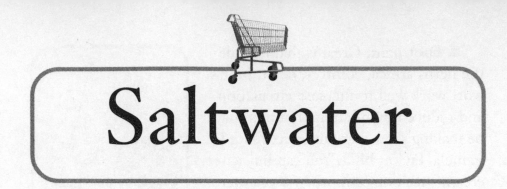

Saltwater

HEALING WITH SALINE

Just because most of the Earth's surface is awash in salty oceans doesn't mean you should take saltwater—or saline, as doctors call it—for granted. Take a look at this.

■ **Skin conditions.** Seawater can kill fungi, dry up poison ivy blisters, and relieve almost any other skin condition. And it's readily available even to land-lubbers: Just convert your tub into a mini-ocean by adding salt to your bathwater. The recipe is 2 tablespoons of salt for each pint of water. Soak for 5 to 10 minutes at a time.

Beach Sore Feet

If you live on a seacoast, take a barefoot walk along the edge of the water and let the surf wash over your feet when they're rashy or sore. The highly saline environment has a cleansing effect and can hasten the cure of your soles.

■ **Sore throat.** Gargling with salty water helps dissolve mucus, cleanse your throat, and add some astringency to your body chemistry to reduce swelling and inflammation when you have a sore throat. It also helps minimize postnasal drip. Simply mix 1 teaspoon of salt into 8 ounces of warm water and gargle four or five times a day.

■ **Earache.** According to Andrew Weil, M.D., gargling promotes healing of an ear infection by bringing more blood to the Eustachian tube. Gargle several times a day with 1 teaspoon of salt dissolved in a glass of water that's as hot as you can tolerate.

■ **Gum pain.** Plain salt is a wonderful gum healer. Stir ¼ teaspoon of salt into ¼ cup of warm water and use the solution as a mouthwash two or three times daily.

■ **Canker sores.** If you have painful canker sores, try an antiseptic mouth rinse. Dissolve ½ teaspoon of goldenseal powder and ¼ teaspoon of salt in a cup of warm water, then swish and spit. Repeat up to four times a day.

■ **Sinusitis.** Irrigating your nose with saltwater is the best way to relieve both acute and chronic sinusitis. Simply mix ½ teaspoon of table salt into a glass of warm water. Put the solution in a spray bottle or an ear syringe, then lean over a sink and turn your head so your

Just What the Doctor Ordered!

A Cure for Glum Gums

Here's a nearly instant way to take away denture pain: Mix ½ teaspoon of salt in a cup of warm water. Take a mouthful of the solution, swirl it around in your mouth, and spit it out. The soreness will disappear like magic, and it probably won't come back for at least an hour or two. You can repeat the saltwater rinse as often as necessary to get relief.

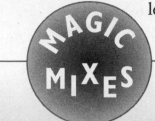

MAGIC MIXES

SALTY SKIN SAVER
According to research from the Dead Sea Mor Clinic in Israel, soaking in a special blend of salts scooped from the Dead Sea clears 90 percent of lesions in a majority of psoriasis patients. You can buy the salts over the Internet, then soak for at least 45 minutes three times a week.

left nostril is lower than your right, keeping your head tilted so your nose is higher than your mouth. Spray or squirt the solution into your right nostril, allowing the water to drain from your left nostril and your mouth. Gently blow your nose, then repeat with the other nostril.

■ **Pneumonia.** When you're battling pneumonia, your nose and throat may be intensely irritated. Sniffing saltwater is a quick way to ease the discomfort because it draws fluid from the tissues and helps reduce inflammation. You can buy ready-made saline solution, or you can make your own by mixing a few teaspoons of salt in a few ounces of warm water. The solution should taste like tears.

■ **Toothache.** For toothache pain, thoroughly rinse your mouth with a saltwater solution made by mixing about ½ teaspoon of salt in a cup of warm water. The relief doesn't last very long, but you can use the rinse as often as necessary.

■ **Throat irritation.** No cough drops or candy handy? Soak half a lemon in saltwater and suck on it for a while to moisten your throat and relieve any soreness.

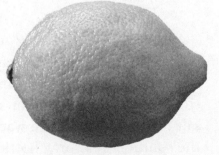

Saltwater

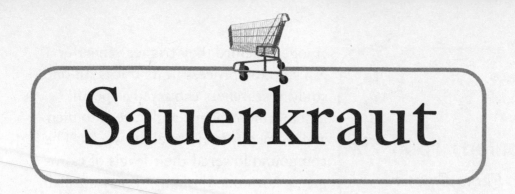

Sauerkraut

PICKLED CABBAGE WITH PUNCH

A lot of people think of sauerkraut as cabbage with a personal hygiene problem. When you combine the fermentation process with the smelly sulfur compounds already present in cabbage—whew! The smell can knock your socks off. But don't let a little odor come between you and the healing benefits. Sauerkraut's tangy (if pungent) taste is accompanied by beneficial chemical compounds that are sweet indeed. Take a gander at what they can do for you.

■ **Heartburn.** Cabbage contains glutamine, an amino acid that appears to promote healing in the digestive tract. If you have frequent heartburn, eating sauerkraut a few times a week may prevent future problems.

■ **Anemia.** The lactic acid in sauerkraut promotes iron absorption, so load up if you're prone to iron-deficiency anemia.

■ **Cancer.** "Cabbage contains at least 11 of the 15 families of vegetable-related compounds found to prevent cancer," says Wendy Demark, R.D., Ph.D. Foremost among those compounds are indoles, which scientists believe can destroy car-

375

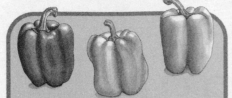

Fabulous Food Fix

Fume Fighter

Sauerkraut contains lots of indigestible dietary sugars, called fructo-oligosaccharides, that feed the "friendly" bacteria in your gut that help digestion. When you take antibiotics, they can wipe out good bacteria along with the bad, causing gassiness. To alleviate this effect, eat sauerkraut or foods such as miso, artichokes, and asparagus.

cinogens before they trigger cancer or can stop the process in its tracks. In one study, researchers extracted a specific indole from cabbage and gave it to men and women for one to eight weeks. The compound lowered their levels of estrogen, a hormone thought to play a role in breast and prostate cancers. In a nutshell, eating more cabbage and sauerkraut will go a long way toward lowering your cancer risk.

■ **Heart disease, stroke, and cataracts.** All of the cruciferous vegetables, including the cabbage that's used to make sauerkraut, may reduce your risk of heart disease, stroke, and cataracts. This is partly because these foods are high in fiber but also because they contain a host of chemical compounds that prevent harmful oxygen molecules in the body from damaging cells. The same compounds help stop the process that causes cholesterol to stick to arteries and possibly block the flow of blood. The more cabbage you put on your plate, the better your circulation is likely to be.

■ **Weak bones.** Some types of cabbage are super high in calcium, so they can help boost bone density. Regular servings of sauerkraut, bok choy, and other types of cabbage—especially after menopause, when bone density declines—can help keep bones strong.

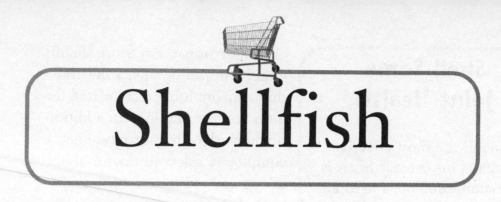

Shellfish

WIN THE SHELL GAME

For a long time, health-conscious eaters avoided shell-fish because these foods contain high amounts of choles-terol. As it turns out, however, the cholesterol in shrimp, oysters, and other shellfish has very little effect on the cholesterol in your blood—and shellfish contain boatloads of other beneficial nutrients. In fact, eating more shellfish is one of the best things you can do to protect your long-term health. Here's why.

■ **Mouth pain.** Low levels of vitamin B_{12} or iron can cause a condition called burning tongue and mouth syndrome, which is just what its name implies. It's easy to beef up your iron supplies by eat-ing more shellfish and meat, or your doc-tor may advise you to take iron supple-ments. If you're low on B_{12}, however, you may need an injection of this vitamin because oral forms are not well absorbed in your stomach.

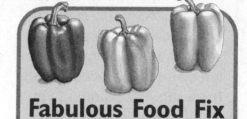

Fabulous Food Fix
Slurp Selenium

Many of us don't get nearly enough of the trace mineral selenium. Like vitamins C and E, seleni-um is a powerful antioxi-dant that appears to play a role in keeping arteries clear. Avoid supplements, but feel free to chow down on oysters and other shell-fish, all of which contain quite a bit of selenium.

Shell Some Joint Health

One of the most effective treatments for osteoarthritis is glucosamine sulfate, a naturally occurring amino sugar that, in supplement form, is produced from shellfish. Not only does it provide pain relief equal to or better than that of nonsteroidal anti-inflammatory drugs, such as aspirin, without the pesky side effects, it also combats cartilage-destroying enzymes and halts cartilage loss in the knee and hip. Since it's made from shellfish, though, you should avoid it if you have a seafood allergy.

■ **Ear noise.** Eat more shellfish to get your fill of zinc, a mineral that may minimize age-related tinnitus and hearing loss. In addition, if you work or play around noisy equipment, ask your doctor about taking 250 milligrams of supplemental magnesium—or just feast regularly on green veggies, whole grains, nuts, and beans, all of which are great sources. Low magnesium levels may constrict inner ear arteries and lead to tinnitus.

■ **Weakened immunity.** Shellfish are outstanding, low-calorie sources of protein, which is needed to maintain every cell in your body and to keep your immune system in top fighting condition. It's especially helpful to put shellfish on the menu during the cold months, when cold and flu viruses are always threatening to pounce.

■ **High cholesterol.** Since shellfish contain almost no saturated fat, you don't have to worry about them raising your blood cholesterol level as you do with fatty meats. True, some shellfish, especially shrimp, pack more cholesterol than beef does, but research tells us that for most people, it's the saturated fat you eat, not the cholesterol in your food, that makes your blood cholesterol skyrocket. So relax and enjoy!

Shellfish

■ **Weak bones I.** To protect your bones, eat more shellfish. They contain a treasure trove of trace minerals, such as magnesium and manganese, that your bones need in small but critical quantities. These trace minerals may be missing from your diet if you eat a lot of processed foods, such as white bread, crackers, pretzels, and cookies.

■ **Weak bones II.** Eating shellfish several times a week is like putting bone in the bank. Mussels are so loaded with manganese that only six steamed mussels pack a whole day's worth. This mineral is especially important to women because it may help reduce calcium loss from bones after menopause. Also, oysters are one of the few food sources of vitamin D, without which you just can't get calcium into your bones.

■ **Poor appetite and night vision.** Oysters may grow on river bottoms, but they're tops when it comes to delivering zinc. In fact, one little oyster delivers 15 milligrams of zinc—a whole day's quota! Zinc is involved with at least 60 different enzymes that interact along complex pathways to affect your appetite, sense of taste, and night vision, as well as your body's ability to fight invaders ranging from cold and flu viruses to carcinogens. In the United States, half of all people over age 50 fail to get enough zinc from their diets. Eating oysters and other shellfish is a great way to ensure that you're not one of them.

Fabulous Food Fix

Energy on the Half-Shell

Some doctors use high-dose B_{12} injections to relieve the fatigue and weakness caused by fibromyalgia. Since B vitamins are crucial for energy, optimal immune function, and mental sharpness, you may help alleviate fibromyalgia symptoms by eating foods rich in these vitamins, such as fortified cereals, eggs, meat, poultry, shellfish, and milk. You might also consider taking a B-complex supplement.

Slippery Elm

MOTHER NATURE'S BALM

The *National Formulary*, a guide for pharmacists, still lists slippery elm as a proven healer, and for good reason: It's been used for centuries to soothe damaged tissues, and new research shows that it's also good in ways that ancient herbalists never imagined. Take a look at some of the amazing things it can do for you.

Freshen Your Feet

You can make your own dusting powder to help reduce odor and keep your feet feeling fresh all day. Combine two parts powdered calendula flowers with one part each powdered slippery elm, lavender flowers, and aluminum-free baking soda. Sprinkle some on your feet before slipping on your socks and shoes.

■ **Sore throat.** Here's a blast of natural relief for a sore throat: First, buy a new plant mister. Next, make a strong tea by adding 3 teaspoons each of dried slippery elm, echinacea, and licorice to 3 cups of water in a saucepan. Bring it to a full boil, then reduce the heat and simmer for 10 to 15 minutes. Strain the solution and pour it into your new spray bottle, then open your mouth, stick out your tongue, and spray the back of your throat. Repeat as often as you need to for relief! Caution: Don't use licorice if you have high blood pressure or kidney disease.

■ **Constipation.** This slippery concoction soothes inflamed intestinal tissues and softens stools so bowel movements are more comfortable. In fact, long before there were powerful laxative drugs, herbalists recommended slippery elm to relieve constipation. Grind equal parts of marshmallow root, flaxseed, and slippery elm (unless you use the powdered form) in a coffee grinder. Stir 1 rounded teaspoon into an 8-ounce glass of water and drink it immediately. Repeat once or twice daily, following each dose with another full glass of water. For even more relief, add some unfiltered apple juice. The pectin in the juice is a type of fiber that absorbs water and makes stools softer and easier to pass.

■ **IBS.** When mixed with water, slippery elm powder makes a drink that will soothe symptoms of irritable bowel syndrome (IBS). This is a good remedy to take first thing in the morning and last thing at night to help your tissues heal 24 hours a day. Pour 1 cup of warm water over 1 teaspoon of slippery elm powder, stir briskly, and drink immediately.

■ **Laryngitis.** Slippery elm is used by professional singers and speakers to recover their voices and keep their laryngeal tissues in tiptop shape. The next time your voice fades to a

Soothing Sips

BANISH THE BURN

Acids that back up into your esophagus can give you miserable heartburn and even cause long-term damage. When you drink slippery elm tea, the slimy herb helps soak up excess acid and soothe any inflammation in your esophagus. To make it, mix 1 teaspoon of powdered slippery elm bark into 1/2 cup of boiling water, let it cool slightly, and sip it two to four times a day.

whisper, steep 1 heaping teaspoon of dried herb in 1 cup of hot water for 15 minutes. Strain, add honey and lemon if desired, and drink three or four cups a day.

■ **Wet rashes.** If you have an oozing rash, try this remedy. First, wash your skin, then dust it with an herbal powder made with equal parts of slippery elm and goldenseal powder to dry up the rash and prevent secondary infections.

■ **Vaginal dryness.** As its name implies, when tissue-soothing slippery elm is moistened, it becomes slick. When you need extra lubrication, simply mix 2 tablespoons of slippery elm powder with enough water to make a paste and add a dab of pure aloe gel. Wash your hands, then spread the mixture over your vulva and inside your vagina.

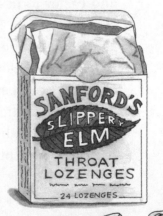

MAGIC MIXES

BOIL BEATER
To treat a boil, buy some slippery elm powder and mix in enough water to make a paste. Put a dab on your finger, then gently apply it to the boil and the surrounding area. Be sure to wash your hands first to reduce the possibility of infection.

■ **Dry throat.** When allergies, a cold, or simply dry air have taken their toll on your throat, slippery elm lozenges can help keep it moist. If your throat's also a little sore, cherry lozenges with benzocaine can numb it temporarily and help with swallowing.

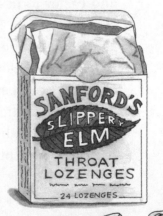

■ **Cold sores.** At the first indication of a cold sore outbreak, take advantage of extracts of slippery elm, calendula, tea tree oil, and myrrh—all of which are either excellent astringents or inflammation and infection fighters. Add several

Slippery Elm

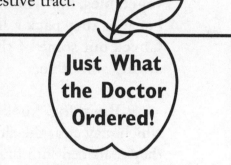

drops of each to a cup of hot water, let it cool, and dab the solution directly onto your cold sore for instant pain relief.

■ **Cranky gut.** Slippery elm and marshmallow root help coat the intestinal tract and are excellent tummy soothers. Both make a great after-dinner tea for any kind of stomach upset. Simply steep 1 to 2 tablespoons of either herb in a cup of hot water for 10 minutes, then strain and drink.

■ **Ulcers.** Tea made with slippery elm forms a sticky, soothing coating on the lining of the digestive tract. This protects small ulcers—sores that can form in the lining of the stomach or intestine—from further acid damage and may help them heal more quickly. Just add a teaspoon of slippery elm powder to a cup of hot water and steep for 10 to 15 minutes. Drink one or two cups daily when ulcers flare up.

■ **Pizza mouth.** Slippery elm is one of the best herbal remedies for pizza mouth—burns caused by scorching-hot cheese. "It's soothing, it reduces irritation and inflammation, and it shortens the healing time for burns," says John Hibbs, N.D. Buy the powdered form and mix it with water. Several times a day, swish the solution around in your mouth, then swallow it or spit it out.

Just What the Doctor Ordered!

Calm the Coughs

If you're coughing so much that your chest and back ache, try slippery elm tea. This time-honored expectorant helps break up the sticky mucus that may be clogging your bronchial tubes. Follow the label directions.

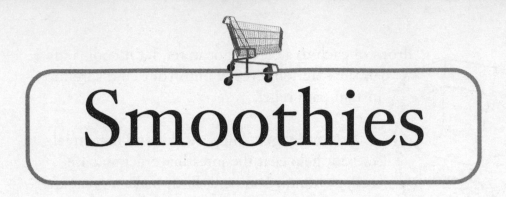

Smoothies

NUTRITION BY THE GLASS

Nutritionists are always telling us to eat more fruits and vegetables, but who has the time? Smoothies can help because they pack a lot of essential vitamins and minerals. Check out some of the other benefits that you'll get from a daily smoothie.

■ **Brain fog.** Look for smoothies loaded with blueberries, which may clear the sludge from your memory banks because they're loaded with brain-protecting chemicals. The berries' blue color comes from a pigment called anthocyanin, an antioxidant. Chug every day!

■ **Vision problems.** Milk thistle is a powerful antioxidant herb that may help protect vision and eye tissues. To use, grind 1 teaspoon of milk thistle seeds and add them to a smoothie once daily.

■ **Dry skin.** Proper nutrition is the first step in building supple skin. Doctors often advise bedridden patients to eat fish at least once or twice a week for their omega-3 fatty acids. If you're not a fish lover, you can get plenty of omega-3's by adding a tablespoon of ground flaxseed to your smoothies a few times a week.

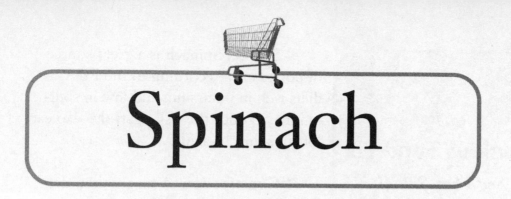

Spinach

THE NUTRITIOUS GREEN MACHINE

If you asked 100 doctors to list the foods that everyone should eat to be healthier, most of them would probably mention spinach. Along with other leafy greens, it's a veritable powerhouse of phytonutrients, plant chemicals that scour the arteries, protect the heart, and lower blood pressure—and that's just for starters. What else can spinach do for you? Take a look.

■ **Hot flashes.** If you eat more fruits and vegetables, you'll have fewer blasts from your internal furnace. Their ability to relieve hot flashes comes from naturally occurring plant sterols called phytoestrogens, which aren't as powerful as human estrogens but have a similar effect, according to Cornell University researchers. Phytoestrogens are found in spinach, apples, alfalfa sprouts, split peas, and especially soybean products.

A Hearty Green

Spinach is packed with coenzyme Q_{10}, a hardworking compound that appears to help bring oxygen to the heart. It may even prevent damage caused by a lack of oxygen.

385

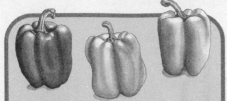

Fabulous Food Fix

See That Salad!

In a small study of men with vision problems, most of those who ate ½ cup of cooked spinach four to seven times a week had improvements in night vision, contrast, and adjustment to bright light.

■ **Stroke.** Spinach is a great source of potassium. According to the FDA, diets rich in potassium and low in sodium may reduce the risk of stroke—so eat lots of spinach salads!

■ **Constipation.** A magnesium deficiency can cause constipation, so make it a point to eat spinach regularly, since it's rich in the mineral. If you have chronic constipation, you may also want to check with your doctor about magnesium supplements.

■ **CFS and fibromyalgia.** You should load up on spinach if you have chronic fatigue syndrome (CFS) or fibromyalgia. It's an excellent source of coenzyme Q_{10}, which provides the spark that fires up ATP in your cells—which may mean less pain, more energy, and much better sleep, says Jacob Teitelbaum, M.D.

■ **Macular degeneration.** Green leafy vegetables such as spinach are like nature's sunglasses—just what you need if you spend a lot of time outdoors. They're rich in a chemical called lutein, which is also part of the pigment in the macula of the eye. This pigment helps filter out the light implicated in macular degeneration, and it also fights the destructive effects of oxidation. A study by the National Eye Institute found that foods rich in lutein and another chemical called zeaxanthin were associated with reduced risk of macular degeneration, a leading cause of vision loss.

■ **Angina.** Vitamin E is an antioxidant, meaning it prevents what's called oxidative damage in cells—including those in the arteries. As a result, low blood levels of E are associated with higher rates of angina, chest pain due to impaired circulation to the heart. It's tough to get enough vitamin E from foods, but spinach is a good source, so eating some daily will help keep your ticker humming right along.

■ **High blood pressure.** Spinach provides lots of magnesium, a mineral that relaxes smooth muscles, including those that encircle blood vessels. To keep your blood pressure in check, have plenty of greens and other produce every day.

■ **Memory loss.** Spinach and strawberries are loaded with plant chemicals that can help restore memory, according to researchers. To help keep your mind sharp, put both on the menu several times a week.

■ **Cancer.** Nature has created a remarkable array of anticancer compounds, and they're free for the taking—as long as you put fruit and vegetables on your plate. The brighter the colors, the greater the anticancer power. In fact, whether you're coping with cancer or want to take steps to prevent it, you can choose healing foods just by looking at their colors. Dark green vegetables such as spinach and broccoli lead the pack.

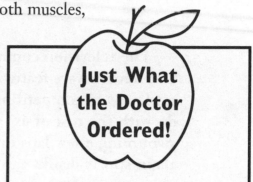

Just What the Doctor Ordered!

Spinach Cuts Cramps

The greener your midnight snack, the less likely you are to be rudely awakened by middle-of-the-night cramps. Leafy green vegetables such as spinach are chock-full of cramp-stopping electrolytes—especially magnesium, potassium, and calcium. A daily salad or stir-fry that includes these ingredients should keep cramps at bay.

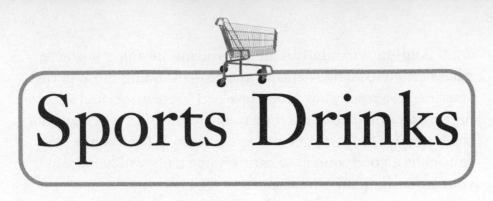

Sports Drinks

TAKE A SWIG FOR HEALTH

The television commercials for sports drinks such as Gatorade always feature hard-driving athletes at the highest levels of competition—as though that has anything to do with the rest of us. Whether your idea of exercise is swimming a few laps or walking to the mailbox, the minerals in sports drinks can help keep you healthy. Here's how.

■ **Muscle pain.** When your body isn't well hydrated, muscle aches feel worse. Filling your tank helps your body get rid of toxins that contribute to muscle pain, so when you're exercising or working hard, keep a sports drink nearby and sip it frequently.

■ **Vomiting.** If your stomach's been upset, you should keep a few bottles of sports drinks on hand in case you need to restore electrolytes—the sodium, potassium, and other chemicals that keep body fluids in balance—that you may lose through vomiting. Drink as much as your stomach can comfortably handle.

■ **Dehydration.** You can make your own sports drink by mixing equal parts of dandelion leaf, nettle, ginger, peppermint, and oatstraw. Steep 1 heaping teaspoon in 1 cup of hot water for 15 minutes, then strain. Pour the tea into a 1-liter jug along with the juice of one lemon and 1 tablespoon of pure maple syrup, then fill to the top with water. If you take diuretics or potassium supplements, talk to your doctor before using dandelion leaf, and remember to wear gloves when handling fresh nettle to avoid its stinging hairs.

■ **Hangover.** If your stomach is roiling after a night of drinking, sip a sports drink, which packs lots of electrolytes.

■ **Diarrhea.** Because diarrhea can quickly deplete your body of essential fluids and electrolytes, it's essential to replace both as soon as possible. Drinking water or sports drinks is one way to do it. It's also helpful to drink soup, broth, or fruit or vegetable juice.

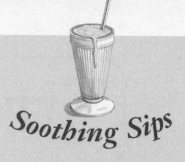

Soothing Sips

NATURE'S GATORADE

Watermelon is like a natural sports drink. It boosts your energy and keeps your blood sugar (your brain's only food) at normal levels, so you'll be physically coordinated and able to think straight. Scoop a cup of seeded watermelon into a sports water bottle, freeze, then take it to the gym. By the time you work up a sweat, it'll be a cool slushy you can sip.

■ **Exercise fatigue.** Sports drinks such as Gatorade help during events that last more than 60 to 90 minutes by fueling your brain to keep you well-coordinated, providing electrolytes to help your muscles perform, and delivering easily absorbed fluids.

■ **Muscle cramps.** Your muscles need minerals to function properly. If you have cramps that may be due to a lack of nutrients, taking a swig of a sports drink before and during exercise could prevent them from occurring (or recurring).

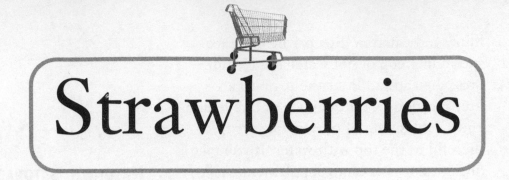

Strawberries

THEY TAKE THE CAKE

If you think of strawberries mainly as a juicy topping for shortcake, you'll want to take another look at these lusciously rich fruits. They're jam-packed with healthful chemicals—and the berries themselves are among nature's best sources of healing fiber. Here are the main reasons doctors say you should beef up your consumption of berries.

Make a C Change

If you have Raynaud's disease and a sweet tooth, you're in luck. Two of the sweetest fruits, strawberries and papaya, are full of vein-strengthening vitamin C, which is helpful if you have this circulatory disorder. Once a day, slice up a cup of each and make a tasty fruit salad.

■ **Cancer.** Want a good reason to slice some strawberries on your morning cereal? A Harvard study of more than 1,200 people concluded that strawberry lovers were 70 percent less likely to develop cancer than those who rarely ate the fruit.

■ **Constipation.** Native American healers believe that eating fresh strawberries clears up constipation. The theory makes sense since fruit provides soluble fiber, which eases the passage of waste through the colon.

■ **Anemia.** Foods high in vitamin C, such as citrus fruits, strawberries, and tomatoes, help your body absorb iron from food. Basically, the vitamin moves the iron through the gastrointestinal system and into your bloodstream so it doesn't pass through to be eliminated. If you have iron-deficiency anemia, you should definitely pop a few berries now and then.

■ **High blood pressure.** The fiber in fruit apparently works even better than the fiber in vegetables and grains to lower systolic blood pressure, studies show. Strawberries, blueberries, and peaches are especially good examples, and in some studies, strawberries lowered diastolic pressure, too. If your pressure is on the high side, get in the habit of polishing off a few strawberries after meals.

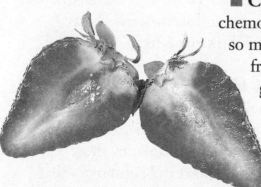

■ **Chemo side effects.** If chemotherapy upsets your stomach so much that even the sight of a fruit or vegetable makes you gag, try juicing these nutrient powerhouses into a drinkable pulp. It's a great way to get a high concentration of antioxidants and chlorophyll, both of which may help neutralize toxins from cancer treatments. Just toss some sweet strawberries in with a few beta-carotene–rich carrots for a nutrient-dense alternative to O.J.

Fabulous Food Fix

Berry Shiny Teeth

An old-time remedy for removing fresh coffee stains and the like calls for rubbing the teeth with crushed slices of fresh strawberries. Let the pulp sit on your teeth for 5 minutes, then rinse thoroughly.

■ **Carpal tunnel.** Birds sit for hours with their talons wrapped around small branches, but as far as we know, they don't get "carpal claw syndrome." What are they doing that we aren't? It may be that they fill up on berries. Blueberries, blackberries, strawberries, and boysenberries all contain natural compounds called bioflavonoids, which are nature's remedies for pain and inflammation. Eating more berries may help make wrist pain a thing of the past.

■ **Memory loss.** Is your mind a little less sharp than it used to be? Berries may help. According to early animal studies at Tufts University, eating ½ cup of antioxidant-rich blueberries a day may help sharpen memory, and strawberries have nearly the same effect.

■ **Heart disease.** When it comes to heart protection, strawberries are tops. That's because they're loaded with antioxidants, those amazingly powerful substances that gobble up free radicals, the bad guys that cause the damage to cells that may lead to heart disease. Eat them every day if you can.

Believe It or Not!

Hands down, the most famous antioxidant in strawberries is none other than vitamin C. Consider this: A single medium strawberry boasts 19 milligrams of vitamin C—approximately 25 percent of the recommended daily intake for women and 17 percent for men. And who can stop at eating just one? Vitamin C is touted for boosting immunity, making wounds heal faster (some dentists recommend it to their patients before gum surgery), and fending off heart disease and cancer. And strawberries taste a heck of a lot better than vitamin pills!

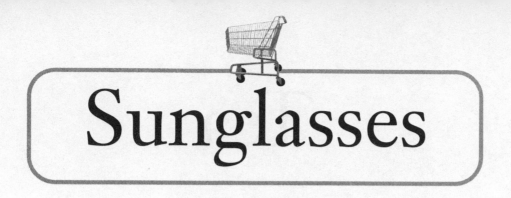

Sunglasses

GIVE UP THE GLARE

We all know people who think they look so cool in sunglasses that they never take them off, even at night. That's a little silly, but wearing sunglasses during the day is probably the best thing you can do to protect your vision. And believe it or not, it can make you look better, too. Take a peek at what a good pair of shades can do.

■ **Wrinkles.** The skin around your eyes stays relaxed when you shade your eyes with sunglasses, and stopping those constant muscle contractions helps reduce wrinkles. Wraparound styles and those with wide sidepieces offer extra protection against crow's-feet.

■ **Macular degeneration.** Many cases of macular degeneration, a leading cause of vision loss, could be prevented if people wore sunglasses to block the sun's damaging rays. Brown and tan lenses offer the best balance of comfort and protection, with gray and green second best.

■ **Pinkeye.** Protecting your eyes from glare can reduce the irritation of pinkeye, a painful (and unsightly) infection.

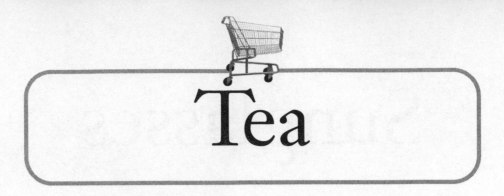

Tea

BETTER HEALTH IS IN THE BAG

Coffee is the favored pick-me-up in this country, but worldwide, green and black teas are by far the most popular beverages—and not only because they offer such a variety of different tastes. Hundreds of scientific studies have shown that tea can play a key role in stopping heart disease and dozens of other common health threats. It even helps prevent wrinkles! Check out the latest findings.

■ **Overweight.** Preliminary studies show that green tea gives the body a metabolic boost. In other words, it helps your "engine" run faster so it burns more calories. If you're trying to lose weight, you may want to drink a few cups of tea daily.

■ **Cavities.** Green tea contains tannins, chemical compounds that kill decay-causing bacteria and stop them from producing glucan, the sticky substance that helps acid-generating

Soothing Sips

TEA TAMES THROAT PAIN

Green tea is among the best sore throat remedies because it's loaded with chemical compounds called bioflavonoids, which help quell irritation and inflammation. If green's not your cup of tea, try chamomile—it's a traditional remedy for sore throat pain.

394

bacteria stick to your teeth. Drink a cup after every meal.

■ **Weak bones.** Drinking even a single cup of black or green tea a day may preserve bone density, especially if you sip it daily for 10 years, according to studies that looked at the tea-drinking habits of women ages 65 to 76. In contrast to coffee, which increases calcium loss in urine, the natural phytoestrogens in tea may help bones remain thicker.

■ **Digestive upset.** Bee balm leaves contain a compound called thymol, which helps ease nausea, vomiting, and even embarrassing flatulence. Simply combine 1 teaspoon of dried bee balm leaves with 1 teaspoon of black or green tea leaves. Put 1 teaspoon of the mixture into 1 cup of boiling water and steep for 5 to 10 minutes, then strain. Sweeten with 1 teaspoon of honey and enjoy.

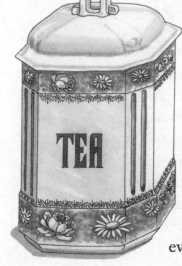

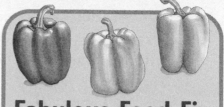

Fabulous Food Fix

Oust Foot Odor

Black tea contains tannic acid, which helps close the sweat glands, thus starving odor-causing bacteria. If you have problems with sweaty, smelly feet, simply brew two tea bags in 2 cups of boiling water for 15 minutes, add the tea to 2 quarts of cool water, and soak your feet for 20 to 30 minutes. Do this for 10 days straight, and your feet will turn out sweet.

■ **Allergies.** Sneezers and wheezers may soon be carrying a new beverage to the grassy playing fields—iced green tea. Green tea contains epigallocatechin gallate, a compound that studies show blocks the allergic response in human cells. While researchers don't know how much you need to drink to stop the reaction, you might try downing a glassful even before heading outside.

■ **Cancer I.** Green tea leaves are rich in polyphenols, special cancer-battling compounds that help cancer drugs attack bad cells and spare healthy ones, says Paul Riley, N.D.

■ **Cancer II.** A while back, epidemiologists, the scientists who compare health risks from one large group of people to another, noticed that in countries where people drink lots of green tea, folks rarely get certain kinds of cancer. They started giving green tea to mice and found that it protected them against cancers of the skin, lung, esophagus, stomach, small intestine, colon, bladder, liver, pancreas, prostate, and mammary glands. It sure sounds like a good idea to get into the habit of drinking a few glasses daily to keep your cells in tiptop shape.

■ **Weak liver.** Green tea protects the liver so it's able to function optimally as your body's detoxification center. Try to drink three to five cups daily.

■ **Leg pain.** If you have intermittent claudication, leg pain caused by poor circulation, make your tea the green kind. Its bioflavonoids make blood vessels stronger and less vulnerable to blockages and pain, so try to have a cup or two every day.

■ **Sunburn.** If you have a sunburn, green tea may help stave off cellular damage and ease pain. Cooled tea bags are especially helpful for sunburned eyelids, notes Jeanette Jacknin, M.D. She recommends steeping four tea bags in a quart of boiling water for several minutes, then letting them cool until they're lukewarm. Squeeze the liquid from the tea bags and apply them to your eyelids, then soak a small towel in the tea and place it over other sunburned areas.

Tea

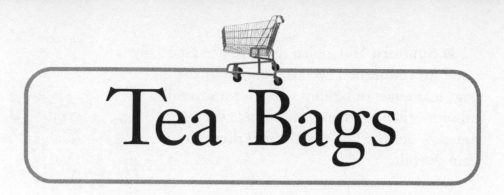

Tea Bags

DUNK 'EM

Our British cousins, with their passion for deportment and the ritual of afternoon tea, tend to look down their noses at the tea bags used in America. They don't know what they're missing. Nothing is more convenient than dunking a tea bag in a cup of hot water—and the used bags themselves provide a surprising range of benefits. Take a look at some of the ways you can bag good health.

■ **Rashes.** The simplest relief for an angry rash? Squeeze out a cooled tea bag and hold it on your tortured skin.

■ **Sunburn I.** Black tea contains tannins that help change the skin's protein structure and assuage sunburn. Brew two tea bags in a cup of water for 5 minutes. Chill the bags and wring them out, then place them on sunburned areas. Strawberry leaves and witch hazel, both of which are also rich in tannins, are also effective.

Doggy Delight

Here's something that can help Fido if he ever breaks out in those ugly skin eruptions known as hot spots. Take him to the vet as soon as you can, but in the meantime, relieve his discomfort with a poultice of cool, moist green tea bags. Apply them directly to the spots and keep them on for as long as his patience holds out.

■ **Sunburn II.** Cooled tea bags are especially good for sunburned eyelids. Steep four tea bags in a quart of boiling water for a several minutes, then let them cool to lukewarm. Squeeze out the liquid and apply them to your eyelids.

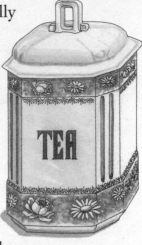

■ **Canker sores.** Every type of tea imaginable can help numb the pain of canker sores. Brew a cup of your favorite, let the tea bag cool, and squeeze it to reduce its size as much as possible, then tuck it into your mouth to cover the sore area.

■ **Boils.** You can also use tea bags to treat a boil, says Lisa Arnold, N.D. Soak the tea bag in hot water just long enough to soften it. Let it cool slightly, then hold it on the boil for about 10 minutes.

■ **Injection trauma.** You can comfort a child who's just had a shot by applying a wet green tea bag to the "scene of the crime."

■ **Stress.** Try this relaxing soak at the end of a tough day. First, put a few chamomile tea bags in a piece of gauze or a leg cut from a pair of pantyhose. Next, slice an orange thinly. Hang the tea pouch under your bathtub spigot as the warm water runs into the tub. Float the orange slices in the water, climb in, and let your cares drift away.

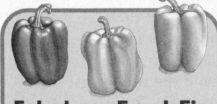

Fabulous Food Fix

Soothe a Shiner

The tannins in black and green teas help reduce swelling, making a tea bag one of the quickest ways to soothe a black eye. After brewing a cup of tea, let the tea bag cool for a few minutes, then squeeze out the excess moisture. Lie back, close your eyes, and hold the tea bag against the injured area for 10 minutes or so.

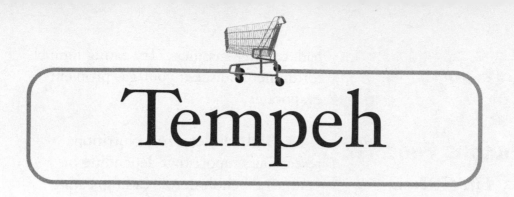

Tempeh

TOFU WITH ATTITUDE

Everyone knows about the health benefits of tofu, but it's hard to get excited about those bland white bricks. Tempeh, a form of soy with a meatier texture and a smoky taste, is a good alternative. It provides all the same benefits as tofu in a more appealing package. Unless you have breast cancer, check out what it can do for you.

■ **Cancer.** Scientists are fairly certain that soy lowers the risk of some types of cancer—especially prostate cancer. That's great news for guys. "For men, eating soy foods should be a no-brainer," says Bill Helferich, Ph.D.

■ **Gas.** Tempeh, along with miso, artichokes, asparagus, and sauerkraut, is a great source of indigestible sugars called fructo-oligosaccharides, which feed the natural bacteria in your gut that facilitate digestion. If you're taking antibiotics, they can wipe out the good bacteria along with the

Bone Builder

A three-year study showed that a diet rich in soy lowers the rate at which you lose the mineral density that keeps your skeleton strong. Researchers have to do more work to confirm the connection between soy and your bones, but at this point, it looks promising.

bad, causing gassiness. Try eating tempeh for dinner and see if your gas problem evaporates.

■ **High cholesterol.** Nutrition researchers report that depending on your actual cholesterol reading, eating two or three servings of soy foods daily can lower your numbers and reduce the risk of heart disease by about 15 to 30 percent. Evidence such as this has led the FDA to allow food manufacturers to claim heart health benefits on the label of any soy product that contains at least 6.25 grams of soy protein per serving, and the American Heart Association has added soy to its list of ticker-friendly foods.

■ **Menopausal discomforts.** Soybeans contain plant sterols, which have an affinity for estrogen receptor sites in your body. This means that they have a slight estrogenic effect and can help reduce symptoms of menopause, such as night sweats. In addition, a daily serving or two of soy products such as tempeh can give you a low-fat, high-protein boost that may be just the thing for relieving hot flashes.

■ **Heart disease.** Tempeh and other soy foods contain chemical compounds that act as antioxidants. They gobble up compounds

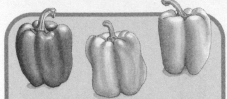

Fabulous Food Fix

Lift the Iron

Tempeh, along with yogurt and sauerkraut, contains lactic acid, which promotes iron absorption. If you're one of the millions of American women who periodically have iron-deficiency anemia, put tempeh and other soy foods on the menu more often. The extra iron you absorb will help keep your energy at peak levels.

called free radicals that can cause cell damage that leads to heart disease. Eat a serving or two of soy daily to keep your heart and arteries in good shape.

■ **Heart attack.** Tempeh, tofu, and other soy foods can help inhibit blood clotting, reduce inflammation, and promote widening of blood vessels when they're under stress so blood flows normally. Barry Goldin, Ph.D., says it's a good idea to eat soy foods in place of other foods that aren't so healthy for the heart, such as fatty meat or whole-fat dairy products.

■ **Weak bones.** Soy foods contain a hefty amount of calcium—up to 250 milligrams per serving. As a bonus, tofu is rich in two major types of isoflavones, compounds that act like weak forms of estrogen and may inhibit bone breakdown. Eating a serving or two of tempeh or other soy foods daily may help prevent bone fractures later in life. Keep in mind, though, that antacids with aluminum can interfere with calcium absorption, as can red meat, soft drinks, alcohol, caffeine, and phosphorus-rich foods. So don't follow your tempeh main course with a cup of high-test coffee or a large cola.

■ **Brain fog.** After menopause, supplies of an important brain chemical called acetylcholine dwindle, decreasing the ability of mem-

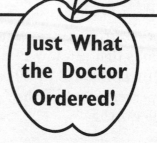

Just What the Doctor Ordered!

Tame PMS with Tempeh

Tempeh contains magnesium, which stabilizes mood, normalizes blood sugar metabolism, and reduces water retention and bloating. Some researchers also speculate that a deficiency of the mineral may be behind the classic PMS craving for chocolate. Unlike chocolate, however, tempeh won't give you that short-lived "sugar high."

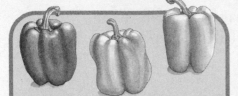

Fabulous Food Fix

Isoflavones Cut Blood Fats

Soy contains isoflavones, estrogen-like compounds that can lower LDL cholesterol by 10 to 15 percent, says Michael Miller, M.D.

ory cells to communicate with each other. High-protein foods such as tempeh contain choline, a component of lecithin used to make acetylcholine, so adding them to your diet can help make up for the loss. Another choice is to take soy-extracted isoflavone tablets (55 milligrams) twice daily, which research from the University of California, San Diego, has shown to help verbal recall. If you have breast cancer or are at risk for it, check with your doctor before supplementing, since isoflavones may have an estrogenic effect on tissues.

■ **Weak heart.** Soy is packed with coenzyme Q_{10}, a substance that appears to help transport oxygen to the heart and may even reduce damage caused by a lack of oxygen. Eating more tempeh or other soy foods may help keep your heart strong.

■ **Vitamin B_{12} deficiency.** Vitamin B_{12} is found only in animal sources and a few fermented foods derived from soybeans, such as miso and tempeh. If you're a vegetarian, be sure to include these foods as well as dairy products and eggs in your diet to avoid a deficiency of this important vitamin. If you are a vegan and avoid all animal products, ask your doctor about taking a B_{12} supplement.

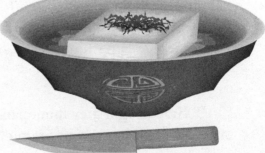

Tempeh

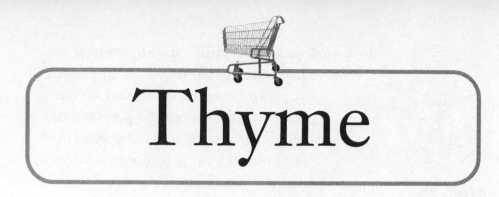

Thyme

AN AROMATIC ALLY

This pungent kitchen spice is the backbone of literally hundreds of recipes, from spaghetti and meatballs to oven-roasted chicken. It's also the backbone of dozens of kitchen cures because it contains powerful chemicals that work just as well on the outside of your body as on the inside. Here are a few of the reasons to make time for thyme.

■ **Athlete's foot.** A Native American remedy for athlete's foot is soaking your feet in hot water with a few drops of oil of thyme added to relieve the itching and burning. Then dust your feet with a mixture of powdered myrrh and goldenseal in any proportion and put on a pair of heavy cotton socks. Repeat daily for several days.

■ **Stuffy nose.** When cold or allergy congestion is making you miserable, whip up this nose-clearing remedy. First, measure ¼ cup of petroleum jelly and put it

---

Soak Away Back Pain

Ease your aching back by tossing a handful of dried thyme into the tub as you run the bathwater. Soak for 10 to 15 minutes and let the aromatic oils in this herb take your aches and pains down the drain.

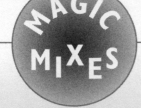

MAGIC MIXES

LUNG-LOVING RUB

To protect your lungs during a cold or the flu, make your own chest rub with I teaspoon of olive oil and three or four drops of thyme oil. The warming vapors will keep your respiratory passages open and moist as they fight infection with their antiseptic action.

in a small saucepan. Warm it until it melts, then remove from the heat and add 10 drops each of peppermint, eucalyptus, and thyme oil. Let it cool to room temperature and pour it into a clean jar. Apply a small amount to your sore nose up to three times a day. The petroleum jelly is soothing, and it keeps the oils from being absorbed into the skin so you can inhale their penetrating vapors longer.

■ **Laryngitis.** An herbal steam can help soothe your respiratory passages and alleviate laryngitis pain. Boil a pot of water, carefully remove it from the stove, and add three or four drops of thyme oil. Drape your head with a towel, bend over the pot—not too close!—and breathe deeply.

■ **Weakened immunity.** The next time you're under the weather from any kind of illness, support your recovery with nature's pharmacy of immunity-supporting, nutrient-dense foods. Make sure your diet includes plenty of garlic; dark leafy greens, such as collards, chard, and kale; orange and yellow vegetables, such as squash and pumpkin; and tonic herbal seasonings, such as thyme.

■ **Weak lungs.** Tone up your lungs with a "thyme-out tonic." Combine equal parts of thyme, ginkgo, aniseed, rose-

404

Thyme

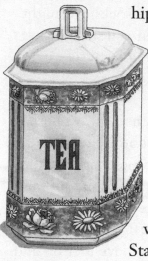

hips, and ginger. Use 1 heaping teaspoon per cup of boiling water, cover, and steep for 15 minutes. Strain and drink two or three cups a day. Omit the ginkgo if you regularly take aspirin or blood thinners.

■ **Chest congestion.** Teas containing thyme, fennel seed, mullein, colt's-foot, marshmallow root, or aniseed are excellent for opening the bronchial passages when you're congested, says Jamison Starbuck, N.D.

■ **Nail fungus.** Fungicidal plants such as thyme, black walnut hulls, pau d'arco, spilanthes, goldenseal, and oregano can help eliminate nail fungi with no side effects, says Daniel DeLapp, N.D. He suggests mixing several drops of tincture of each herb in a quart of warm water, then soaking your feet twice daily. Dry your feet well, then dust them with antiperspirant sage powder and put on clean cotton socks.

■ **Yeast infections.** When you're battling a yeast infection, use fungus-fighting herbs, such as thyme, oregano, and rosemary, generously in your recipes.

■ **Ingrown toenail I.** To reduce the risk of infection from an ingrown nail, change your socks two or three times a day. For additional protection, add a few drops of thyme oil to

Soothing Sips

THYME OUT FOR GERMS

If you're trying to oust an infection, you need look no further than your spice rack for some thyme, which contains a germ-killing compound. Add a teaspoon to a cup of boiling water and steep for 10 minutes. Strain out the herb, let cool slightly, and drink. Have one or two cups a day until the infection is history.

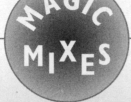

MAGIC MIXES

a basin of water and soak your socks overnight. The oil's germ-killing action will help ensure that infection-causing bacteria can't thrive in your socks.

■ **Ingrown toenail II.** An herbal foot massage can soothe the pain of an ingrown nail and protect against the development of a potentially serious infection. Combine 1 ounce of infused calendula oil with 10 drops each of thyme, oregano, and lavender oil and apply the mixture all over your foot. The hands-on attention will make the area feel a lot better, and the oils will help reduce swelling and pressure around the sore nail.

■ **Chafing.** If you're concerned about infection due to chafed skin, you can relieve your worries with two strong antiseptic herbs that you probably have in your kitchen, says Lisa Arnold, N.D. Add a tablespoon each of thyme and rosemary to a cup of hot water and steep for about 10 minutes. Let the liquid cool to room temperature, strain it, and pour some on a cloth. Hold the cloth against the sore area for about 20 minutes once or twice a day until your skin heals.

FIGHT THE FLAKES

If you'd like to try an herbal approach to dandruff control, dab some thyme oil diluted in olive oil (four drops of thyme oil per teaspoon of olive oil) on your scalp 1 hour before washing your hair. After shampooing, use an anti-dandruff rinse made by boiling a handful of dried thyme leaves in a quart of water. When the solution is cool, strain and pour over your hair.

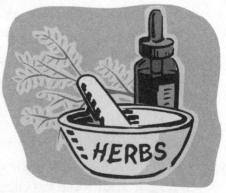

HERBS

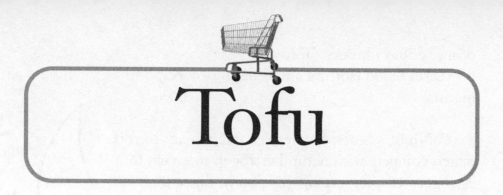

Tofu

THE JOY OF SOY

It's only in the past few decades that Americans have discovered what Asian cooks have known all along—tofu, a processed form of soy, is a versatile meat substitute that soaks up flavors and adds texture to vegetarian recipes. Although those with breast cancer should avoid it, the fact is that tofu is one of the most healthful ingredients you can use. Here's why.

■ **PMS.** The magnesium in soy foods is helpful for PMS symptoms because it stabilizes mood, normalizes the metabolism of blood sugar, and helps minimize bloating. If you make it a point to add tofu to stir-fries and other dishes in the week or so before your period, you'll boost your intake of this mineral, which may also eliminate those premenstrual chocolate cravings.

■ **Heart disease.** Compounds in tofu act as antioxidants, gobbling up renegade oxygen molecules called free radicals that can cause cell damage that contributes to heart disease and can increase the risk of stroke, Alzheimer's disease, and dozens of

407

other serious illnesses. Tofu also decreases blood clotting and inflammation.

■ **Night sweats.** Soybeans contain plant sterols, which compete with natural estrogen to attach to estrogen receptor sites in your body. Since their slight estrogenic effect can help reduce symptoms of menopause, such as night sweats, many doctors advise eating one or more servings of tofu daily to minimize discomfort.

■ **High cholesterol.** According to studies, eating two or three servings of soy foods daily may lower cholesterol and reduce your risk of heart disease by about 15 to 30 percent. Although the amount of reduction largely depends on your initial cholesterol levels, the FDA was impressed enough with this evidence to allow food manufacturers to claim heart health benefits on the label of any soy product that contains at least 6.25 grams of soy protein per serving. The American Heart Association also includes soy in its list of heart-friendly foods.

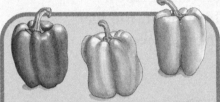

Fabulous Food Fix

Tofu for Men

Scientists are fairly certain that tofu lowers the risk of prostate cancer. Because of that benefit and the preventive effects of soy on heart disease, Bill Helferich, Ph.D., says that "for men, eating soy foods should be a no-brainer."

■ **Hot flashes.** If you're among the millions of American women who have hot flashes, consider adding soy to your menu. Researchers have found that some women get a lot of relief from soy foods such as tofu, while others don't. To see if you're one of the lucky ones, you'll just have to try it.

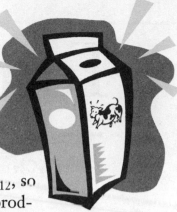

■ **B$_{12}$ deficiency.** If you're a vegetarian, you may be at risk for a deficiency of vitamin B$_{12}$, which is found mainly in animal foods. A few foods derived from soybeans, such as tofu, also supply B$_{12}$, so include these foods as well as dairy products and eggs in your diet.

■ **Osteoporosis.** Tofu may help out with thinning bones, one of the most serious effects of menopause. One study showed that a diet with lots of soy reduces the loss of bone density that characterizes osteoporosis. More studies are needed to confirm the connection between soy and bone strength, but things look promising right now, so you may want to eat one or more daily servings of tofu and other soy foods just to be safe.

■ **Memory loss.** When estrogen levels fall after menopause, so do levels of acetylcholine, a brain chemical that's necessary for communication between memory cells. To make up for the loss, eat more high-protein foods such as soy, which supply choline, a component of lecithin used to make acetylcholine. Alternatively (as long as breast cancer doesn't run in your family), you could take soy-extracted isoflavone tablets (55 milligrams) twice daily to help verbal recall.

The Soy Switch

Barry Goldin, Ph.D., encourages his patients to eat a serving of soy foods in place of something that isn't as heart healthy, such as fat-laden cream sauces and meats.

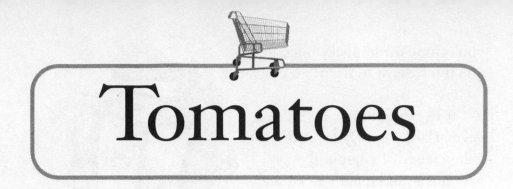

Tomatoes

REACH FOR THE REDS

It's hard to get excited about most supermarket tomatoes, which some have likened to cardboard with a little juice. If you stock up on vine-ripened varieties, though, you'll get more juice and flavor than you know what to do with—along with a chemical bonus that can literally add years to your life. What else can you get from the fruit of the vine? Take a look.

■ **Allergies.** Some people call tomatoes love apples, and like regular apples, they contain a powerful bioflavonoid-antihistamine called quercetin that may help knock out allergy symptoms, says Connie Cantellani, M.D. During allergy season, eating tomatoes every day may reduce your need for brain-fogging antihistamines.

■ **Anemia I.** The vitamin C in tomatoes, citrus fruits, and strawberries helps your body absorb iron from other foods by helping it move through the digestive system and into your bloodstream so it's

A Slice against Cancer

Here's great news from the American Institute for Cancer Research: A single tomato contains hundreds, possibly thousands, of phytochemicals that perform different functions to prevent cancer. Pizza, anyone?

not eliminated. The more iron you retain, the lower your risk of iron-deficiency anemia.

■ **Anemia II.** To take advantage of the iron in tomatoes, cook them in a cast-iron pan. The reaction of the acids in tomatoes with the metal in the pan can more than double the amount of iron you take in. For example, 4 ounces of tomato sauce has 0.7 milligram of iron, but cooking it in an iron pan gives you 5 milligrams more! Although it won't affect their taste, iron cookware may discolor some foods, and experts say the iron from cast iron isn't absorbed quite as well as iron from foods.

Fabulous Food Fix

Get the Red Out

The lycopene in tomatoes can help repair damage from too much sun. Eating these scarlet veggies cooked with oil—in other words, eating foods made with prepared tomato paste—has been shown to help protect the skin from sun damage and redness. Apparently, the oil helps boost the uptake of lycopene in the body.

■ **Heart disease.** Eat more tomatoes if you want to protect your heart. They're rich in lycopene, a carotenoid that's believed to have powerful antioxidant properties. That is, it helps prevent harmful molecules in the body from damaging healthy cells in the arteries—the "trigger" that causes cholesterol to stick to artery walls and impede circulation to the heart. High levels of cholesterol also increase the risk of blood clots in the arteries, the cause of most heart attacks. The chemicals in tomatoes (and other produce) will go a long way toward stopping this dangerous cascade.

■ **Gum disease.** Tomatoes, oranges, and broccoli are practically dripping with vitamin C, a nutrient that toughens gums, reduces swelling, and squelches infection. Its partner antioxidant, vitamin E, which is found in nuts and seeds, fights cell damage caused by renegade oxygen molecules called free radicals. Eating plenty of tomato-based foods, such as spaghetti sauce, and popping daily multivitamins with vitamin E will help keep your gums healthy. These strategies can also save your teeth, because gum disease is the leading cause of tooth loss, and protect your heart, since gum infections can damage it. So tank up on tomatoes!

■ **Cancer.** A growing pile of research shows that the lycopene found in tomatoes and tomato products, such as tomato sauce, can cut the risk of certain cancers by up to 40 percent. During a six-year study in which Harvard researchers diagnosed 812 cases of prostate cancer among study participants, they wanted to see if there were differences between the diets of the men who developed this all-too-common cancer and those who remained healthy. Of the more than 40 foods examined, they found only 4 that protected against prostate cancer. Of those foods, 3 were good sources of lycopene—tomato sauce, tomatoes, and pizza. Eating tomatoes or tomato products twice a week, the researchers concluded, could lower the risk of prostate cancer by 20 to 40 percent. The bottom line, guys? Eat at least two weekly servings of tomatoes and tomato-based foods.

Just What the Doctor Ordered!

The Power of Potassium

If you experience monthly bloating, you may want to spend more time in the produce department. That's where you'll find piles of tomatoes—potassium-rich veggies that send puffiness packing.

Toothpaste

YOUR MAIN SQUEEZE

Sure, toothpaste freshens your breath and makes your teeth shine, but that's not all it does. Brushing your teeth often, and with the right paste, can make a real difference in how you feel as well as in how you look. Here are a few ways to use toothpaste to make your life shine!

■ **Sensitive teeth.** If you're thinking of having a bleaching treatment, and your teeth are extremely sensitive, you may need to prime them first. Ask your dentist about tooth primers such as Gluma, which can be painted on your teeth to desensitize them. Or you can opt for the less expensive route and simply brush your teeth with a toothpaste such as Sensodyne, which contains potassium nitrate, for six weeks before your treatment.

■ **Plaque.** "Coenzyme Q_{10} is a potent antioxidant that helps tighten gum tissue so plaque can't become trapped in it," says Darin Ingels, N.D., and studies show it also

Tame the Pain

Toothpastes made for sensitive teeth often work, but not right away. "It may take a tube or two before you notice results," says Richard Price, D.M.D. "Pastes for sensitive teeth have different ingredients, so you may have to experiment until you find the one that works for you."

speeds healing and repairs tissue. Some brands of toothpaste contain CoQ_{10}.

■ **Gum disease.** Goldenseal powder should be in everyone's medicine cabinet because it not only reduces inflammation and fights bacteria, it also contains a host of minerals, including calcium, phosphorus, potassium, and vitamins that keep gums healthy. You can mix 1 tablespoon of powdered goldenseal with enough water to make a paste and apply it directly to tender gums or add 1 tablespoon of powder and 1 teaspoon of baking soda to 1 cup of warm water, then swish and spit. Check the toothpaste aisle for brands that contain goldenseal, too.

■ **Dragon breath.** A dehydrated mouth is an ideal spawning ground for bacteria—and mouth bacteria, as you know, are the leading cause of bad breath as well as gum disease. There's even evidence that bacteria in the mouth can increase your risk of heart disease. If you have serious dry mouth from medications, look for Biotene toothpaste and mouthwash. Both contain natural salivary enzymes that can be helpful.

■ **Canker sores.** The mucous membrane of the gastrointestinal tract, which begins in the mouth, is very vulnerable to chemotherapy drugs, which can cause acutely painful canker sores. But there is an ancient solution: myrrh, the herb carried to Bethlehem by one of the biblical Wise Men. Long prized for its astringent properties, myrrh soothes sore mouth tissues and works as a fluoride alternative. Look for it in toothpastes or buy an extract and make your own rinse by mixing 20 drops in 1/4 cup of water.

Toothpaste

Turmeric

A VERY NICE SPICE

The next time you whip up an Indian meal or a savory pot of beef stew, go heavy on the turmeric. Like many other kitchen spices, it contains a bevy of chemical compounds with wide-ranging benefits. Here's a sample of what it can do for you.

■ **Arthritis.** Instead of taking aspirin the next time arthritis pain flares, try turmeric. The same spice that gives curry its distinctive flavor makes an excellent pain reliever, in part because it breaks down bits of pain-causing protein that circulate in damaged tissue. Mix ½ teaspoon of turmeric with enough water to make a paste and apply it to the painful spots.

■ **Shoulder pain.** The next time your shoulder is out of whack—after too many hours on the tennis court, for example—take turmeric, a potent anti-inflammatory. Stir ½

Spice Up Circulation

Turmeric, along with ginger and red pepper, inhibits arterial inflammation that may lead to or worsen angina, chest pain caused by diminished blood flow to the heart.

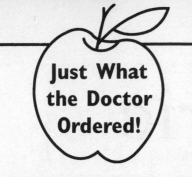

Just What the Doctor Ordered!

Gallstones, Be Gone!

If you enjoy the cuisine of India, you're in luck. Turmeric, commonly used in Indian cooking, is a traditional gallstone remedy. If you don't care for the taste of turmeric but still want the benefits, you can take 50 to 100 milligrams in capsule form three times a day, preferably with meals.

teaspoon into a glass of water and drink it twice a day. Unlike nonsteroidal anti-inflammatory drugs such as aspirin and ibuprofen, turmeric is safe to use long term.

■ **Stuffy nose.** Using turmeric and other pungent spices in recipes can help reduce nasal and sinus congestion and promote drainage when you have a cold.

■ **Bronchitis.** If you have bronchitis due to allergies, spice up your dinner. Turmeric is a great source of quercetin, a bioflavonoid-antihistamine combo that can calm reactivity in the airways. You can also simply supplement with three 200- to 300-milligram capsules of quercetin a day, suggests Michael DiPalma, N.D.

■ **Radiation side effects.** If you're being treated for cancer, use more turmeric in your recipes. Studies indicate that curcumin, a component of turmeric, can both strangle tumors by cutting off the blood vessels that feed them and protect against burns and blisters that can occur due to radiation treatments.

■ **Sciatica.** People with sciatica who like spicy foods should definitely seek out recipes that contain turmeric, since this fragrant herb has powerful anti-inflammatory effects that help counteract sciatica flare-ups. You'd have to eat a lot of turmeric to get enough of the active ingredient, though, so a more practical approach is to take turmeric capsules. Check with your doctor first, then start with about 250 milligrams three times daily, preferably with food.

■ **Heartburn.** Turmeric can break down fatty foods and reduce the stomach acidity that causes heartburn. Get some empty gel capsules at the drugstore, fill them with turmeric powder straight from your spice rack, and take one capsule after meals.

■ **Sore throat.** Turmeric is one of nature's strongest antibacterials. Simply mix ½ teaspoon of turmeric and ½ teaspoon of salt in a cup of hot water, let it cool slightly, and gargle with it morning and evening until your sore throat is better.

■ **Calf pain.** Turmeric is a traditional remedy for reducing pain and inflammation. If you have a calf cramp, first give your leg a quick massage by reaching down with both hands and massaging the muscle thoroughly, working across the muscle fibers rather than up and down. Then apply a spicy herbal salve made by mixing about a teaspoon of dried turmeric with enough water to make a paste. Spread it on the affected area and leave it on for about 20 minutes.

■ **Chest congestion.** Here's a potent spread that can get mucus flowing and help clear chest congestion. James A. Duke, Ph.D. suggests making a paste with small amounts of garlic, ginger, mustard, turmeric, chopped chile peppers, and horseradish. Spread a bit on some crackers and eat them in very small bites. You'll find that your eyes, your nose, and the thick mucus gunking up your bronchial tubes will all start to run, and you'll soon feel better.

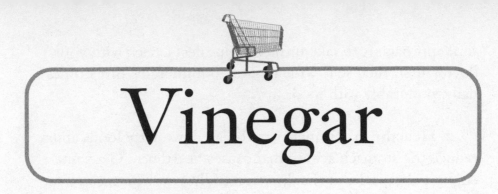

Vinegar

BE A SOURPUSS

Vinegar isn't just for salads, as every grandmother knows. It's a traditional remedy for dozens of different conditions, and it really does seem to work. Here are some of its best uses.

■ **Weight loss.** Trying to lose weight? Here's a trick that may help: Before each meal, mix 1 teaspoon of apple cider vinegar in a glass of warm water (make sure it's warm!), and drink up. If you're like most folks, the elixir will decrease your appetite, so you'll just naturally want to eat less.

■ **Leg pain.** If you're prone to charley horses, here's a homemade liniment that you can whip up in advance. In a small container with a lid, combine ½ ounce of powdered cramp bark, 1 cup of apple cider vinegar, and a pinch of red pepper. Keep the mixture in a cool, dark place for a week, shaking the container every day. When the week's up, transfer the solution to a clean glass bottle. Then, the next time a charley horse strikes, rub your affected calf with the liniment.

Sour Is Sweet

Immerse your smelly feet in a solution of one part warm water and one part vinegar for 10 minutes twice a day for three weeks. Vinegar soaks can often eradicate an offensive odor for good.

418

■ **Shin pain.** Moist heat is a great treatment for shin pain, and adding vinegar to the mix increases the anti-inflammatory power. Heat a mixture of equal parts of vinegar and water, soak a small towel, wring it out, and apply it where you hurt.

■ **Insect stings.** When you've been targeted by a stinging critter, try a sage poultice to reduce pain and swelling. First, crush some fresh sage leaves between your fingers and simmer them in a saucepan with a little vinegar until they're soft. Remove them from the pan and let them cool, then put them on the sting and cover the area with a warm, moist washcloth. Leave it in place for about 15 minutes.

Fabulous Food Fix
Hot Pepper Vinegar

This culinary staple packs a big health-giving wallop. Research says it helps to prevent heart disease by stimulating cortisone production. Plus it's a snap to make! Pack 12-15 clean hot peppers and a pinch of parsley in a sterilized 10-ounce jar. Cover with white-wine vinegar and seal with a tight lid. Steep at room temp for a week, then use it as you wish.

■ **Age spots.** To help fade age spots, mix 1 teaspoon of vinegar, 1 teaspoon of grated horseradish, and 1 teaspoon of lemon juice with three drops of rosemary oil. Don't be put off by the strong odor; this stuff really works!

■ **Sore throat.** Gargling with apple cider vinegar may not sound very appetizing, but it's worth it. Add 2 tablespoons to a glass of warm water, gargle and spit until you finish the glass, then repeat the sequence. Your throat should feel better within 3 to 4 hours.

■ **Chest congestion.** The volatile oil allicin in onions can relax and open your airways. Warm some oil in a cast-iron skillet and add a teaspoon of apple cider vinegar, a handful of chopped onions, and a bit of cornstarch. Cook over low heat to make a paste, then let it cool and place it on a cloth. Make a layered poultice by putting the cloth on your bare chest, covering that with plastic wrap and another cloth, and topping everything with a heating pad set on low. Lie down and set a timer for 20 minutes. Limit this to once a day.

■ **Defeat Diabetes.** To reduce the effect of potatoes on your blood sugar, try potato salad made with unpeeled potatoes and vinaigrette dressing. The acid in the vinegar slows the conversion of the carbohydrates in the potatoes to blood sugar. You can also douse French fries with vinegar as the British do.

Pulverize Joint Pain!

Creaky knees? Hurtin' hips? Aching fingers? This remarkable remedy provides soothing relief: Mix equal parts of apple cider vinegar and honey, and store the mix in a lidded glass jar at room temperature. Once a day, stir 1 teaspoon of the combination and 1 teaspoon of Knox® orange-flavored gelatin powder (don't use sweetened Jell-O®) into 6 ounces of water, and drink up. Before you know it, your joints will be jumpin' again!

■ **Keep your cool in hot weather.** The prickly heat rash that pops up when hot, humid weather clogs up your sweat glands responds well to the acidity in vinegar. For quick relief, add a teaspoon of apple cider vinegar to a cup of water and sponge the solution over the affected area.

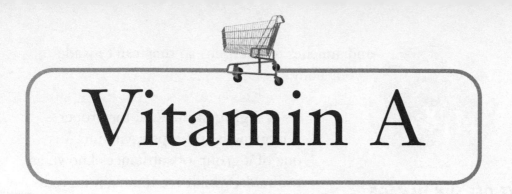

Vitamin A

PUT IT ON YOUR A-LIST

All vitamins are sold in supplement form, and vitamin A is no exception. In most cases, though, you can get all the vitamin A you need from foods. It's worth doing because this essential nutrient deserves a solid "A" for all the hard work it does. Take a look at the latest research.

■ **Dull skin.** Apricots, with their ample vitamin A, can be blended into a cream to moisturize and revitalize dull skin. They soften it, too. Look for creams containing apricot oil or add 1 tablespoon of apricot oil to 1 cup of your favorite skin cream.

■ **Vision problems.** Since your eyes soak up vitamin A, be sure to regularly include carrots in your diet. They're rich sources of beta-carotene, the plant-based building block for vitamin A.

■ **Allergies.** If you're plagued by allergies, eat more tuna, salmon, and other cold-water fish. They provide vitamin A, which boosts IgA, a beneficial antibody that's released in saliva

421

and attaches to allergens so they can't invade your body.

■ **Aging skin.** Vital for proper skin growth and repair, vitamin A is one of a group of substances known as retinoids, which are the main ingredients in many anti-aging prescription drugs, such as tretinoin (Retin-A). To get nearly the same protection without the high cost of the drugs, just fill your plate with beta-carotene–rich foods, such as cantaloupe, carrots, and apricots.

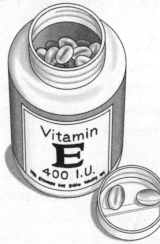

■ **Sinus headache.** Vitamins A, C, and E are among the best weapons against sinus headaches during the high-risk cold and allergy seasons. Unless you're pregnant or planning to become pregnant, take 5,000 IU of vitamin A daily to strengthen your mucous membranes.

MAGIC MIXES

STAVE OFF SUN DAMAGE
For mild sunburn, you can make a soothing oil by adding the contents of six capsules each of vitamin A and vitamin E to ¼ cup of flaxseed oil or aloe vera juice, then apply it frequently to the sunburned areas.

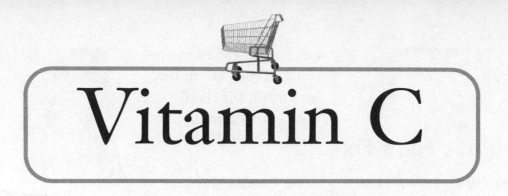

Vitamin C

NATURE'S HEAVY HITTER

There probably isn't a single nutrient that does more for the body than vitamin C. Whether you're talking about heart disease, skin injuries, or cataracts, the first words out of your doctor's mouth just may be "Get more vitamin C"—but don't forget to ask his advice before using supplements, especially if you have stomach or kidney problems. Here's why C is so versatile.

■ **Stubbed toe.** You need extra vitamin C when you've stubbed your toe. This all-purpose nutrient (which could have been voted "most likely to succeed" in high school) is essential for skin repair, so take 500 milligrams four times a day for a few weeks.

■ **Cataracts.** Bilberry, a close relative of the blueberry, may help prevent cataracts, or at least slow their growth. This shrubby plant is high in bioflavonoids, nutrients that enhance the action of vitamin C. Because the lens of the eye naturally contains so much vitamin C, some scientists believe a deficiency

Good for the Gut

Vitamin C can beat back *Helicobacter pylori*, the bacterium that causes ulcers. Look for the coated kind, such as Ester-C, that doesn't promote acid production.

423

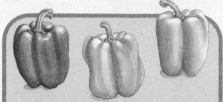

Fabulous Food Fix

Get Your Iron Here!

Citrus fruits, strawberries, tomatoes, and other foods high in vitamin C help your body absorb iron by moving the mineral into your bloodstream so it's not eliminated during the digestive process.

can lead to cataracts. You can find bilberry in tincture form; the usual dose is 1 to 2 milliliters twice a day.

■ **Colds.** You probably suck down gallons of orange and other citrus juices when you have a cold. Perhaps it's the vitamin C in citrus that feels so cleansing, or maybe just the idea of C—even if it's a placebo effect—does the trick. There's no proof that vitamin C can actually cure a cold, but some experts say it acts like interferon, a natural body chemical that halts the growth of viruses. For best effect, up your intake of C at the first sign of a sniffle.

■ **Gallstones.** One study examined data from 13,000 people and found that women with low levels of vitamin C were more likely to get gallstones, according to Joel Simon, M.D. That's one important reason to add foods rich in vitamin C to your diet. Citrus fruit and juices are the best sources—a whole orange, for example, offers 70 milligrams of C.

■ **Sinus headaches.** During the cold and allergy seasons, you can fight sinus headaches with vitamins A, C, and E. Together, they can strengthen your mucous membranes and

Vitamin C

your immune system, reduce congestion, and help protect against cold- and flu-causing germs. Check your supermarket for a combination vitamin, then ask your doctor about the dosage that's right for you.

■ **Razor bumps.** To keep your bikini line smooth, apply shaving gel, leave it on for a few minutes, and then shave with a wet razor. This will soften the hair so you can shave closer and reduce the chance of ingrown hairs. Next, smooth on a cream with alpha hydroxy acids (AHAs), which can also reduce ingrown hairs and minimize bumps, suggests J. Michael Maloney, M.D. Finally, apply a vitamin C–based cream to reduce redness.

■ **Rosacea.** The flushing caused by rosacea means that the blood vessels in your face dilate frequently, which can leave them flabby and less likely to constrict the way they should, notes Jeanette Jacknin, M.D. She suggests taking vitamin C along with bioflavonoids to help tone the blood vessels; take 500 milligrams three times a day.

■ **UTIs.** Some experts believe that taking vitamin C helps acidify the urine, which prevents bacteria from clinging to the bladder and causing urinary tract infections (UTIs). Others say its biggest benefit is that it acts as a powerful antioxidant to help fight infection. Either way, the best form to take is Emergen-C, says Melody

C for Sciatica

Vitamin C has been shown to help repair muscle damage that can lead to tightness as well as nerve pain. You'll want to take up to 3,000 milligrams of vitamin C a day if you have sciatica caused by a back injury. That's a lot more than the usual daily dose, so it's a good idea to take it in several smaller doses throughout the day.

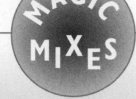

Wong, N.D. It's a powdered formula that provides 1,000 milligrams of C along with electrolytes such as potassium, which may be flushed away if you're also using diuretics.

■ **Arthritis.** Vitamin C has antioxidant properties that help prevent harmful molecules called free radicals from damaging your joints. It also promotes the growth of collagen, a type of tissue that helps keep joints healthy, says Gerald J. Murphy, D.D.S. He tells people to take 3,000 milligrams daily. Since doses this large may cause diarrhea or other side effects and may be harmful for people with stomach or kidney problems, check with your doctor before you start. You can minimize digestive side effects by dividing the amount into two or three doses and taking them at different times during the day; taking the supplements with food also helps.

■ **Herpes.** If you have herpes, downing 600 milligrams each of vitamin C and bioflavonoids three times daily for three days from the moment you detect the first telltale tingling could cut your outbreak short. For milder, less frequent flare-ups, take 25 milligrams of zinc and 250 milligrams of vitamin C twice daily for five weeks.

■ **Headache.** Vitamin C has powerful anti-inflammatory properties, which is important because inflammation

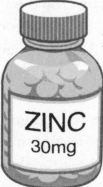

ZINC
30mg

SALVE FOR OL' SOL
Vitamin C is an anti-inflammatory that can boost the soothing effects of aloe when you have sunburn. Mix 2 tablespoons of vitamin C powder into ½ cup of commercial aloe juice, pour the mixture into a small spray bottle, and spritz your skin twice a day until it's healed.

Vitamin C

plays a role in some tension headaches. You can try taking 1,000 to 2,000 milligrams of vitamin C at the first sign of a headache; if it's going to work, you should feel the benefits within an hour or two.

■ **Angina.** If you're trying to control angina, chest pain caused by impaired circulation to the heart, plan on taking at least 500 milligrams of vitamin C daily. Vitamin C helps keep free radicals from damaging artery walls and helps prevent chemical changes in cholesterol that make it more likely to stick to the arteries. Because angina is a serious problem, it's especially important to let your doctor know that you're taking supplements, since they can potentially interact with other drugs that you may be taking.

■ **Bruises.** Your body uses vitamin C to repair damaged capillaries. Since a bruise is the result of injury to dozens or even hundreds of them, you need as much of this nutrient as you can get, so eat plenty of C-rich fruit (especially citrus fruits) and vegetables. It's also helpful to take 2,000 to 3,000

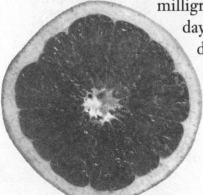

milligrams of vitamin C supplements for a day or two. To avoid stomach upset or diarrhea, divide the dose into smaller amounts taken several times a day with food.

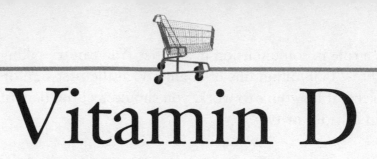

Vitamin D

THE SUNSHINE VITAMIN

Vitamin D is so essential that your body has developed two ways of getting enough: from the foods you eat and from exposure to sunlight. Still, millions of Americans don't get enough, which is unfortunate because this nutrient is essential for your health. Take a look at the critical roles it plays.

■ **Arthritis.** One study showed that people with too little vitamin D in their diets were more likely to develop osteoarthritis and three times more likely to have existing arthritis get worse. Be sure you get enough D—from fortified milk, for example, or a multivitamin.

D Builds Bones

Your body needs vitamin D to absorb calcium, the mineral that keeps bones strong. Take 400 IU of D each day if you are over age 50 or 600 IU if you're over age 70.

■ **The blues.** Vitamin D helps the body maintain higher levels of serotonin, a brain chemical that helps regulate mood. Check your daily multivitamin to be sure it contains at least 400 IU of vitamin D.

428

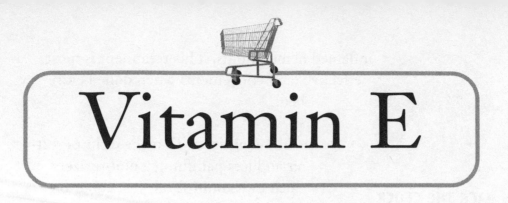

Vitamin E

BET YOUR LIFE ON IT

Vitamin E may prove to be the most important nutrient ever discovered. Whether you get it from foods or supplements, it acts as a shield between your body's cells and free radicals, the "toxic" molecules in your body that greatly increase the risk of cataracts, cancer, and heart disease. Vitamin E can even make scars almost disappear! Read on to see what this "miracle vitamin" can do for you, but check with your doctor before taking supplements if you're taking any other medication, especially blood thinners.

■ **Vaginal dryness.** When vaginal lubrication decreases, intercourse is the pits. If you find yourself a bit drier than usual, prick a vitamin E capsule with a pin and insert the capsule into your vagina. Do this every night before bed for two weeks, then three times a week thereafter.

■ **Hemorrhoids.** Break open a vitamin E capsule and apply the oil to your freshly washed anal area to help heal and soothe

Brain Booster

In one study, vitamin E slowed mental decline in Alzheimer's patients. Just one caveat: Vitamin E supplementation may not be advisable for people who are taking aspirin, garlic, or blood-thinning medication.

429

inflamed hemorrhoids. This treatment is most effective (and convenient) when done before bed.

■ **Calluses.** To make calluses softer and less painful, try moisturizers such as vitamin E oil. Just rub it on the callus after bathing or showering and before you go to bed.

■ **Dementia.** As reported in the journal *Neurology*, doctors at New York's Weill Cornell Women's Health Center concluded that supplements of vitamins E and C had a significant protective effect against vascular dementia (loss of thinking ability due to atherosclerosis). The study subjects performed better on tests, too. Check with your doctor to see if taking extra C and E could help keep your mind sharp.

TURN BACK THE CLOCK
This simple treatment will make your face look younger. Just mash a peeled medium banana, mix it with ¼ cup of heavy whipping cream, and stir in the contents of one vitamin E capsule. Smooth the concoction onto your face and neck, wait 10 to 15 minutes, and wipe it off with a damp washcloth.

■ **Hot flashes.** Vitamin E often helps relieve the severity and frequency of hot flashes and other menopausal discomforts, according to Lila Nachtigall, M.D. Check with your doctor first to see which dose is right for you.

■ **Itchy scalp.** Here's a time-tested remedy for an itchy scalp: In a small pan, warm a few drops of vitamin E oil, then gently comb it through your dry hair. Wrap a towel around your head and leave it on for at least 15 minutes, then sham-

Vitamin E

poo. The oil will help loosen dry scales and make your hair shiny, not greasy.

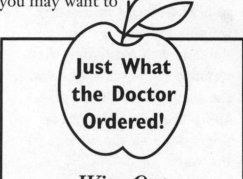

■ **Gum disease.** To protect your gums, you need plenty of antioxidant vitamins E and C. Vitamin E, which is found in nuts and seeds, fights cell damage caused by renegade oxygen molecules. Its partner vitamin C toughens gums, reduces swelling, and squelches infection; get your daily quota from foods such as oranges, broccoli, and tomatoes.

■ **Burns.** If you have a serious burn, your body's supply of vitamin E may be diminished, so you may want to take a daily supplement until the burn heals; check with your doctor about the appropriate dose for you. Once the burn starts to heal, you can also break open a vitamin E capsule and apply the contents directly to the burn twice daily to help fight cell damage.

■ **Tendinitis.** You wouldn't think that what you eat would have much effect on tendinitis, but diet really does make a difference. Top a salad with hard-boiled eggs for vitamin A, red peppers for vitamin C, and sliced almonds for vitamin E. These nutrients are all excellent anti-inflammatories that may help reduce the swelling in your tendons that's causing your pain, says Andrew Lucking, N.D.

Just What the Doctor Ordered!

Wipe Out Workout Pain

Want to stop muscle pain before it starts? Take vitamin E before you exercise. This powerful antioxidant can offset muscle damage caused by exertion. Ask your doctor how much is right for you.

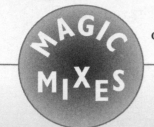

MAGIC MIXES

WHIP WARTS
Yellow cedar, also called thuja, is an excellent wart remedy. Fill a small jar with thuja leaves and add enough oil to cover, along with the contents of a vitamin E capsule. Put the jar in a sunny window for 10 days and shake it well every day, then strain out the herb and store the jar in a cool, dark place. Apply the oil two or three times daily to the surface of the wart.

■ **Wrinkles.** As an ingredient in lotions or as oil, topical vitamin E—particularly the form known as alpha tocopherol—reduces skin roughness, the length of facial lines, and wrinkle depth. Combining it with topical vitamin C in the form of ascorbic acid (which seems to help promote the growth of collagen, the skin's underlying support) may enhance those restorative effects. Check the health and beauty aisle for a product that includes both and follow the package directions.

■ **Lupus.** Vitamin E helps fight organ damage caused by inflammation, and people with lupus tend to be deficient in it. To be sure you're getting plenty, take a multivitamin supplement daily and snack on E-rich sunflower seeds whenever you can.

■ **Psoriasis.** To help heal psoriasis lesions, bathe the areas twice daily, pat them dry, and immediately rub in a generous amount of vitamin E oil. Within a week, at least 80 percent of the plaques should be gone, says David Cohen, N.D.

■ **Leg pain.** Millions of Americans have intermittent claudication, leg pain caused by poor circulation. People who take vitamin E can often walk farther without pain because E is a vasodilator that opens narrowed blood vessels and allows more blood to flow through. The recommended dose is 400 IU daily, but check with your doctor before supplementing.

■ **Cuts and scrapes.** If you have a minor skin injury, vitamin E oil can encourage healing without scarring. Wait two or three days to let the healing process get started, then break open a vitamin E capsule and apply a little of the oil a few times a day.

■ **Dry skin.** If your skin is desert dry, nourish and soften it with an aromatic facial mask. Combine two drops of vitamin E oil, 2 tablespoons of mashed strawberries, and 1 tablespoon each of coconut oil, olive oil, and light vegetable oil in a bowl. Smooth the mixture sparingly onto your face and go about your normal routine for a few hours. Then rinse with warm water, put some witch hazel on a cotton pad, and pat it on your face. Store any remaining moisturizer in a covered container in the refrigerator and use it within a week.

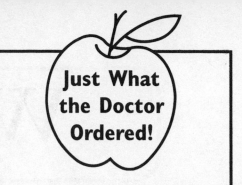

Just What the Doctor Ordered!

E-ase Away Cold Sores

An application of vitamin E is just the thing for cold sores. Open a capsule and spread the oil on the sore and the surrounding area. It's a good moisturizer, and it may help cold sores heal more quickly.

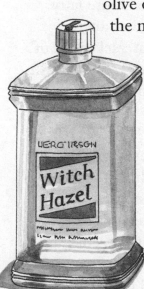

Witch Hazel

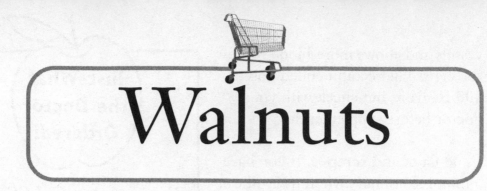

Walnuts

GO A LITTLE NUTS

Unless you buy them shelled, walnuts aren't the easiest (or neatest) snack in the house, but they're definitely one of the healthiest. Studies have shown that people who eat a lot of walnuts feel better and maybe even live longer than those who don't. So go ahead—get crackin'!

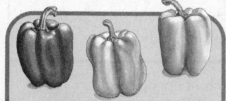

Fabulous Food Fix

Say "Nuts" to Dry Skin

If your skin is dry, especially in the winter, it could be that you're not getting enough fat—the right kind of fat. Make sure your diet includes one or more servings a day of the omega-3 fats found in walnuts.

■ **Itchy skin.** If your skin gets itchy in water, you probably need more fatty acids. Walnuts are loaded with these valuable fats, so dig the nutcracker out of the drawer and enjoy a few. Your skin will probably feel better within a few weeks.

■ **High cholesterol.** Scientists report that people who eat walnuts tend to have lower cholesterol and healthier hearts. The theory is that the monounsaturated fat in nuts can protect against heart disease, but their mineral content—magnesium and copper—may guard the heart as well. About ¼ cup of nuts per day is the recommended amount.

■ **Heart disease.** Doctors have known for a long time that the Mediterranean diet, which is brimming with fat (along with boatloads of fish, fruit, and vegetables) is very good for the heart and arteries. Now there's evidence that you can make a good diet even better by substituting a handful of walnuts (8 to 11 a day) for some of the oil in that diet. According to a study reported in the *Annals of Internal Medicine*, walnuts can lower cholesterol even more than olive oil, and they reduced the risk of coronary heart disease by 11 percent, reported lead researcher Emilio Ros, M.D. In other research, walnuts incorporated into the Mediterranean diet reduced bad cholesterol by almost 6 percent more than the basic Mediterranean diet did. A handful of nuts a day is enough to provide critical protection.

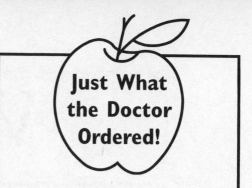

Just What the Doctor Ordered!

Boost Your Brain Power

Brain cells are 60 percent fat, which is needed to transmit the impulses that carry thought. In a healthy brain, omega-3 fatty acids predominate. Where do you get these healthy fatty acids? They're plentiful in walnuts.

■ **Brain fog.** Regularly eating tuna, walnuts, Brazil nuts, soybeans, and flaxseed is a great way to enrich your diet with omega-3 essential fatty acids, which reduce the inflammation that can impair focus and memory. In fact, unless you're taking blood thinners, your doctor may advise taking about 2 grams of omega-3 supplements a day to ensure you get enough.

Walnuts

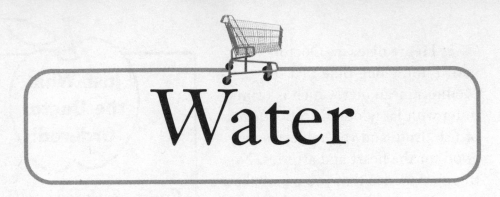

Water

IT FLOATS YOUR BOAT

The Earth's surface is mainly water. Most of your body weight is water. The skin, heart, and other organs are awash in water. Get the picture? Without water, your body simply can't function—and even a short-term drought caused by not drinking enough can have long-term consequences. Here's why doctors say we should all chug a little more.

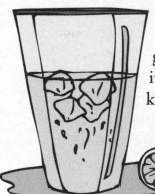

■ **Toothache.** A toothache can get a lot worse when your mouth is dry. Until the pain is gone, it's important to drink a lot of water to keep it lubricated. Have a glass handy at all times and keep taking small sips.

■ **Diarrhea.** According to the Centers for Disease Control and Prevention, if you have severe diarrhea, you should take in only fluids (such as water or sports drinks) and salty crackers until it's under control.

■ **Pneumonia.** You should never be more than arm's length from a glass of water while you're recovering from pneumonia, says Norman H. Edelman, M.D. "We suggest that people drink plenty of fluids, at least eight glasses a day," he says. Drinking lots of water dilutes all the mucus your lungs produce when you have pneumonia, so if you stay hydrated, you'll breathe easier, and your lungs will recover more quickly.

■ **Dehydration.** When you exercise, drink lots of water to prevent dehydration and replenish the fluids and nutrients you lose during workouts. Have a glass of water before you begin and take a break every 20 to 30 minutes for more. This workout wisdom is especially important for people with diabetes.

■ **Cranky gut.** You'll need to give up milk and other dairy products when your intestines are under the weather. Likewise, you'll want to avoid citrus and vegetable juices, alcohol, and caffeine, which also make things worse. Instead, drink plenty of water—as much as you can hold.

■ **Dry eyes.** When you're in a dry, dusty climate, rinse your face and eyes often with cool, clean water. This will ease irritation and add some moisture to offset the effects of the arid atmosphere.

■ **UTIs.** The more water you drink, the more bacteria will be flushed from your bladder, which can help prevent urinary tract infections (UTIs) or help you feel better if you already have one. In addition to flushing out bugs, water helps dilute pain-causing substances in the bladder. Drink at least 2 quarts a day, doctors advise.

Just What the Doctor Ordered!

Wash Away Cramps

The abdominal cramps that often accompany constipation can be excruciatingly painful. A fast way to get relief is to soak in a warm bath for 15 to 20 minutes. The warm water relaxes the muscles and helps reduce painful pressure and spasms.

■ **Dry skin.** You need lots of water to keep all parts of your body working well, including your skin. It's really quite simple: The more water you drink, the more water is available to pump up and out to your epidermis, so don't be stingy. Drink at least 8 to 10 glasses a day and carry a water bottle with you when you're exercising or out in the heat.

■ **Constipation.** All experts agree that the simplest way to wake up your colon when you're constipated is to drink water—lots and lots of it. When stools in the colon absorb water, they become larger, softer, and easier to pass, so try to down 10 glasses within 24 hours. Need to get things moving now? Drink a large glass of water every 10 minutes for 1 hour to soften your stools and force elimination.

■ **Vaginal dryness.** An excellent but exceedingly simple way to help increase vaginal lubrication is to drink water throughout the day.

■ **Anal pain.** No matter what's making your bottom hurt, soaking in a warm bath for 10 to 20 minutes will almost certainly make you feel better. "It helps soothe the area and relaxes tight muscles," says Michael P. Spencer, M.D.

More Fiber, More Water

Doctors advise nearly everyone to add more fiber to their diets. After all, fiber promotes digestive health, lowers cholesterol, and reduces the risk of heart disease and stroke. Keep in mind, though, that a high-fiber diet requires lots of liquids, according to the Mayo Clinic. Fiber acts as a sponge in your large intestine, so if you don't drink enough, you could become constipated. Aim to drink at least eight glasses of water a day.

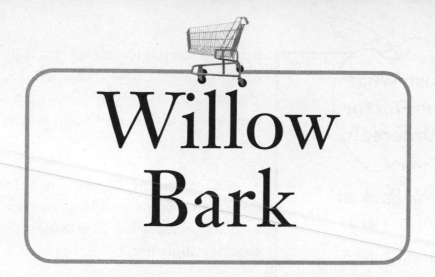

Willow Bark

BARKIN' UP THE RIGHT TREE

Long before doctors discovered aspirin, people used willow bark for its anti-inflammatory and painkilling effects. Even today, a lot of people prefer the traditional approach because it's a lot less likely to cause "aspirin stomach"— and it may work just as well as newfangled pills for all kinds of problems. (You shouldn't use it in any form, however, if you are allergic to aspirin or take aspirin regularly, and never combine it with alcohol.) Check it out.

■ **Back pain.** Willow bark is a super treatment for back pain because you can take it for a long time without experiencing stomach irritation, says Glen Rothfeld, M.D. To make a tea, pick up some willow

Chew on This

Willow bark contains salicin, which metabolizes in the body like aspirin, its synthetic sister. To ease a headache, chew some fresh willow twigs or, if there's no willow tree nearby, try the more powerful tea or tincture (30 drops of tincture every 4 to 6 hours).

439

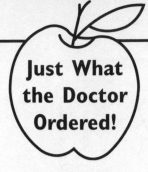

Just What the Doctor Ordered!

Bark Back at Joint Pain

Don't let arthritis keep you down. White willow bark helps reduce pain as well as swelling. As long as you're not taking any other form of aspirin or blood-thinning medication, take two 200- to 400-milligram capsules three times a day between meals.

bark and steep 2 teaspoons in a cup of boiling water, then strain and sip. You can also take capsules or apply willow bark ointment directly to your back.

■ **Sore throat.** Douse your sore throat with willow tea. It can reduce pain and swelling while providing soothing moisture.

■ **Carpal tunnel.** Black willow has long been used as an anti-inflammatory and pain reliever, so it's perfect for treating carpal tunnel syndrome. Make a tea by simmering 1 heaping teaspoon of black willow bark in 1 cup of water for 10 minutes. Strain and sip one or two cups a day. Within a few days, you should notice the swelling decreasing, which is important because swelling and inflammation can significantly increase healing time.

■ **Headache.** Like coffee or any other caffeinated drink, black tea can constrict your blood vessels and chase away a throbbing headache, but it can also be dehydrating. White willow bark tea has no caffeine, which means it will rehydrate you. Plus, it contains salicin, which is similar to the pain reliever in aspirin. The only difference between the two is that willow bark is easier on the stomach than aspirin. Buy some powdered white willow bark tea, then follow the package directions. Drink three cups a day.

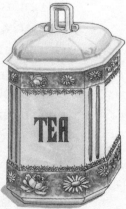

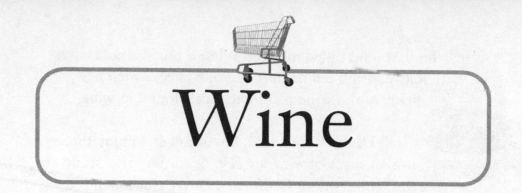

Wine

MAKE A TOAST TO GOOD HEALTH

All you beer drinkers, listen up: Wine, especially red wine, is loaded with substances that can knock years off your arteries, strengthen your heart, and even help you get over a bad cold. Here are some of the best reasons to lift your glass for a healing sip.

■ **Acne.** Did you know you can control acne breakouts by dabbing a little wine on your skin? Do it once or twice a day after washing your face. Use white wine for fair skin, red for darker complexions.

■ **Heart disease.** Light to moderate consumption (up to one glass a day for women or two for men) of wine reduces your risk of developing heart disease or of dying from it. Red wine is more effective than white because certain chemicals it contains have antioxidant and anti-clotting properties. Experts believe that the pigment in red grape skins contains a powerful

No More Chlorine Green

Has swimming in a chlorinated pool given your blonde hair a greenish tinge? Pour yourself a glass of red wine— but don't drink it! Instead, pour it on your head. Work it through your hair, follow up with your normal shampoo, and that'll be the end of the green-hair blues!

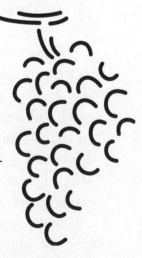

bioflavonoid called quercetin. For a nonalcoholic alternative, drink red or purple grape juice, which has many of the same plant chemicals found in wine.

■ **High cholesterol.** Go ahead and enjoy three to six glasses of wine a week. According to a study at the University of California, Davis, this much red wine lowers levels of low-density lipoprotein (LDL) cholesterol, possibly due to wine's relatively high concentration of saponins. These plant compounds—believed to bind to cholesterol and prevent its absorption—are 10 times more plentiful in red grapes, especially those used to make red zinfandel, than in white. If you have elevated triglycerides (which may be boosted by alcohol's high sugar content) or diabetes, if you're pregnant, or if alcoholism runs in your family, stick to another red drink, such as grape juice or unsweetened cranberry juice.

■ **Chemo side effects.** The anthocyanins in wine are cancer-fighting antioxidants and may help correct an imbalance of B vitamins, which can be a result of cancer treatments and may cause a sore mouth, anemia, and nerve problems. Red wine also contains an antifungal compound that's converted in the body into a powerful cancer-fighting agent. Unless your doctor says otherwise or you have breast cancer, you can enjoy a glass of wine a day during treatments. Eating red grapes, though, is a good choice for anyone.

■ **Cataracts.** The quercetin in red wine is associated with a lower risk of cataracts. If this vision-robbing condition runs in your family, or you've spent a lot of time in the sun, sipping a little wine may help protect your vision.

■ **Dull hair.** Want to add golden highlights to your hair? Try this time-honored trick: Heat 2 cups of white wine (but don't let it boil), add 3 tablespoons of chopped rhubarb stems, remove it from the stove, and steep for 10 minutes. Shampoo as usual, rinse with the solution, and partially dry your hair with a towel, then sit in the sun to finish the job. Repeat the process until your tresses reach the desired shade of pale. Be sure to give your hair a good rinse with clear, warm water afterward.

■ **Dull skin.** Here's a simple skin freshener that your face will love: Put 1 cup of white wine and 1 sliced lemon in a glass or enamel pot and bring it to a boil over medium heat (or put it in a microwaveable bowl and microwave on high until it boils—about 1½ minutes). Boil for a full minute, remove the pan from the heat, and stir in 1 tablespoon of sugar. Let the mixture cool, strain it, and store it in a tightly capped bottle. Whenever you feel the need for facial refreshment, just dab the lotion onto your skin with a cotton ball.

■ **Sunburn.** To use white wine for sunburn relief, just spritz it directly onto the stricken skin, but don't rub! When the liquid has evaporated, apply a moisturizing lotion. Of course, you may smell a little odd, but your skin will feel much better.

Soothing Sips

CALM YOUR COUGH

Sipping hot red wine with lemon, cinnamon, and sugar added is a traditional cough remedy. Alcohol is a component of many cough medicines, and it can help you relax and sleep, but use it cautiously. Too much will weaken the immune response, which you need to fight infection.

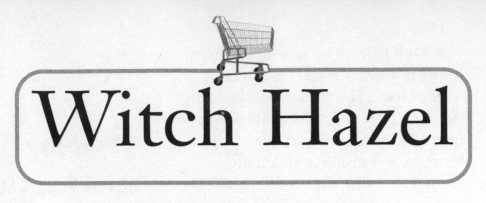

Witch Hazel

DON'T DITCH THE WITCH

A traditional remedy for skin problems, witch hazel is probably among the most common herbal treatments in American medicine chests. It costs less than most skin products, and it produces a tingling, cooling sensation that's just what the doctor ordered. Plus, it works for dozens of common complaints. Take a look at what it can do for you.

■ **Poison ivy and bug bites.** To stop the itch of poison ivy and insect bites, make a paste of witch hazel and baking soda, then smooth it onto the itchy area for fast relief.

Shave and Soothe

Want a really simple alternative to commercial aftershaves? Just mix one part witch hazel and one part apple cider vinegar, then slap it on your face. It's refreshing!

■ **Hemorrhoids.** Most people get hemorrhoids from time to time. They can really hurt—and when they're not hurting, they're itching like crazy. There are a few products that can ease the

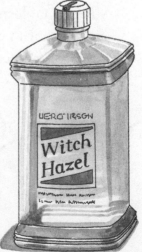

itch, such as zinc oxide ointment and

Preparation H, but in a pinch, witch hazel can help. Moisten a cotton ball with witch hazel and dab it onto the swollen vein or, if you have access to fresh witch hazel, place a leaf on the sore spot and literally sit tight. Replace the leaf a couple of times a day.

■ **Rashes.** The angrier your rash, the more you need a natural astringent such as witch hazel. The tannins in this botanical help constrict tissues and control inflammation.

■ **Shiners.** You were standing in the wrong place when the wind caught the door, and you wound up with a shiner the size of a saucer. Now what do you do? Just soak a washcloth in witch hazel and hold it over your eye. The pain and swelling will vamoose. Be sure you don't get any in your eye, though, because it will sting like crazy!

■ **B.O.** To banish body odor of any kind, combine five drops each of oil of sage (which dries perspiration), sweet-smelling coriander, and lovely lavender with 2 ounces of distilled witch hazel (a great source of tannins, which help close sweat glands so odor-causing bacteria are starved) in a spray bottle. Shake well, then spritz your problem areas.

■ **Acne.** Sweaty workouts are great for your body, but they increase sebum production—which is not so great for your face if you have acne. To get rid of the extra oil gently, swab your

MAGIC MIXES

NATURAL SKIN SAVER
This tonic tightens pores and soothes minor burns. Mix 1 cup of witch hazel, 3 tablespoons of coarsely chopped cucumber, and the juice of one lemon in a jar with a lid. Set it aside for two days, then strain out the cucumber and pour the liquid into a bottle. Keep it in the refrigerator and dab it on with a cotton ball whenever the need arises.

face with tannin-packed witch hazel, suggests Kathlyn Quatrochi, N.D. Commercial witch hazel products contain few tannins, so it's best to whip up your own. Simply steep 5 to 10 grams of witch hazel bark in a cup of boiling water for 10 to 15 minutes. Strain the solution, let it cool, and pour it into a plastic bottle for spot treating pimples after exercise.

■ **Varicose veins.** If you have varicose veins, mix 1 part horse chestnut tincture (look for a tincture with 50 milligrams of aescin per dose) with 10 parts distilled witch hazel (a vessel strengthener in its own right) and apply the solution to your problem veins once a day. You'll need to be patient, though, since it could take three months to see an effect.

Keep Your Cool

When the weather turns steamy, keep your cool by misting your skin with this elixir. Mix 2 teaspoons of witch hazel, 10 drops of peppermint oil, and 12 drops of lavender oil in an 8-ounce spray bottle, then fill the rest of the bottle with water. Keep it in the refrigerator and reach for it anytime you feel too darn hot.

■ **Skin ulcers.** For a skin ulcer that's still in the red, painful stage, apply a little witch hazel to a cotton ball and dab the sore once or twice a day to cool inflammation and help the sore heal more quickly. You'll feel a moment of pleasant coolness while the witch hazel evaporates, and the pain will usually diminish right away.

■ **Abrasions.** Distilled witch hazel is helpful when an abrasion continues to bleed, says Priscilla Natanson, N.D. "It's a styptic that slows blood flow," she explains. It stings a little, she adds, but only for a few seconds.

■ **Saggy skin.** You can make a healthful skin toner by mixing 1 teaspoon of green tea leaves in ½ cup of witch hazel. Gently dab the mixture onto your face and neck with a cotton pad. There's no need to rinse.

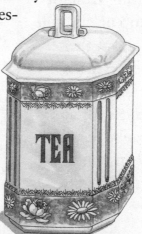

■ **Sunburn.** Stick a bottle of witch hazel in the fridge, then slather it on when you have a sunburn. Its tannins will help cool your skin.

■ **B.O.** Make a spray deodorant by mixing ½ cup of witch hazel with 2 tablespoons of vodka, 1 tablespoon of glycerin, and ½ teaspoon of liquid chlorophyll. Pour the solution into a hand-held spray bottle and spritz your underarms morning, noon, and/or night.

■ **Strains or sprains.** Doctors usually recommend RICE (rest, ice, compression, and elevation) for strains or sprains, but witch hazel can also help to shrink the swelling. Brew a tea by adding 1 teaspoon of dried leaves or 2 inches of root to 1 cup of boiling water. Steep for 10 to 15 minutes, then strain. Drink two or three cups a day.

Drain the Oil

Witch hazel, an excellent oil remover, is a standby in locker rooms because dabbing it on the skin keeps it sweat- and oil-free.

Witch Hazel 447

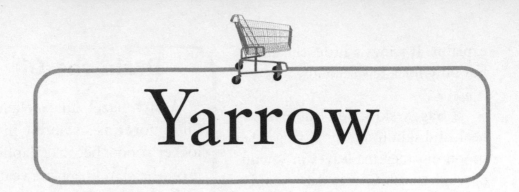

Yarrow

MOTHER NATURE'S BANDAGE

This attractive, feathery-leaved perennial was traditionally used to stop bleeding, but that's not all it can do. Research shows that yarrow is also good for balancing hormones, improving circulation, and even helping hair grow. But check with your doctor before using yarrow, and don't take it at all if you are pregnant or breastfeeding or have pollen allergies. Here are some other benefits of this herbal helper.

Blister Relief

You can help a blister heal faster by applying yarrow, an herb that naturally draws out fluid. If you're using fresh or dried yarrow, chop or crumble it as finely as you can, then add enough water to make a paste. Apply the paste to the blister and cover it with an adhesive or gauze bandage. Replace the dressing once a day until the blister is gone.

■ **B.O.** Sluggish or poor elimination sometimes causes body odor, but you can use gentle herbs to help clean your body on the inside. First, combine equal parts of red clover, yarrow, cleavers, calendula, and peppermint, then add 1 heaping tablespoon of the mixture to 1 quart of warm water. Steep for 15 minutes, strain, and drink throughout the day.

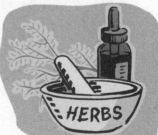

■ **Colds.** Immune-stimulating and astringent herbs can help ease the discomforts of a cold. For a healing tea, combine equal parts of yarrow, lemon balm, licorice root, ginger, eyebright, and rosehips and add 1 heaping teaspoon of the mixture to a cup of boiling water. Steep for 10 to 15 minutes, then strain. Drink two or three cups per day. If you have high blood pressure or kidney disease, skip the licorice root.

■ **Leg swelling.** If fluid retention makes your legs swell, this remedy will refresh them and help discourage fluid buildup. First, make a strong infusion of yarrow and peppermint by steeping 2 tablespoons of each in 1 pint of hot water. Strain out the herbs and put the solution in the fridge to chill. Meanwhile, prepare several lengths of gauze, muslin, or cheesecloth. When the infusion is cold, soak the cloths in it and wrap them around your lower legs. Sit or lie down, elevate your legs, and chill out for 20 minutes or so.

■ **Hemorrhoids.** Yarrow, horse chestnut, butcher's broom, and rose hips can help strengthen your blood vessels and may relieve hemorrhoids. Mix equal parts of each herb, then measure 1 heaping teaspoon of the mixture into 1 cup of hot water and steep for 10 minutes. Strain and drink two or three cups per day.

■ **Thinning hair.** Yarrow, elder, nettle, and prickly ash are nutrient-rich herbs that help increase circulation—necessary for healthy hair

Soothing Sips

BRAIN BOOSTER

This lovely tea will give your brain a healthy workout. Combine two parts ginkgo with one part each rosemary, yarrow, and hawthorn. Add 1 heaping teaspoon of the mixture to a cup of hot water and steep, covered, for 15 minutes. Drink one or two cups per day. If you take aspirin or blood-thinning medication, consult your doctor before using ginkgo.

growth. Steep 1 heaping teaspoon of any of the herbs in 1 pint of hot water for 10 to 15 minutes, then strain. Drink the warm tea throughout the day.

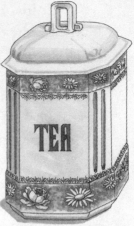

■ **Poor circulation.** To increase circulation, combine equal parts of yarrow, oatstraw, horsetail, meadowsweet, and peppermint. Use 1 heaping teaspoon per cup of boiling water, cover, and steep for 10 to 15 minutes, then strain. Drink a cup twice daily.

■ **Endometriosis.** Yarrows helps balance hormones, which makes it especially useful for women with endometriosis who may have excess estrogen. To prepare a tea, steep 1 to 2 teaspoons of dried yarrow flowers in a cup of boiling water for 10 to 15 minutes, strain, and drink one to three cups a day.

■ **Varicose veins.** Herbal formulas that include the classic blood vessel strengtheners yarrow, butcher's broom, horse chestnut, and stoneroot may help tone veins and reduce painful inflammation. Follow the package directions.

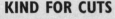

MAGIC MIXES

KIND FOR CUTS
Yarrow is an excellent choice for healing minor wounds. It acts as both an astringent to stem the flow of blood and an anti-inflammatory to calm the pain. Simply rinse some fresh yarrow leaves, chew them into a paste, and spit the mashed poultice directly onto your wound. The fresher the leaves, the more quickly the bleeding will stop.

Yarrow

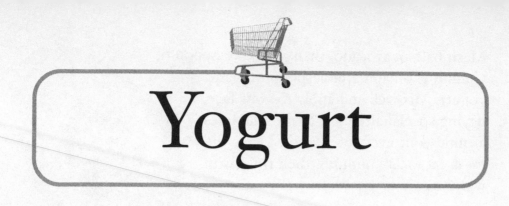

Yogurt

CAN'T BEAT THOSE BUGS!

The tangy taste of yogurt makes it a perfect snack when you're in the mood for something light. It's also perfect for helping you stay healthy. Why? Because apart from its load of essential nutrients, yogurt contains beneficial bacteria that not only keep you healthy but also can reverse diseases that have already taken hold. Here are a few reasons that doctors advise eating more yogurt.

■ **Vaginitis.** The *Lactobacillus acidophilus* organisms in yogurt crowd out the bad bugs that cause vaginitis and restore the acid-alkaline balance (pH) of the vagina. Eat more yogurt to help prevent future infections.

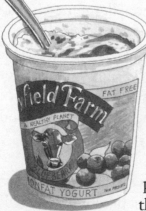

■ **Gas.** Live-culture yogurt can reduce gas because it breaks down milk sugars and keeps a balance of healthy bacteria in the digestive tract. Eat it often for better digestive health.

■ **Wrinkles.** You'd be hard-pressed to find a better facial mask than avocado combined with yogurt.

451

Mash half an avocado, then add ½ teaspoon of vitamin E oil and 1 tablespoon of plain yogurt. Mix well and apply to your face, paying special attention to the fine lines around your eyes and mouth. Leave the mask on for 20 minutes, then rinse with warm water.

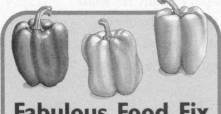

■ **Lactose intolerance.** Traditional nomadic peoples, who continued to use dairy products as a food source beyond infancy, cultured milk products to make them more easily digestible. If you're lactose intolerant, you may be able to use fermented dairy products such as yogurt and kefir without problems.

■ **Anemia.** Yogurt contains lactic acid, which promotes iron absorption from other foods. It's a good choice if you have iron-deficiency anemia.

■ **Vaginal dryness.** If you need a lubricant right away and can't dash off to the store, you may find help in the fridge. Yogurt is an excellent vaginal lubricant that's nonallergenic for most women.

■ **IBS.** Yogurt helps balance bacteria in the digestive tract and reduce the cramps, diarrhea, and other symptoms of irritable bowel syndrome (IBS).

■ **Weak bones.** When calcium is needed to accomplish certain bodily functions, such as cell

Fabulous Food Fix

Spoon Up Yeast Protection

Eating a cup or two of live-culture yogurt daily can help prevent vaginal yeast infections. One study reported that eating 8 ounces of yogurt containing the bacterial culture *Lactobacillus acidophilus* reduced the risk of yeast infections threefold.

Yogurt

regeneration, your body searches for it. If you haven't consumed enough, it's withdrawn from your bones, so you can see why it's important to take in ample amounts. The daily calcium requirement for adults is 1,200 milligrams, or 1,500 milligrams for postmenopausal women. One cup of yogurt provides 275 to 325 milligrams.

■ **Sunburn.** A dab of cold yogurt feels great on scorched skin.

■ **Diarrhea.** "Beneficial bacteria—so-called good bugs—are incredible healing agents that literally wipe out the bad bugs that may be causing your diarrhea, usually within a day or so," says Skye Weintraub, N.D. Look for brands of yogurt that contain active cultures of beneficial *L. acidophilus*, or take acidophilus in liquid or capsule form.

■ **Yeast overgrowth.** If you're taking an antibiotic for chlamydia or gonorrhea, you can offset the side effects—namely, an overgrowth of yeast—by eating a cup of yogurt that contains live cultures of "good" *L. acidophilus* bacteria daily.

■ **Surgical side effects.** A common side effect of surgery is the loss of beneficial types of bacteria that live in your digestive system. Anesthesia destroys them, and the

MAGIC MIXES

CLEAN AND MOISTURIZE
For a great facial cleanser, try this tangy recipe. First, grind lemon peels in a blender or coffee grinder, then mix about 1 tablespoon of the grounds with enough plain yogurt to make a paste. Wash your face with the mixture, rinse with cool water, and pat dry. If your skin is on the dry side, substitute vegetable oil for the yogurt.

Do the Fade

The enzyme activity of horseradish and yogurt may help fade age spots. Mix 1 tablespoon of grated horseradish with ¼ cup of plain yogurt. Keep the mixture refrigerated and dab it on your spots daily until they fade. Follow each application with a smear of vitamin E oil or wheatgerm oil.

antibiotics that people often take after surgery can also kill them. Protect yourself by eating a serving or two of live-culture yogurt daily.

■ **Weakened immunity.** Yogurt may rev up your entire immune system. A review of studies at Tufts University suggested that people with compromised immune systems, especially older folks, may increase their resistance to certain diseases by eating yogurt. If you find that you get sick more often than you'd like, get into the habit of starting the day with yogurt.

■ **Cancer.** Animal research suggests that the organisms in yogurt may decrease the risk of breast, colon, and liver tumors triggered by carcinogens. "Although we have to conduct clinical human trials, the relationship between active cultures in yogurt and the reduced risk of breast and colon cancers looks very promising," says Ian Rowland, Ph.D. To stay healthy year after year, get in the habit of eating yogurt at least several times weekly.

■ **Queasiness.** To quiet a roiling stomach, try eating ½ cup of plain yogurt to which you've added 2 pinches of cardamom and ½ teaspoon of honey, suggests Vasant Lad, M.A.Sc.

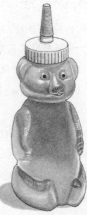

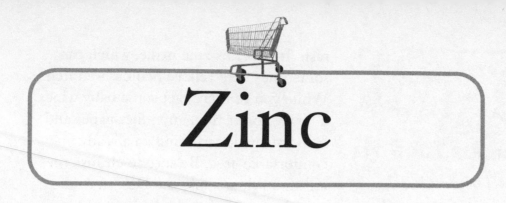

Zinc

ALL-PURPOSE PROTECTION

Zinc is one of those minerals that are involved in so many of your body's functions that it's hard to imagine you could ever get enough. It plays a crucial role in cell replication, male fertility, and wound healing. As if that weren't enough, it's also an immunity-boosting mineral that bolsters your defenses day after day. Check out some of its amazing effects.

■ **Dandruff.** For really stubborn dandruff, look for anti-dandruff shampoos containing zinc pyrithione and selenium sulfide—and purchase both. These two minerals scruff up the scalp, initiate cell turnover, and can break cornflake-size flakes into less noticeable ones.

■ **Hemorrhoids.** The pain and itch of hemorrhoids can make a baby out of anyone, so even if you're a big bruiser, be bold and venture into the baby products aisle to pick up some Desitin, an over-the-counter remedy for diaper

Zinc about This

The mineral zinc is among the most potent immune boosters, and it helps prevent headache-causing sinus infections. Take 30 milligrams of zinc daily for up to six weeks during sinusitis season. To maintain your mineral balance, you should also take 2 to 4 milligrams of copper a day while you're taking zinc.

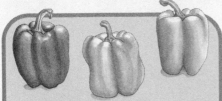

Fabulous Food Fix

Think Zinc

Are oysters really an aphrodisiac or simply a sexual placebo? Men who slurp them off the half-shell in the hope of extra sexual vigor may find that the strategy succeeds just because they believe it will. It's interesting to note, though, that oysters are rich in zinc, which the prostate needs to manufacture seminal fluid.

rash. It contains zinc oxide, which can sometimes help relieve hemorrhoid itch. While you're there, get some baby wipes. They're softer than any toilet paper and help you avoid irritating an already uncomfortable area. Be sure to cleanse the area first, then apply the Desitin in the morning and before bed.

■ **Itchy skin.** When you have a miserable itch anywhere on your skin, an ointment such as zinc oxide can provide relief.

■ **Colds I.** Try zinc the next time you have a cold. A Cleveland Clinic study found that people who began taking zinc lozenges within 24 hours of when their symptoms began were free of cold symptoms after about 4½ days.

■ **Colds II.** A zinc nasal spray may cut the duration of colds by about two days by acting as a physical barrier that keeps viruses from entering the cells that line the nose and throat. All you have to do is spritz some over-the-counter zinc spray in each nostril four times a day within 48 hours of the first inkling of a cold.

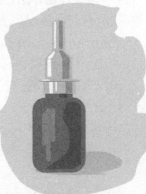

■ **B.O.** Pumpkin seeds provide a good, concentrated supply of zinc, a deficiency of which can prompt body odor. If you're not keen on the seeds, you can take 30 to 50 milligrams of zinc in tablet form daily to help reduce body and foot odor—but not without your doctor's guidance. If taken continuously, zinc can

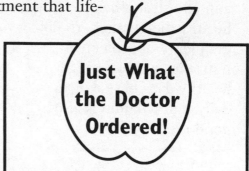

deplete copper and other minerals, and it could be toxic.

■ **Weak nails.** If your nails bend or break easily, you could have a zinc deficiency. Try popping a daily multivitamin/mineral supplement and see if your nails improve.

■ **Cuts and scrapes.** Zinc helps wounds heal more quickly, so try to get more of this mineral when you have a cut, scrape, or other skin injury.

■ **Cold sores.** The same white ointment that lifeguards use on their noses to protect against sunburn may heal cold sores in 5 days instead of the usual 10. The catch, according to research, is that you have to apply zinc oxide four times a day—and perhaps every hour—and start it within 24 hours of the first hint of an outbreak.

■ **Hangover.** The next time you wake up regretting the vodka-and-tonics you had the night before, take a multivitamin/mineral supplement that contains 15 milligrams of zinc. It assists the enzymes that break down alcohol.

■ **Restless legs.** A high-potency supplement that contains zinc and folic acid can help relieve the tingling and jumping sensations of restless legs. These ingredients help

Just What the Doctor Ordered!

In the Pink with Zinc

If you've been tiptoeing through the poison ivy patch, you may find yourself with a wet, ugly rash. After washing it well and patting it dry, apply zinc oxide ointment. That should help put those itchy nerve endings into a coma.

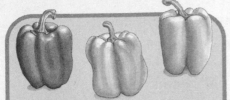

Fabulous Food Fix

Eat Away Cankers

To battle canker sores, you need extra nutrients, especially folic acid, vitamin A, and zinc, which your body uses to maintain and strengthen healthy membranes. You'll get plenty of protective nutrients just by eating a healthy diet, but taking a daily multivitamin is also a good idea.

ensure that your nerves get the nutrients they need to function properly, says Andrew Weil, M.D. He also recommends taking a calcium/magnesium supplement at bedtime to help calm your nerves and muscles. Ask your doctor about the dose that's right for you.

■ **Herpes.** For occasional mild herpes outbreaks, take 25 milligrams of zinc and 250 milligrams of vitamin C twice daily for five weeks. If you start this regimen within 24 hours of the first telltale tingle, you may be able to completely suppress eruptions, but don't take this amount of zinc for longer than the recommended time.

■ **Underactive thyroid.** Selenium and zinc are crucial for thyroid function because they help convert thyroid hormone into a more active form. If tests show that you're not producing enough of the hormone, ask your doctor about helpful dosages of both minerals.

■ **Pale lips.** Eating more green vegetables is a great way to keep your lips in the pink. They're rich in zinc, essential fatty acids, and riboflavin—everything your lips need to retain moisture and stay healthy, says Priscilla Natanson, N.D.

■ **Ear noises.** If you're annoyed by the ghost noises of tinnitus, eat more lean meat and shellfish. They're rich in zinc, a mineral that may minimize age-related tinnitus and hearing loss.

Zinc

Trademarks and Disclaimers

The brand names of products mentioned in this book are registered trademarks. The companies that own these trademarks do not endorse, recommend, or accept liability for any use of their products other than those uses indicated on the package label or in current company brochures. When using any commercial product, always read and follow label directions.

Advil and Preparation H are registered trademarks of Wyeth Consumer Healthcare Inc.

AIM Herbal Fiberblend is a registered trademark of Aim International, Inc.

Allegra is a registered trademark of Aventis Pharmaceuticals Inc.

ArginMax is a registered trademark of the Daily Wellness Company.

Bactine is a registered trademark of the Bayer Corporation.

Beano is a registered trademark of GlaxoSmithKline.

Benadryl, Desitin, Dramamine, and Listerine are registered trademarks of Pfizer Inc.

Biochem Aller-Max is a registered trademark of Country Life Vitamins.

Cheerios is a registered trademark of General Mills, Inc.

Claritin is a registered trademark of Schering-Plough HealthCare Products, Inc.

Clear-Ease is a registered trademark of Health Solutions Medical Products Corp.

Excedrin is a registered trademark of Bristol-Myers Squibb.

Feverall is a registered trademark of Alpharma USPD.

Gatorade is a registered trademark of Stokley Van Camp, Inc.

HeartBar is a registered trademark of Unither Pharma, Inc.

Jarrow Formulas is a registered trademark of Jarrow Formulas.

Kellogg's All-Bran, Kellogg's Bran Buds, and Kellogg's Guardian are registered trademarks of the Kellogg Company.

Kira is a registered trademark of Lichtwer Pharma.

Menastil is a registered trademark of Claire Ellen Products.

Metamucil, Vicks, and VapoRub are registered trademarks of Procter & Gamble.

Migrahealth is a registered trademark of HealthAssure, Inc.

Milky Way is a registered trademark of Mars, Inc.

Motrin is a registered trademark of McNeil-PPC, Inc.

Nature Made is a registered trademark of Pharmavite LLC.

Nature's Plus is a registered trademark of Natural Organics, Inc.

Nurofen is a registered trademark of the Boots Company PLC.

Old Bay is a registered trademark of McCormick & Co., Inc.

Orabase is a registered trademark of the Colgate-Palmolive Company.

Pernod is a registered trademark of Pernod Ricard USA.

PMS Escape is a registered trademark of Back Bay Scientific.

Proflex is a registered trademark of Novartis Consumer Health.

Promensil is a registered trademark of Novogen.

RemiFemin is a registered trademark of GlaxoSmithKline.

Replens is a registered trademark of Lil' Drug Store Products, Inc.

Starbucks is a registered trademark of the Starbucks Corporation.

Styrofoam is a trademark of the Dow Chemical Company.

Tabasco is a registered trademark of the McIlhenny Company.

Twinlab is a registered trademark of the Twinlab Corporation.

Tylenol is a registered trademark of McNeil-PPC, Inc.

Water Pik is a registered trademark of Water Pik, Inc.

459

Acknowledgments

We are deeply grateful to the following health practitioners, who generously gave their time and expertise in the preparation of this book.

Crystal Abernathy, N.D., a naturopathic physician in Charlotte, North Carolina

Daniel Amen, M.D., medical director of the Amen Clinics in southern California and Washington State

Jeremy Appleton, N.D., chairman of the National College of Naturopathic Medicine in Portland, Oregon

Lisa Arnold, N.D., a naturopathic physician in Orleans, Massachusetts

Karen Barnes, N.D., a naturopathic physician in Burlington, Ontario, Canada

Leslie Baumann, M.D., associate professor of dermatology at the University of Miami School of Medicine in Tampa

Judith Boice, N.D., a naturopathic physician in Portland, Oregon

Robert Bonakdar, M.D., director of pain management and heart health at the Scripps Center for Integrative Medicine in La Jolla, California

Bradley Bongiovanni, N.D., a naturopathic physician in Atlanta

Christine Boorean, N.D., a naturopathic physician in Portland, Oregon

David Borenstein, M.D., a Washington, D.C.–based rheumatologist

Cristopher Bosted, N.D. a naturopathic physician and faculty member at Bastyr University near Seattle

Stephanie Brooks, R.D., a registered dietitian and San Francisco–based nutrition consultant

Beth Burch, N.D., a naturopathic physician in Gresham, Oregon

Connie Cantellani, M.D., an internist who specializes in integrative medicine in Skokie, Illinois

Hyla Cass, M.D., assistant clinical professor of psychiatry at the University of California, Los Angeles, School of Medicine

Bernard Cohen, M.D., professor of dermatology at the University of Miami School of Medicine in Tampa

David Cohen, N.D., a naturopathic physician in New York City

Terri Dallas-Prunskis, M.D., codirector of the Illinois Pain Treatment Institute in Chicago

Daniel DeLapp, N.D., instructor in dermatology at the National College of Naturopathic Medicine in Portland, Oregon

Wendy Demark, R.D., Ph.D., researcher at the Duke University Comprehensive Cancer Center in Durham, North Carolina.

Michael DiPalma, N.D., a naturopathic physician in Newtown, Pennsylvania

Christian Dodge, N.D., a naturopathic physician and faculty member at Bastyr University near Seattle

Rob Dramov, N.D., a naturopathic physician in Tigard, Oregon

Ryan Drum, Ph.D., a medical herbalist in Washington State

James A. Duke, Ph.D., president and CEO of Duke's Herbal Vineyard in Fulton, Maryland, and a former specialist in medicinal plants for the USDA

Magdalena Dziadzio, M.D., a faculty member in the department of internal medicine at the University of Ancona, Italy

Norman H. Edelman, M.D., scientific consultant for the American Lung Association and dean of Stony Brook School of Medicine in New York

Orli Etigen, M.D., director of the Center for Women's Healthcare and vice chairman of the department of medicine at Weill-Cornell Medical College in New York City

Richard N. Firshein, D.O., medical director of the Firshein Center for Comprehensive Medicine in New York City

Kathleen Flewelling, N.D., a naturopathic physician in Seaside, Oregon

Victoria Franks, N.D., a naturopathic physician in Cornwall, Ontario, Canada

Kim Galeaz, R.D., of Galeaz Food and Nutrition Communications in Indianapolis

Gary Gitnick, M.D., chief of the division of digestive diseases at the University of California, Los Angeles, School of Medicine

Barry Goldin, Ph.D., professor of family medicine at Tufts University in Boston

Jerry Gore, M.D., medical director of the Center for Holistic Medicine in Riverwoods, Illinois

Susan L. Greenspan, M.D., professor of medicine at Beth Israel Deaconess Medical Center in Boston

Murray Grossan, M.D., a consultant in the department of otolaryngology at Cedars-Sinai Hospital in Los Angeles

Sara Grossi, D.D.S., director of periodontal disease research at the University of Buffalo in New York

John Hahn, N.D., D.P.M., a naturopathic physician and podiatrist in Bend, Oregon

Rowan Hamilton, Dip.Phyt., professor of botanical medicine at Bastyr University near Seattle

Mary Hardy, M.D., director of the Integrative Medicine Medical Group at Cedars-Sinai Medical Center in Los Angeles

Bill Helferich, Ph.D., associate professor of food science and human nutrition at the University of Illinois in Urbana

Robert Henry, D.M.D., associate professor at the University of Kentucky School of Dentistry in Lexington

James Herndon, M.D., chair of the department of orthopedic surgery at Brigham and Women's Hospital in Boston

John Hibbs, N.D., a naturopathic physician and professor at Bastyr University near Seattle

Alan Hirsch, M.D., director of the Smell and Taste Treatment Foundation in Chicago

Jane Hopson, N.D., a naturopathic physician in Hillsboro, Oregon

John W. House, M.D., president of the House Ear Institute in Los Angeles

Tori Hudson, N.D., a naturopathic physician and director of A Woman's Time clinic in Portland, Oregon

Darin Ingels, N.D., a naturopathic physician and director of New England Family Health in Southport, Connecticut

Robert Ivker, D.O., assistant clinical professor of otolaryngology at the University of Colorado School of Medicine in Denver

Jeanette Jacknin, M.D., a dermatologist in Scottsdale, Arizona

Joseph Keenan, M.D., of the University of Minnesota Medical School in Minneapolis

Kathi Keville, an herbalist in Boulder, Colorado

Alan Kristal, Dr.P.H., of the Fred Hutchinson Cancer Research Center in Seattle

Manfred Kroger, Ph.D., professor emeritus of food science at Pennsylvania State University in University Park

Vasant Lad, M.A.Sc., director of the Ayurvedic Institute in Albuquerque

Carol Leonard, a certified nurse-midwife and chair of the New Hampshire Council of Midwifery in Hopkinton

Erica LePore, N.D., a naturopathic physician in Wakefield, Rhode Island

Suzanne M. Levine, D.P.M., a podiatrist in New York City

Marcus Loo, M.D., clinical associate professor of urology at Weill-Cornell Medical College in New York City

Andrew Lucking, N.D., a naturopathic physician in Minneapolis

Kathy McManus, R.D., of Brigham and Women's Hospital in Boston

J. Michael Maloney, M.D., a Denver-based dermatologist

Christine Matheson, N.D., a naturopathic physician with the Women's Pelvic Health Center at Sunnybrook Women's College of Health Sciences in Toronto

Chris Meletis, N.D., chief medical officer of the National College of Naturopathic Medicine in Portland, Oregon

Michael Miller, M.D., director of the Center for Preventive Cardiology at the University of Maryland Medical Center in Baltimore

Dixie Mills, M.D., cofounder of the Breast Cancer High-Risk Clinic at the Dana Farber Cancer Institute in Boston and a gynecologist in Yarmouth, Maine

Anil Minocha, M.D., chief of gastroenterology at Southern Illinois University School of Medicine in Chicago

Mary Ellen Mortensen, M.D., executive director of medical affairs at McNeil Consumer Healthcare

Gerald J. Murphy, D.D.S., director of publications for the American Academy of Craniofacial Pain

Lisa Murray-Doran, N.D., a naturopathic physician in Whitby, Ontario, Canada

Dana Myatt, N.D., a naturopathic physician in Phoenix

Lila Nachtigal, M.D., professor in the department of obstetrics and gynecology at New York University

Jana Nalbandian, N.D., a naturopathic physician and faculty member at Bastyr University near Seattle

Priscilla Natanson, N.D., a naturopathic physician in Plantation, Florida

Gail L. Nield, M.D., a dermatologist in Woodbridge, Ontario, Canada

Gary Null, Ph.D., host of the "Natural Living" radio show and author of *Secrets of the Sacred White Buffalo*

Ralph Ofcarcik, Ph.D., nutritionist and guest education manager at the Red Mountain Health Resort in Ivins, Utah

Grace Ornstein, M.D., medical director and scientific advisor for Himalaya USA, a marketer of herbal formulas based in Houston

Annette Fuglsang Owens, M.D., Ph.D., a counselor at the Charlottesville Sexual Health and Wellness Clinic in Virginia

Andrew Parkinson, N.D., a naturopathic physician and faculty member at the Bastyr Center for Natural Health near Seattle

Richard Price, D.M.D., a dentist in the Boston area and consumer advisor for the American Dental Association

Robert Pyke, M.D., Ph.D., a physician and pharmacologist specializing in digestive diseases in Ridgefield, Connecticut

Kathlyn Quatrochi, N.D., a naturopathic physician in Oak Glen, California

A. V. Rao, Ph.D., professor of nutrition at the University of Toronto

John Reed, M.D., a physician in Arlington, Virginia

Jennifer Reid, N.D., a naturopathic physician at the Columbia River Natural Medicine Clinic in Troutdale, Oregon

Martin Resnick, M.D., chairman of urology at Case Western Reserve University School of Medicine in Cleveland

Paul Riley, N.D., a naturopathic physician at the Seattle Cancer Treatment and Wellness Center

Emilio Ros, M.D., head of the Lipid Clinic at the Hospital Clinic of Barcelona, Spain

Glen Rothfeld, M.D., clinical assistant professor of medicine at Tufts University School of Medicine in Boston

Ian Rowland, Ph.D., of the University of Ulster in Ireland

Susan W. Ryan, D.O., an osteopathic physician in Denver

Ralph Sacco, M.D., a stroke researcher at Columbia University in New York City and a spokesperson for the American Heart Association

Sean Sapunar, N.D., a naturopathic physician and clinical faculty member at the Bastyr Center for Natural Health near Seattle

Donald Schwartz, M.D., associate clinical professor of ophthalmology at the University of California, Irvine

Michael D. Seidman, M.D., director of neurotologic surgery at Henry Ford Hospital in Detroit

Samuel Selden, M.D., assistant professor of clinical medicine at Eastern Virginia Medical School in Chesapeake

Joel Simon, M.D., assistant professor of nutrition at the University of California, San Francisco

David A. Sirois, D.M.D., Ph.D., chair of the department of oral medicine at New York University College of Dentistry in New York City

Michael P. Spencer, M.D., a colon and rectal surgeon and assistant professor of surgery at the University of Minnesota, Twin Cities

Jamison Starbuck, N.D., a naturopathic physician in Missoula, Montana

Margaret Stearn, M.D., an internist in Oxford, England

Ronald Steriti, N.D., Ph.D., a naturopathic physician in Naples, Florida

Anna Szpindor, M.D., director of Allergy and Asthma Care in Oak Park, Illinois

Maida Taylor, M.D., associate clinical professor of obstetrics, gynecology, and reproductive sciences at the University of California, San Francisco

Nadine Taylor, R.D., a registered dietitian and chair of the women's health council of the American Nutraceutical Association in Birmingham, Alabama

Pamela Taylor, N.D., a naturopathic physician in Moline, Illinois

Jacob Teitelbaum, M.D., director of the Annapolis Research Center for Effective FMS/CFS Therapies in Maryland

Cynthia Thompson, R.D., Ph.D., assistant professor of nutritional sciences at the Arizona Cancer Center in Tucson

Sharol Tilgner, N.D., a naturopathic physician and director of the Wise Acres Herbal Education Center in Eugene, Oregon

Lila Wallis, M.D., a New York–based internist

Claire Warga, Ph.D., a midlife health psychologist in New York City

William Warnock, N.D., a naturopathic physician in Shelbourne, Vermont

Andrew Weil, M.D., director of the Program in Integrative Medicine and clinical professor of internal medicine at the University of Arizona in Tucson

Michael E. Weinblatt, M.D., codirector of clinical rheumatology at Brigham and Women's Hospital in Boston

Heidi Weinhold, N.D., a naturopathic physician in the Pittsburgh area

Skye Weintraub, N.D., a naturopathic physician in Eugene, Oregon

Linda White, M.D., a pediatrician in Golden, Colorado

Thomas Wolever, Ph.D., professor of nutritional science and medicine at the University of Toronto

Melody Wong, N.D., a naturopathic physician in Sausalito, California

Phoebe Yin, N.D., a naturopathic physician and faculty member at Bastyr University near Seattle

David Zeiger, D.O., a family physician in Chicago

Index

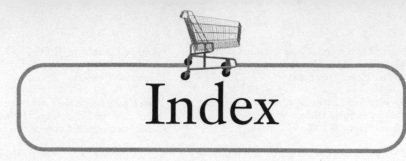

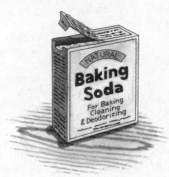

Index

Index